Doctors in a Strange Land

Doctors in a Strange Land

The Place of International Medical Graduates in Rural America

Leonard D. Baer

LEXINGTON BOOKS
Lanham • Boulder • New York • Oxford

LEXINGTON BOOKS

Published in the United States of America
by Lexington Books
A Member of the Rowman & Littlefield Publishing Group
4720 Boston Way, Lanham, Maryland 20706

PO Box 317
Oxford
OX2 9RU, UK

British Library Cataloguing in Publication Information Available

Library of Congress Cataloging-in-Publication Data

Baer, Leonard David.
Doctors in a strange land : the place of international medical graduates in rural america / Leonard D. Baer.
p. cm.
Includes bibliographical references and index.
ISBN: 978-0-7391-0493-4
1. Physicians, Foreign—United States. 2. Medicine, Rural—United States. 3. Social medicine—United States. I. Title.
R697.F6 B344 2002 2002010337

Printed in the United States of America

∞™ The paper used in this publication meets the minimum requirements of American National Standard for Information Sciences—Permanence of Paper for Printed Library Materials, ANSI/NISO Z39.48-1992.

Contents

List of Figures vii

Acknowledgments ix

Part 1: Overview

1 Introduction 3

2 Theoretical Framework 17

Part 2: Case Study on Quincy

3 Background on Quincy: Across the Unclear Boundaries 35

4 Mechanisms and Quincy: Tipping Points For and Against Acceptability 49

5 Contexts and Quincy: "Breaking that Ice" 67

Part 3: Case Study on Hamilton

6 Background on Hamilton: Tapestry on a Different Fabric 113

7 Mechanisms and Hamilton: Exclusions and Uncertainties 133

8 Contexts and Hamilton, Part I: Issues and Nonissues 185

9 Contexts and Hamilton, Part II: Peering into the Hologram 229

Part 4: Conclusions

10 Conclusions 271

Appendix 291
Bibliography 295
Index 303
About the Author 307

Figures

Figure 1.1	International Medical Graduates per 100,000 Population, 1996	8
Figure 1.2	International Medical Graduates of Asian Indian Origin per 100,000 Population, 1996	8
Figure 2.1	A Realist Framework Contexts of (Structures), Mechanisms, and Events	23
Figure 10.1	Concept Map	293

Acknowledgments

This book is based on a dissertation that I completed for my Ph.D. in geography at the University of North Carolina at Chapel Hill. Wil Gesler served as my advisor, and I cannot thank him enough for his input on this and so many other projects. It would be impossible to find enough high praises to sing about his place in geography, or about his contributions to my growth as a researcher. My sincere thanks also go out to Bob Konrad, a sociologist at the Sheps Center for Health Services Research. Through rambling conversations about any issue on almost any day, we would consider geography in offbeat ways on offbeat topics. As a result, I saw more of the links between sociology and geography, and how such links could be useful in my research. I am also grateful to Altha Cravey, particularly for her contributions to my considerations of social theory, and to John Florin and Leo Zonn for their continued interest in this study. I also wish to thank Tom Ricketts for helping me develop my initial interest in the issue of the role of international medical graduates in rural America. Thank you also to Don Pathman for his time and energy in providing feedback while my work was in the planning stages. I also want to acknowledge the Agency for Healthcare Quality and Research, which provided funding for this study through a pre-doctoral fellowship.

I am grateful to Pat Carroll of Medscribe for her help with transcription, and her patience while I learned about audio quality. Thank you also to Neil Thakur and Samruddhi Thaker for reviewing a few of the anonymous transcripts to cross-check our impressions of individual interviews. Thanks also go out to Chris Beacock for help with graphics and to Steve Fleetwood for his input. Last but by no means least, there were literally hundreds of people in small towns who went out of their way to help me conduct this study. I cannot list any of their names here because of confidentiality but I am so grateful to them for their insights in making this study work. My sincere thanks go out to all of them for their help.

Part One

OVERVIEW

Chapter One

Introduction

"He wants to know what we think of the foreign doctors." That was how some people in rural areas described this research project to one another. In less colloquial terms, I considered whether and to what extent international medical graduates (IMGs) are accepted in rural America. Acceptability is a complicated issue but at its core, in this study, is the inclusiveness of a place in receiving IMGs in the medical and nonmedical communities.

A simple scenario can help personalize a key problem addressed by this study. Suppose that you are one of many physicians who immigrated to the United States. Imagine this, too: Policy makers in Washington, D.C., and in every state are talking about you. They are holding meetings and proposing strategies on the best way to include or exclude you. Academic researchers are gathering composite data about you and other physicians, crunching the numbers, and writing articles about your strengths and weaknesses. Many of the policy makers and researchers claim that you do not go where you are most needed. They have reached a broad consensus that you are a "problem" and that the number of people like you should be reduced. The arguments appear rational, data-driven, and persuasive, but they tell only part of the story.

This scenario is not far-fetched for IMGs—physicians who received their medical degrees outside of the United States and Canada. The issue of the role of IMGs within the U.S. health care system elicits conflicting views from policy makers, researchers, and health professions educators. Many policy makers consider IMGs a "problem" that adds to a presumed physician oversupply, while others see IMGs as a badly needed resource in places that have difficulty recruiting U.S. medical graduates. Residents of a particular town may view some IMGs as the "other," as outsiders belonging to somewhere else and yet practicing in their community (see Valentine, 1999; Rose, 1993;

Sibley, 1992, 1995; Jackson, 1989; Said, 1978). By merely counting the number of physicians situated in rural and needy areas, researchers have made a case that IMGs do reduce physician shortages (e.g., Baer et al., 1998, 1999a; Mick and Lee, 1997a; Mick et al., 2000). Yet we need to look beyond the numbers and find out what really takes place in local communities.

Quantitative studies have their place, but numbers can mask the human dimension of the health workforce, even in well-designed studies. A patient's thoughts about seeing a physician, and a physician's thoughts about living in a rural town, can lie hidden beneath *r* squares, Gini coefficients, and policy discussions. Contexts such as race, gender, or foreignness are perceived differently from one place to another, with depth in meaning that cannot possibly be included in an equation or a map.

A nongeographer may seem puzzled at this point, as might a geographer focused primarily on spatial analysis. At first glance, the issue of IMG acceptability may seem largely a consideration of sociology, psychology, or anthropology, and unrelated to geography. However, everything has a geography, and acceptability is no exception. Acceptability can be related to the core geographic notion of place. Some places may be more weakly or strongly classified as homogeneous in terms of acceptability (Sibley, 1992; Said, 1978). People may consider some places as having a particular character or nature of being less or more open to outsiders. People who fit in well in one place may be "othered" in another. Meanwhile, the identities of any place change over time, as different events occur, but people who live in a place—any place—may have a static view of what that place should be or what it is. IMGs may inadvertently challenge such place identities by bringing in language, customs, social networks, and mores that are perceived as Other. Moreover, rural residents—or anyone, for that matter—experience shifts in the size of their social worlds through exposure to different ideas, places, and people. Even within a place, different communities shrink or expand in their external connections because of travel, the media, shifts in social networks, and countless other contacts with people and places. The clash or melding of multiple worlds coming together—across multiple scales from the local to the global—might result in some resistance to change. Within places, IMGs are part of such change, and resistance to them could limit perceived or real access to health care.

THE RESEARCH QUESTION AND STUDY AREA

The following question is the primary focus for this study: Are IMGs accepted in rural America? As mentioned earlier, acceptability is defined here as the inclusiveness of a place in receiving IMGs in the medical and nonmedical communities. As part of that definition, I consider places to be most inclusive if IMGs have a sense of belonging in the medical and general communities where they practice. Acceptability is a two-way process, involving both IMGs' perceptions toward the inclusiveness of a town, and the town's perceptions toward IMGs.

The extraordinary complexity of such issues makes precise subcategorizations of acceptability seem naïve. Moreover, in conducting this study, I developed research questions that served primarily as a tool to help guide data collection; each question that I developed blurs with the other questions and leads to many finer points of discussion. Nonetheless, such questions help lay the groundwork for more detailed discussion about each town:

1. Do IMGs have difficulty overcoming status as outsiders when living or practicing in a rural area? An aspect of this question is, how might people's views of IMGs as outsiders vary in the medical and nonmedical communities?
2. How well do the medical community and patients accept IMGs as clinicians, compared with the acceptance of U.S. medical graduates? Similarly, do IMGs or others in the medical community perceive any differences in patients' acceptability of IMGs (e.g., by race, education, income, or rurality)?
3. Do IMGs have difficulty communicating with patients? Similarly, are there local or regional expressions that pose problems for IMGs in caring for patients?
4. Are there any indications of discrimination toward IMGs in the towns where they practice?

The above questions are not typical research questions in the sense that I make no effort to analyze them in separate, contained boxes. Instead, the research questions helped in conducting in-depth interviews that included many different angles and ideas (see the appendix). Research and interview questions evolved through the course of the study, since I did not know which questions should guide my interviews until I talked with study participants in rural communities. It would be relatively easy to arrive at other research questions within the confines of my office; the downfall would be that some questions would be less applicable than others in rural health care.

In addressing the above questions, this study focuses on two rural towns in the Southeastern United States as case studies ("Quincy" and "Hamilton"). In both towns and their nearby areas, I talked with selected residents and medical personnel to learn about the acceptability of IMGs. I learned from townspeople of all walks of life who were kind enough to open up their thoughts, their hospitality, and their experiences to me. Both towns are in rural areas with relatively high levels of poverty and large minority populations and have similar population sizes. The two towns are also similar in driving distance from my own location during fieldwork[1] and have contrasting IMG percentages and physician specialty mixes.

The names of all towns and counties within and around the study areas have been changed, based on guarantees of confidentiality made to participants. This applies also within study participants' quotations in order to provide a continuous flow in the narrative.

In order for the findings and questions to be more meaningful beyond the two selected towns, this study also includes numerous considerations of broader contexts for IMG acceptability. Social or spatial issues (e.g., race, gender roles, religion, globalization) serve as contexts for place-specific findings (e.g., acceptability within Quincy or Hamilton). Such contexts are considered through the words and ideas of rural Americans in and near Quincy and Hamilton, and through my own observations.

POLICY CONTEXT: INTERNATIONAL MEDICAL GRADUATES IN THE UNITED STATES

A report about IMGs aired on the U.S. news program *60 Minutes* at the time of my field work (CBS News, 1999). As correspondent Lesley Stahl reported, "If the question used to be 'Is there a doctor in the house?' today it's more likely to be, 'Where are you from, doctor, and how did you end up in the United States?' Not a bad question considering that doctors from abroad now account for 25 percent of all our M.D.s." As the national media turns its attention to doctors from abroad, a number of observers have expressed a concern that the United States should have fewer IMGs (American Association of Colleges of Osteopathic Medicine et al., 1997; Mullan, 1997; Council on Graduate Medical Education, 1998; CBS News, 1999). At the same time, recent studies indicate that IMGs reduce physician shortages by practicing in rural and inner city areas where U.S. medical graduates are less likely to practice (Baer et al., 1998; Mick and Lee, 1997a, 1999a, 1999b). Although many IMGs tend toward urban-based practices (Politzer et al., 1998), IMGs who practice in rural areas are more likely to practice in underserved than non-underserved counties (Baer et al., 1998). Moreover, many community health centers have become dependent on IMG staffing so that they can remain open to provide care for the poor and underserved (Baer et al., 1999a).

However, the issues involved are far from straightforward. The role of IMGs is complicated by many factors: altruistic concerns about distributing health providers in needy areas; concerns about a physician oversupply; economic concerns; immigration laws; the potential for personal or political biases against or for IMGs; the unique complexity of each place served by an IMG; and concerns about national security after the tragic events of September 11, 2001.

As of 1996, there were approximately 550,000 physicians in the United States, including over 123,000 IMGs (American Medical Association, 1996). Approximately 3 percent of all physicians in the United States were US-IMGs—i.e., American citizens who left the country to pursue an M.D. Approximately 20 percent of all physicians in the United States were foreign-national (FN) IMGs (Mullan et al., 1995). These data largely reflect other authors' ideas about the distribution of IMGs in the mid-1990s. The fact is though that most secondary data sources cannot be used to distinguish between US-IMGs and FN-IMGs, so we cannot be absolutely certain how many IMGs are actually "FN."

A distinction between US- and FN-IMGs is important in this study for at least two reasons: (1) the policy debate primarily concerns FN-IMGs, since immigration pathways and laws have less relevance to US-IMGs; and (2) the overwhelming majority of IMGs are FN-IMGs, so their experiences warrant some study. Therefore, my focus in this study is on FN-IMGs (in colloquial terms, "the foreign doctors"), even if the quantitative data do not enable such specificity.

The map in Figure 1.1 shows that the geographic distribution of IMGs is widespread throughout the country's nonmetropolitan counties.[2] Figure 1.1 cannot be used to distinguish between FN-IMGs and US-IMGs because of data limitations of the American Medical Association Physician Masterfile. As indicated by the darker shadings in Figure 1.1, some counties have a substantially higher number of IMGs per 100,000 population. One reading of the map could be that western counties have the fewest IMGs. This finding is supported by research showing that the western United States has less dependence on IMGs than do other parts of the country (Baer et al., 1998). However, the smaller size of counties in the eastern part of the country obscures the fact that many counties, particularly in the Midwest, also have relatively few or no IMGs.

The map can be redrawn to reflect the geographic distribution of IMGs from specific countries of origin. Figure 1.2 shows the geographic distribution of IMGs who received their medical degrees in India, which represents the largest proportion of IMGs in the United States (19.5 percent) and, more specifically, in nonmetropolitan counties in the United States (22.7 percent) (American Medical Association, 1996; American Medical Association International Medical Graduates Section, 2000). From the map in Figure 1.2, further detail about the geographic distribution of IMGs from India is evident, particularly in comparing western and eastern counties in the United States. Substantial portions

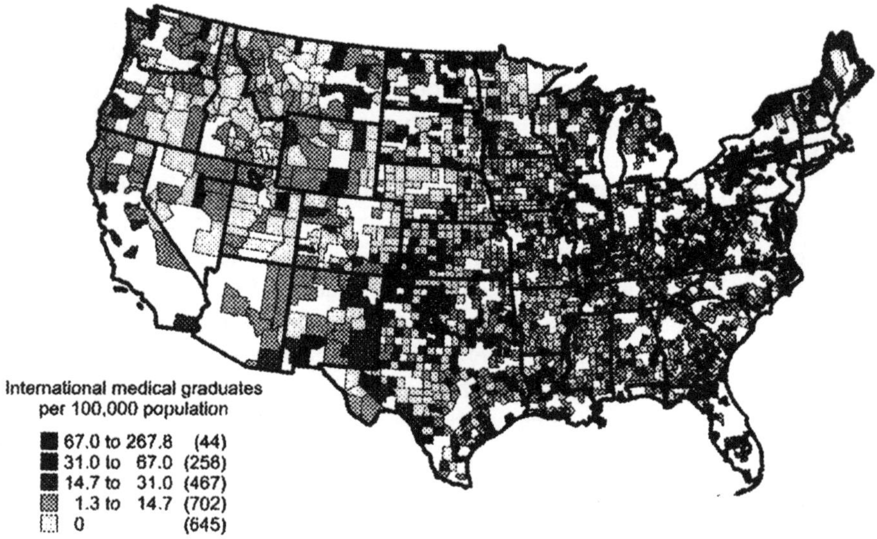

Note: Limited to physicians in direct patient care. Metropolitan counties are aggregated into white areas on the map.
Source: American Medical Association Physician Masterfile, 1996; Area Resource File, 1998.

Figure 1.1. International Medical Graduates per 100,000 Population in Nonmetropolitan Counties, 1996

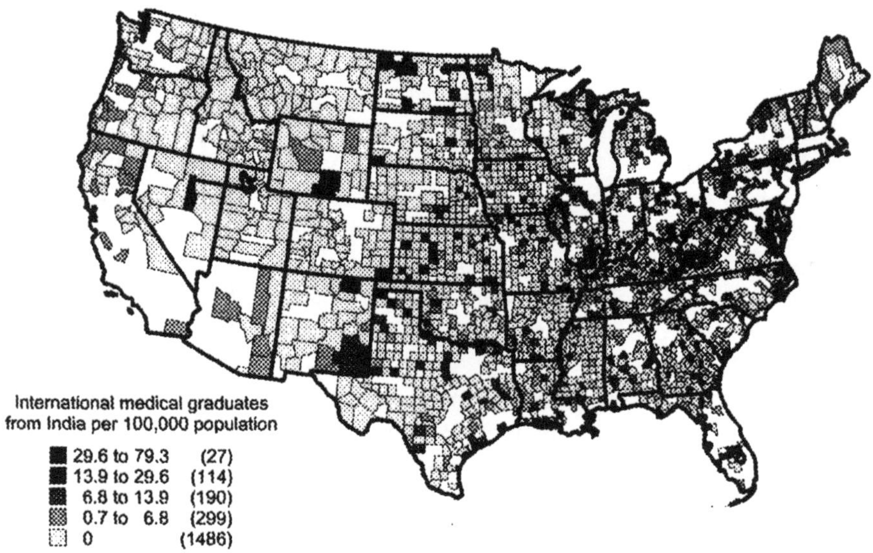

Note: Limited to physicians in direct patient care. Metropolitan counties are aggregated into white areas on the map.
Source: American Medical Association Physician Masterfile, 1996; Area Resource File, 1998.

Figure 1.2. International Medical Graduates of Asian Indian Origin per 100,000 Population in Nonmetropolitan Counties, 1996

of most western states have no IMGs from India in nonmetropolitan counties. By contrast, the eastern United States has several clusters of nonmetropolitan counties that have a relatively high number of IMGs per 100,000 population. For example, IMGs from India have a dense concentration in the Appalachian region, including many counties in West Virginia and Kentucky.

In and of themselves, geographic clusters raise questions. For example, why are there clusters of IMGs in some parts of the country? Similarly, why are there clusters of IMGs within specific towns, or in specific medical practices? The answers could have something to do with acceptability, and therefore warrant some attention in this work. Clustering of IMGs is shaped at least indirectly in many ways, including but not limited to: state laws and policies, international social networks, a global economy in which physicians practice medicine outside of their country of origin, and the viewpoints of people from other countries toward the United States, and toward a region or state in the United States.

What may have seemed an easy exercise—studying the geographic distribution of people in different counties or regions—is now considerably more complex because acceptability does not take place in a vacuum. Events and ideas at far broader scales of analysis cannot be cut off easily from perceptions in a place. Thus, Figures 1.1 and 1.2 help lay the national groundwork for considering IMG acceptability locally.

There can also be differences in the acceptability of IMGs of different countries of origin. IMGs are a heterogeneous group. As of 1996, nearly half of all nonmetropolitan IMGs came from three countries: India (22.7 percent), the Philippines (18.4 percent), and Mexico (7.3 percent). Pakistan (5.2 percent) and South Korea (3.3 percent) are also among the countries that contribute to the supply of nonmetropolitan IMGs (American Medical Association, 1996). Country of origin for IMGs can vary widely; Mullan et al. (1995) reported that, in 1995, the Educational Commission for Foreign Medical Graduates (ECFMG) certified credentials for medical schools in 130 countries. Somewhat related, many IMGs have special cultural and linguistic competencies that make them an asset in some places more than in others (Magdalena Miranda, Educational Commission for Foreign Medical Graduates, personal communication, January 5, 1999). For example, IMGs who speak Spanish can care for some non-English speaking populations without any need for interpreters and may be able to relate on a personal level to similarities in cultural background. Also, the experience of growing up or treating patients in less developed countries can familiarize physicians with poverty beyond what is expected in the United States. Considering such competencies and experiences, it becomes especially useful to learn more about the acceptability of IMGs in underserved areas.

Yet another major consideration for IMGs is immigration law. FN-IMGs are at various stages of the immigration process, including being naturalized

U.S. citizens, permanent residents, and temporary visitors. As part of a larger, complicated process of immigration and health policy, IMGs must undertake U.S. residencies in order to be licensed, the exact length of which varies by state (Mullan et al., 1995). The number of IMGs in U.S. residencies more than doubled between 1988 and 1995, while the number of U.S. medical graduates in U.S. residencies remained relatively stable (Mullan, 1997; Council on Graduate Medical Education, 1998). However, the number of IMGs in U.S. residency programs has leveled off since then, including a slight decrease in recent years, from 25,531 in 1997 to 25,403 in 2001 (JAMA, 2002). The proportion of residents who are IMGs has remained relatively stable since 1995, around one-fourth of all physicians (Miller et al., 1999). Medicare pays for much of graduate medical education, which adds to policy concerns about how many IMGs should be trained.

The increase that occurred in the number of IMGs becomes more evident when considering exchange visitor visa waivers. An IMG can enter the United States for work or training with a temporary visa known as the "J-1" visa, which may be requested through state governments or specific federal agencies, including the Appalachian Regional Commission. Once the visa expires, the IMG is required by law to return to the home country. However, a waiver can be granted for the return home requirement if the IMG practices in an underserved area. Waivers may also be requested for direct employment within a federal facility, such as Veterans Administration hospitals, and for academic research of national importance (Chehrazi et al., 1999). The annual number of J-1 visa waiver requests to practice in underserved areas increased from 70 in 1990 to 1,374 in 1995, which raised further concerns among policy makers about the impact of IMGs on physician oversupply (U.S. General Accounting Office, 1996). In a complex immigration process, waiver physicians can seek an H-1B visa, which can be followed by application for a green card, which enables permanent entry into the United States (Chehrazi et al., 1999; Mullan et al., 1995). Despite its roots as a way of helping other countries improve the training and quality of their physician workforce, the J-1 visa has become part of the immigration pathway for permanent entry into the United States as an IMG (U.S. General Accounting Office, 1996).

There is considerable interstate variation in policies toward requesting J-1 waivers, and, in several states, substantial changes have been made in restrictiveness toward the placement of waiver physicians from one year to the next (Chehrazi et al., 1999). Beginning October 1994, each state could request up to twenty waivers per year (P.L. 103-416). As of 1999, eleven states—primarily in the western United States—had no program to request waivers (Chehrazi et al., 1999). The U.S. General Accounting Office (1996) reported that in 1995, most waivers were requested through federal agencies, and states generally did not request all twenty waivers.

States vary in the contractual length of time waiver physicians must practice in underserved areas. Typically, the contract term is three years, but a few states require a four year commitment (Chehrazi et al., 1999). Some employers require longer commitments than states, so an IMG can be obligated to practice in an underserved area after the waiver is over. An added issue is that employers can file petitions for an H-1B visa, which is another temporary exchange visitor visa that is often pursued by physicians on a J-1 visa waiver. The U.S. Immigration and Naturalization Service (INS) places a cap on how many H-1B visas can be issued annually, with some exemptions under specific legal criteria. The H-1B visa can be issued to people from a broad variety of different professions that require a college degree, such as computer scientists, architects, engineers, mathematicians, accountants, theologians, and physicians (Maggio, 1998). At this writing, the U.S. Senate is considering a bill to increase the total number of H-1B visas from 115,000 to 200,000 over each of the next three years. Without passage of the bill, the number of H-1B visas for all occupational groups would fall to 107,500 in the next fiscal year beginning October 1, and 65,000 in the year after that (Jansen, 2000). Failure to receive an H-1B visa would limit the ability of an IMG to stay in the country, much less remain in a rural, underserved area after completion of the waiver obligation.

As IMGs steer through complicated immigration pathways, observers have expressed a concern that the United States already has too many physicians. Many policy makers and health planners believe that a physician surplus leads to unnecessary expenditures, including extra diagnostic tests, referrals, prescriptions, and medical procedures. As government expenditures rise for Medicare and Medicaid, one could argue that it is in the taxpayers' interests to reduce the supply of physicians. However, there is no benchmark to indicate how many physicians is too many.

Critics of IMGs have contended that it makes no policy sense to continue importing so many physicians if the United States already has a physician surplus. Moreover, some observers contend that IMGs can contribute to future underemployment and unemployment of U.S. medical graduates (Mullan et al., 1995). However, the policy dynamic has changed since the events of September 11, 2001. The economic concerns about a possible physician oversupply that seemed urgent only a few years ago are no longer as pronounced. Now, national security is a driving force behind policy maker's concerns about the influx of IMGs, and it would be an overstatement to say that there is a movement for an IMG cutback (Stephen S. Mick, personal communication, August 22, 2002). Yet it would be unwise to forget that, only a few years ago, policy makers were calling for a cutback on the number of new IMGs.

The Council on Graduate Medical Education (1998, 2000) had called for the elimination of new J-1 visa waivers to practice in underserved areas, expansion of the return home requirement from two to five years, and capitation of residency training at 110 percent of the total number of 1993 graduating U.S. medical graduates. A joint consensus statement by a number of prominent health professions associations, including the American Medical Association, had nearly identical suggestions about restrictions on IMGs in the U.S. physician workforce (American Association of Colleges of Osteopathic Medicine et al., 1997). However, there may have been a softening of the language used by some advocates of an IMG cutback. For example, a report by the Council on Graduate Medical Education (1999) indicated that the marketplace could be effective in reducing the number of IMGs entering U.S. residency programs. Only a few years later, the U.S. Department of Agriculture (2002) withdrew from the waiver program because of security concerns about ensuring adequate background checks after the events of September 11, 2001. Thus, there are swings that can move relatively quickly, from IMG increases to calls for cutbacks, with the pendulum still in motion.

Theoretically, an increase in the supply of IMGs would lead to an increase in the number of physicians practicing in underserved areas. However, an increase in physician supply cannot be expected to lead to more equitable distributions of physicians. As indicated by the inverse care law, places with the greatest need have the lowest availability of good medical care, and places with the least need have the greatest availability of good medical care (Tudor Hart, 2000, 1971; Jones and Moon, 1987; Joseph and Phillips, 1984). By way of analogy, an increasing supply of physicians can be likened to large "sandpiles" or strong concentrations of physicians. Some of the sand may eventually spill into places that have no sandpiles, but simply piling on more sand is a very expensive process of filling empty spaces. In financing medical education that helps produce lopsided distributions of physicians, government may be using taxpayer money inefficiently.

Yet another concern in health workforce policy has been that the number of IMGs in the United States could add to bloated resident trainee numbers. Since it is less expensive to employ a resident than house-staff, some inner city teaching hospitals employ physicians who have already undergone residencies. Such physicians agree to have further residency or fellowship training in order to remain employed, and thus receive a markedly lower wage relative to other physicians with comparable training. Meanwhile, the resulting, bloated number of resident trainees is financed, in part, by Medicare expenditures. Again, national policies (e.g., Medicare) have different impacts at the local level, influenced by numerous factors such as need, opportunity, economics, and the use of IMGs in specific places.

Meanwhile, physician maldistribution is evident internationally, as when less developed countries lose their most highly educated citizens to practice medicine in the United States. Within local areas, and among countries, there is often an inequitable distribution of physicians. For example, IMGs help alleviate physician shortages in local areas within a number of more developed countries, including the United States, the United Kingdom and New Zealand (Baer et al., 1998, 1999a; Mick and Lee, 1997b; Barnett, 1991a, b, c, d, 1992; Taylor and Esmail, 1999). Such geographic patterns reflect at least some extent larger social processes (e.g., unevenness in employment opportunities, ethnic representation in the medical profession, differences in laws and policies) that push or pull physicians from one locality to another. Thus, it would be naïve to assume that any single issue, such as concerns about a physician oversupply, or national security, is necessarily the sole driving force behind policies toward IMGs. So many different issues are influencing the policy dynamic simultaneously.

Within such a complex policy context, concerns about IMG acceptability pose a particularly striking paradox: Should policy makers seek to funnel IMGs into underserved places that are less accepting of physicians from other countries? Exploring the issue of acceptability in some depth will help in understanding what can be done along several fronts, such as reducing local objections to IMGs, to whatever extent those objections exist; improving the experiences of IMGs; and addressing local concerns about IMGs through changes in policy, medical training, or involvement between communities and physicians in social and professional life.

SOCIAL THEORY AND GEOGRAPHIES OF HEALTH

Until now, social theory has been primarily an implicit consideration in this discussion, and not addressed directly. By "social theory," I mean the construction of social and philosophical frameworks for understanding the world around us. This study builds on ideas from critical realism and yet focuses more on original theory-building than on following a prescribed format or recipe from other scholars. More on the specifics of my theoretical ideas will come later, in the next chapter, but it is important to lay the groundwork first for considering why we should even be thinking about social theory for health geography studies.

In health geography, social theory tended to be overlooked until the early 1990s, with a major exception being the work of Jones and Moon (1987). However, in the broader health services research community, social theory is still a novel and often unknown concept, albeit one that is highly relevant to learning about health care.

Much of the literature in health geography continues to omit a social framework that, in the earliest geographic works in health services research, had been more prominent (e.g., deVise, 1973). For example, in the book, *Geographic Methods for Health Services Research*, Ricketts et al. (1994) discussed geographic contributions to health services research while omitting consideration of social theory altogether. In geography, many quantitative techniques and methods such as location-allocation modeling, Monte Carlo simulations, GIS, and cluster analysis are tremendously useful in advancing technical and scientific contributions of health geographers, but practitioners often pay little attention to the social theories that actually underpin their work. Such inattention to social theory can be likened to a scene from the classic movie *The Wizard of Oz* in which a man behind a curtain tells Dorothy, "Pay no attention to the man behind the curtain." Researchers all too often take for granted that their particular approaches and most basic assumptions make sense, while never really "pulling the curtain" to see what is behind it. Social theory is about questioning authority and, ideally, doing away with dogma, absolutes, and cookbook instructions that (at the risk of mixing metaphors) allow the curtain to stay closed. This point will become clearer in the next chapter on the theoretical considerations that underpin this study.

An inattention to social theory has permeated much of the subdiscipline of health geography (Litva and Eyles, 1995; Mayer and Meade, 1994; Kearns, 1993; Kearns and Joseph, 1993). In reaction to such inattention, Kearns (1993) called for a "reformed medical geography." He wanted health geographers to look beyond mere location and start considering the importance of place. Kearns and Joseph (1993) voiced similar concerns and discussed whether geographers should consider the social construction of place and the meanings and experiences therein. They called for consideration of the connections between place and space, including connections between site-specific findings and human activity at broader scales of analysis.

Prior to such calls for a reformed health geography, Gesler (1992) considered whether health care landscapes are therapeutic. In doing so, he linked the social construction of place with health care. More recently, Gesler et al. (1997) raised the idea that social theory can be extended beyond health services research to disease ecology and, in particular, to studies addressing infant mortality. In 1998, Kearns and Gesler edited a book, *Putting Health into Place*, that further demonstrated the importance of the meanings and social construction of place in health care delivery. In this book, for example, Takahashi (1998) provided lists of places in order of how acceptable they are to health professionals. However, these and other advances in conceptualizing geography within social frameworks have been presented largely to geographers and other academics, but not to policy makers.

Unfortunately, many of the calls for a more informed use of social theory in health geography have been limited to thought papers in academic settings. However, researchers have also done fieldwork that applies more ideas from social theory to research in health geography. For example, Cutchin (1997) adapted the philosophy of pragmatism to theory-building from his fieldwork on the retention of rural physicians in Kentucky. Wilton (1996) wrote about diminishing activity spaces over time for people with AIDS, and Alderman (1997) addressed the importance of place in the construction and location of nineteenth century mental asylums. In these and many subsequent articles that appear in the journal *Health and Place*, contributors often use qualitative methods as part of theory-building in health services research.

Consistent with calls for further use of social theory, the line between social and health geography is often blurred. Social geographers often focus on the complex linkages between social structures (e.g., race, gender) and geographic considerations. Health geographers can apply social geography toward health services research, disease ecology, or disease distribution (Gesler et al., 1997), even without being social geographers. For example, Good (1987) showed the importance of belief systems in ethnomedical health care in Kenya. Among other issues, he considered the psychosocial benefits of traditional health care in sub-Saharan Africa within the broader context of the structure of biomedicine. Yet in depth considerations of social geography are largely missing in the increasing drive for larger and larger data sets and analyses of secondary data in health services research. To accommodate funding constraints, the massive capabilities of computers, and pervasive mindsets, health services researchers often limit their studies through implicit assumptions of separateness between the social and the spatial.

Kearns and others calling for further linkages between social theory, social geography, and health geography have pointed to the ideas of Massey (1984, 1997), Tuan (1974) and others who challenge basic notions of the meaning of place. Entrikin (1991) considered place as context, presenting a complex if not quasi-philosophical overview of how geographers can look at the concept of place. Ideas from other non-health geographers, such as Sibley (1992), have particular usefulness within health geography as well. Sibley (1992, 1995) discussed geographies of exclusion. He wrote about places as open or closed to different people or ideas, with some places more strongly defined as homogeneous than others. Such works demonstrate the growth of the discipline, while still leaving many research gaps in linking applied and theoretical studies.

The challenge now is to build on advances in health geography to highlight their usefulness both inside and outside of academia. It is far too easy to cordon off complex academic ideas and assume that they have no bearing in the "real world." On the one hand, it would be highly unconventional for policy makers to delve into the strengths and weaknesses of different philosophies, such as critical realism, humanism, or structuralism. On the other hand, we cannot let theoretical divides between policy makers and academics hold back our work, either. There is a need to unite the practical concerns of policy makers with the theoretical concerns of academics. The issue of acceptability is far too important and multifaceted to avoid socially useful, theoretically informed work.

NOTES

1. The approximate distance is not given because of confidentiality guaranteed to participants.
2. The term "nonmetropolitan" is one of many designations that can be used in defining what is or is not a rural area (Ricketts et al., 1998; Johnson-Webb et al., 1997).

Chapter Two

Theoretical Framework

Several ideas from critical realism, to be discussed in this chapter, helped form the framework used in this study. At the same time, to describe the philosophical underpinnings of this book as a carbon copy of the critical realist ideas of Andrew Sayer or Roy Bhaskar would be misleading. On the one hand, my research builds heavily on realist ideas that are described below, such as the interplay among structures, mechanisms, and events, and the consideration of open versus closed systems. On the other hand, my (re)interpretation of critical realism is what worked best in my own thinking. It would be simplistic to merely follow a cookbook recipe, as though the main focus of theory is to "fit" a study into predetermined categories, such as structures, mechanisms, and events. It would also be simplistic to act as a reporter to merely summarize ideas from critical realism that have been described far more thoroughly elsewhere (e.g., Sayer, 1992, 2000). It cannot be emphasized enough that "theory" as defined earlier is considered alive and not static. Theory is not used here to follow someone else's rules, but instead to question, and then question some more.

Having said that, I recognize that some readers may still wonder why theory is important at all in research. That is why this chapter is so important. Most people have never heard of the word "positivism," perhaps because it is a term that is rarely used outside of academia. Nonetheless, the appeal of positivism stretches far beyond the walls of the Ivory Tower and into newscasts and everyday conversations. Positivist theory is based on the assumption that human beings behave in a regular manner and that their behavior follows logical, repeatable trends. The aim of positivist research is to find regularities and generate laws. In the social sciences, this often means that researchers quantify various phenomena in order to measure, classify, or predict human behavior. From predicting the winner of a football game to predicting patient satisfaction with physicians, many researchers try to reach conclusions about virtually any aspect of human behavior.

Many researchers do not recognize that their approaches are based on a positivist framework and even call into question the positivist label as unnecessary and derisive. Well-conducted, positivist studies do have numerous benefits, including the perception of precision, repeatability, measurability, conciseness, and power in influencing people's viewpoints, as well as fundability and broad acceptance in the research community. However, there are also several important shortcomings to positivist research or (if positivism is an uncomfortable label) to research that is based on a search for generalizable laws about human behavior.

In physics and other fields that focus on measurable quantities (e.g., temperature, body mass, liters of water), quantification and the generation of laws are obvious resources. But do we know all of the variables necessary to measure social phenomena or to predict what will happen to human beings in the future? Moreover, is it possible to take the same research frameworks used in the natural sciences and apply them to studies on human behavior? This point will be returned to shortly, in considering the ideas of "open" versus "closed" systems.

The issue of causality presents further complex problems for many research studies, particularly considering across-scale linkages, choice of variables, and correlations as a frequent proxy for causation. Obviously, not everything can be quantified, especially not intrinsically qualitative or subjective phenomena that affect human behavior. For example, important information about human behavior can be missed by reducing complex interdependencies among places to a matrix or statistic (see Blalock, 1971).

A CRITICAL REALIST FRAMEWORK

Readers looking for a comprehensive overview of critical realism or of other philosophies are advised to look elsewhere (e.g., Sayer, 1992, 2000). What I am discussing here are ideas *from* critical realism that served as important in my research. Before proceeding any further, consider first a critical realist perspective on the idea of causality.

Causality can be important for positivist researchers trying to learn *why* human beings behave in particular ways. Researchers often take for granted the idea that a *cause* for a problem can be found in an equation. Nonetheless, the issue of causality poses major problems for researchers in search of measurable predictions. Whether in the physical or social sciences, the same spatial form can result from many different processes. For example, a rock slide is not necessarily the result of one factor but possibly of many. Similarly, the geographic distribution of IMGs can arrive from multiple factors, many of which are likely left unstated or overlooked (Baer et al., 1998). As Sayer (1985, p. 162) noted, "what causes something to happen has nothing to do with the matter of the number of times it has happened or been observed to happen and hence with whether it constitutes a regularity."

Much of Sayer's concern is based on the distinction between open and closed systems. The use of quantitative methods to study causality in closed systems requires controls on all possible variables (Sayer, 1992, 1985). However, we live in open systems. Everything exists in some context, and it would be impossible to find complete explanation about causality through selected, quantitative techniques. In fairness, careful statistical analysis involves consideration of confounding variables and interaction terms. Nonetheless, statisticians cannot be expected to know and quantify all relevant variables in every study. Moreover, many variables, such as rurality or race, are far too complex to be captured beyond a superficial level in an equation.

In simplifying complexity to find "predictions," researchers may find that *X* covaries with *Y*, while overlooking the fact that a correlation does not necessarily entail causality. For example, suppose that a drunk has no idea how he actually gets drunk. One day, the drunk drinks soda and scotch, and the next day he drinks soda and rum, and the next day soda and bourbon. On the next day, he does not drink any soda and does not get drunk. The drunk's conclusion is that soda made him drunk (Sayer, 1992). Sayer (1992) asserts that the same general mistake is common in research. Correlations can indicate that a quantitative relationship between two variables exists, but such a relationship might be unimportant in terms of causation.

In contrast to the general mindset in positivist research (e.g., the measurable impact of *X* on *Y*), realists do not associate causality with regularity (Sayer, 1992). Instead, causality is dependent on context and varies by the "mechanism" that triggers the event. What causes a particular spatial form (e.g., a rock slide, or a geographic distribution of physicians) in one place may not be the same in another. Furthermore, the causes of a spatial form can change over time and should not be expected to remain constant. In short, causality is often *contingent* upon other factors being present.

Events, Mechanisms, and Structures

Suppose an event occurs (e.g., a person looking for an apartment, a patient choosing a physician, a plant laying off workers). Why does this or any event occur? In a critical realist framework, it is essential to understand that there are mechanisms, which combine to create causal powers or ways of acting that can lead to events. Sayer (1992) likens mechanisms to gunpowder. There might be a cannon and a cannonball, but without gunpowder, there will be no explosion. In some cases, a mechanism will trigger an event (e.g., an explosion) and, in other cases, it will not.

On its own, a mechanism does not produce a particular event. For example, the mere existence of gunpowder could not possibly be all that is required for an explosion. The firing of the cannonball is *contingent* upon a number of possible mechanisms (e.g., production of the cannon and cannonball, proper maintenance and upkeep of all relevant materials, someone to fire the cannonball). Furthermore, structures are also important in the firing of the cannonball. For example, there may be conflict (e.g., territorial disputes, ideological disagreements); resolution (e.g., agreement among warring factions), sovereignty (e.g., political independence of a country), or oppression (e.g., denial of freedom of assembly, imprisonment of community leaders) that are among other contexts or "structures" for a specific event. A specific event is not always linked with the same mechanisms, and the same mechanisms are not always linked with the same structures (Figure 2.1). Indeed, it can be complicated to consider the various connections within and among structures, mechanisms, and events.

At this point, the term "structure" needs clarification. In discussing critical realism, Sayer (1992) defined structures as *necessary*, internal roles, related objects, or practices. An internal role or relation is considered necessary for

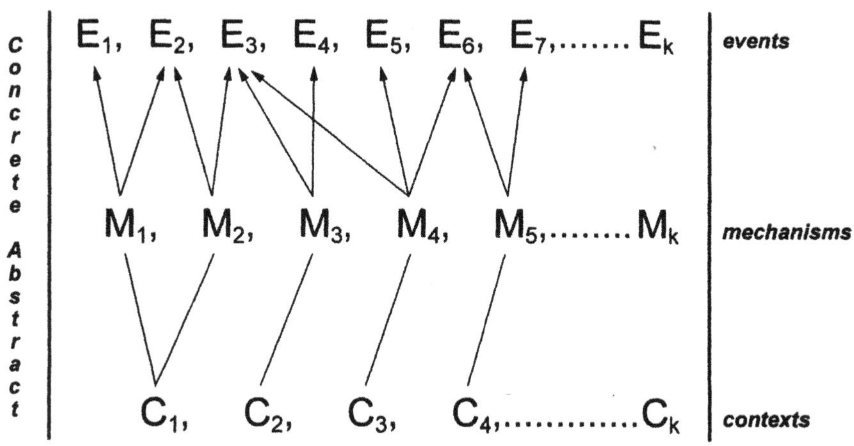

Figure 2.1. A Realist Framework of Contexts (Structures), Mechanisms, and Events. Adapted from Sayer, 1992.

at least one of the actors—e.g., provider-patient, landlord-tenant. Without the health provider, there would be no patient; without the landlord, there would be no tenant. Both roles are necessary in order for at least one of the roles to exist. Such relations also can include objects or ideas, as between discrimination and racial segregation.

A basic idea in critical realism is that there are both "internal or necessary relations" and "external or contingent relations" (Sayer, 1992, pp. 89–90). While I do not take issue with such a breakdown, my consideration of structures and mechanisms differs from the sense used by Sayer. First, consider my use of the term "context" in place of "structure." I am considering contexts as abstract spatial or social considerations that occur at broader scales of analysis than the event in question, much like Giddens's use of the term "structure" in structuration theory.

Meanwhile, the idea of contingency is still highlighted for mechanisms because contexts can be much less tangible in people's minds as potential triggers for an event. For purposes of this work, the main difference between contexts and mechanisms is the level of perceived abstraction. Events are considered in this study to be relatively concrete, mechanisms less so, and structures or "contexts" as the most abstract. In contrast to critical realism, I am not assuming a rigid breakdown between the different layers of analysis. Instead, the variations in abstraction between one layer (e.g., mechanisms) and another (e.g., contexts) can be subtle and open to interpretation in this analysis. This is not a dualistic study in which A is absolutely differentiated from B, or even (in contradiction to critical realism) mechanisms from contexts. Reality and people's views of reality can become entangled. Each exists independently of the other, but the distinctions between them, or between most categories, cannot always fit neatly in a box or diagram. The ideas presented in this work fall within the unclear intersection between reality and our perceptions of it. Therefore, it cannot be emphasized enough that I am not using the terms "mechanism" and "context" in the same sense as critical realists. In fact, the very identification of something as a context or mechanism can be open to question. By this, I mean that there can be ambiguity in determining exactly what is a mechanism and what is not; not everything has to be clearly defined or fit neatly in its place. Thus, what I am considering is not as conceptually tidy a framework as critical realism but, still, builds on it.

Consider the idea of broader structures or "contexts" even further, such as race, gender, and religion. These and all other contexts are socially constructed differently from one place to another (i.e., people create meanings for them, as opposed to the contexts having an inherent meaning). Their meanings vary geographically, as people interpret and reinterpret contexts differently in different places through their own perspectives (Sayer, 1992). The social construction of race, gender, religion, and discrimination might each be examples of contexts for IMG acceptability. Each context will have different meanings and interpretations in one town than in another. In other words, there is a place-specific interpretation of race or religion or gender, since these and other contexts are not constructed the same way in every place.

Amid variation in the abstraction of contexts, each town also has events and mechanisms. In this study, there is one major event under consideration, acceptability, but other events are also of relevance, too, such as the hiring of IMGs, a conversation between a physician and a nurse, a patient seeing a physician, or an IMG attending a community function. Indeed, such events are concrete, consistent with my reconsideration of the realist framework, whereas acceptability is less tangible and not always seen or even expressed. Nonetheless, acceptability can be perceived as if it were a palpable action (e.g., a feeling of being unwelcome; a sense that a place is more open to immigrants). Similarly, a patient's trust in a physician can be seen as an event, too, even if it is not as concrete as some of the other examples.

Mechanisms form an essential role in the relation between events (e.g., acceptability) and contexts (e.g., race, communication). Some examples of mechanisms that can influence acceptability include geographic clustering of IMGs, competence, retention, and the role of schools, hospitals, and medical clinics. For example, a specific hospital can act as a mechanism for an IMG's acceptability in an area, contingent upon other mechanisms (e.g., the competence and work ethic of IMGs in an area; the staffing patterns of individual clinics) and contexts (e.g., local attitudes toward Americanness; concerns about communication).

Even if the events are similar in the two case study towns, there may be some differences in mechanisms and contexts. However, it is often difficult to discuss one part of the context-mechanism-event framework without simultaneously discussing another. Still, for organizational purposes, I will draw my attention mainly to contexts or mechanisms in separate chapters, while discussing one principal event, acceptability.

This is an intensive study, and by "intensive," I mean a particular term used by critical realists. Intensive studies include structures (i.e., contexts), mechanisms, and events, whereas extensive studies include only events. In an extensive study, realists explore generalities among a large number of people in order to make statements about society. By contrast, intensive studies enable more details on a smaller sample (Cloke et al., 1991). For example, in this study, I learn from a limited number of people about the acceptability of

IMGs, rather than trying to be representative about general, abstracted views on society in general.

SIMPLIFICATION AND COMPLEXITY

An issue like acceptability is extraordinarily complex, since it is influenced by different contexts and mechanisms, which take shape differently in different places. Furthermore, each context has different meanings in different places, and each place is unique from all others. In light of so much complexity, categorical statements about acceptability mask considerable depth of meaning that reveal insight into human behavior. Unfortunately, complexity is often relegated to a side role in positivist research as part of an error term, or not regarded at all, in favor of precise measurements on a scale. Indeed, Baer et al. (1999b) constructed a scale of acceptability of nurse practitioners and physician assistants, while Konrad et al. (1999) constructed scales to measure an issue related to acceptability: physician job satisfaction. My contention is that the "noise" that is missing from such scales is often more important than the scales themselves. In other words, it is important to look beyond simplifications toward a fuller, richer consideration of acceptability.

The issues involved in this study cannot be reduced easily to a set list of facts, since it is not always clear in reality what constitutes a fact. Most readers might consider it a truism that "a fact is a fact is a fact." Certainly, basic principles from mathematics (e.g., two plus two equals four), and physics (e.g., gravity) still apply. Yet beliefs, perceptions, or experiences cannot always be simplified into a set list of facts. For example, people often have different views toward other races and often disagree about the characteristics that make someone black or white or Native American. Facts can be socially constructed, viewed through the lens of a person or group of people in a particular place or time (Jackson, 1989). In simplifying human activity into a set list of facts, I would be overlooking complexity that also can be relevant for this study.

Simplification is often unavoidable. For example, any description of any event necessarily entails some description that encapsulates activity into language. My aim is not to take issue with simplification but, rather, to point out that complexity can be embraced, too. For example, the framework used here includes numerous issues (i.e., the various contexts, mechanisms, or events) that can be overlooked in most positivist studies. Thus, in studying IMG acceptability, my concern is with providing new insights that help in gaining a fuller picture of IMG acceptability, which reflect the complexities of life. Exploring such complexity can be the fuel that leads to insightful research in subsequent studies, regardless of philosophical paradigm.

PLACE AND SPACE

Throughout this work, specific geographic concepts will emerge again and again. Two of these key concepts are "place" and "space." Their relevance to my theoretical framework has already been part of the discussion, particularly in relation to the idea of context. For example, I discussed earlier the importance of place in considering how abstract contexts can be considered geographically.

The concepts of "place" and "space" do not hold the same weight or meaning for all geographers. In a number of textbooks, "spatial" is even synonymous with "geographic" (e.g., de Blij and Muller, 2000). Geographers are trained to identify spatial patterns. Thus, we often look at maps of empty polygons, splash colors on them, and postulate why the resulting spatial or "geographic" patterns occur. However, if the aim of research is not to identify regularity but instead to identify complexity, all of the data and splashed-on colors only go so far. Place-oriented research can bring out complexity that might be overlooked in spatial analysis.

This study brings the uniqueness of each place to the forefront since contexts are abstracted differently in different places; mechanisms assume different importance in different places; and different events occur. Amid so much place-oriented complexity, physicians may find it easier to be accepted in some places than in others. The meaning of *place*, as conceptualized by Yi-Fu Tuan and Doreen Massey, is important in laying the groundwork for such complexity.

For Tuan (1974), place has meaning, whereas space does not. His conceptualization of place includes public symbols and fields of care. Public symbols have high imageability; that is, they are well known externally, beyond the place itself. Some of Tuan's examples of public symbols are a holy site, a formal garden, a monument, and an ideal city. Fields of care present a contrast by having low imageability; that is, they are known primarily within the place itself (Tuan, 1974). A few examples of fields of care are a person's home, a corner drug store, a bar, a marketplace, or a small town. A field of care could be any place that is not well known externally but, rather, is familiar internally. For example, a corner drug store is likely to be familiar to most people in a small town, but not to people far away. The drug store and other fields of care help define a place internally, whereas the Washington

Monument, Eiffel Tower, or other public symbols also help define a place externally. Through people's experiences, public symbols and fields of care give a place meaning that is not generalizable to other places (Tuan, 1974).

In contrast to place, Tuan (1974) considered space to be a vacant vessel that has no inherent meaning. Imagine for a moment that a polygon delineates a particular area on a map. The space within the polygon is only important insofar as it falls within drawn boundaries. In interpreting the map, thematic data can be more important than the space represented by the polygon. For example, in previous research on IMGs in underserved areas, my co-authors and I showed that there is substantial variation among states in the extent to which IMGs reduce physician shortages (Baer et al., 1998). We made spatial generalizations about IMGs by breaking the country into empty geometric forms (e.g., states), to be filled with secondary data. Such research contrasts sharply with place-oriented research because places are not empty vessels, places are unique, and places do have meaning.

Whereas Tuan dichotomized places through external and internal meanings, Massey (1997, p. 322) stated that places are "extroverted, which includes a consciousness of its links with the wider world, which integrates in a positive way the global and the local." In her view, each place is a "meeting place," constructed through networks of social interaction. For example, in one street in her hometown in the United Kingdom, there could be a TV made in Japan, a conversation in Urdu, clothes from China, and people originally from Latin America. This convergence of various communities defines the street in her hometown. Through such convergences, the street is linked with other places at far broader scales of analysis, which makes the street a unique place. Since such connections vary over time, place is not static but is a process that changes continuously, as interconnections gain shape, diminish, increase, or vanish. Boundaries are unclear since places do not stop or start at territorial lines. Instead, the boundaries always change along with the changing connections among places. Thus, although a choroplethic map may have a polygon showing the jurisdictional or imposed boundaries on an area, the real meaning of the place is not limited by those boundaries.

Consistent with critical realism, each place for Massey is contextualized within spaces. In order for this statement to have much meaning, there needs to be a different conceptualization of space. Whereas Tuan often considered Cartesian space, Massey considered social space. Space as a "vacant vessel" without meaning is altogether different from social space, constructed through human activity. In practical terms, there can be home space, rural space, ethnic space, medical space, work space, and public space, to name only a few examples. None of these spaces can be found on a map but they have meaning for people. Home space is broader than a single home. Public space is broader than a single public square. Within my theoretical framework, public space can be considered as a context for what happens within a specific location (e.g., within Central Park).

The distinction between place and space can be subtle. According to Kearns and Joseph (1993), the same ideas behind "place" can be used to define "space," and vice versa. The two terms can be differentiated by considering geographic scale of analysis. Place does not have to be defined at a particular scale of analysis, but space necessarily is at a far broader scale than the place being studied (Kearns and Joseph, 1993). Place influences space, and vice versa (Massey, 1996, 1997). For example, crime in Central Park can affect people's views of public spaces, and concerns about safety in public spaces can influence people's views of Central Park.

Put simply, place should not be a peripheral consideration in studying human activity. After all, places are not mere backdrops like settings in a play. Rather, places have personalities that can affect which behavior is appropriate, which people may interact with one another, and who does or does not belong there. The acceptability of newcomers to a town might take place within abstract contexts (e.g., the local abstraction of religion or race) and mechanisms (e.g., the influence of local churches, local politics, local leaders). Furthermore, such contexts and mechanisms are different from one place and time to another. Such issues cannot be considered in each place as an isolated entity, since social networks do not start and stop at clearly defined boundaries.

In my own conceptualization, the idea of "place" can be likened to philosophical and psychological questions about "self." What constitutes the self, or, for that matter, what constitutes a place? Are people defined by their experiences with others, by heredity, or by a complex combination of internally and externally derived factors? The same set of complex questions can be posed about places. Even if two places could have identical interconnections, I do not think that identical interconnections would lead to identical places. For example, the town of Chapel Hill, North Carolina, where I received my Ph.D. in geography, has a particular personality that can be traced back decades, and even to hundreds of years ago. Meanwhile, the town's connections with other places have expanded greatly. Other towns have gone through their own changes over time, too, with different external connections transposed against the personality of each place (Entrikin, 1991).

In my view, each place also has an underlying personality, just as people do. Even if place identities are constantly changing, there are still internal, innate characteristics (e.g., personality, character) that help define each place and help create fields of care and public symbols (Tuan, 1974; Entrikin, 1991).

Building on Massey's call for an extroverted focus on place, an introverted focus also warrants some attention. For example, some places might be more strongly "networked" than other places. There might be overlap in various people's social networks that leads to greater (or less) familiarity with other segments of the population. In a highly networked place, key people could link new physicians with other key people who can help open doors in different communities. In other places, it could be harder to find key people to enable such contacts with different communities. Obviously, such considerations are heavily dependent on the scale used in defining a place. It may be easier to network in a state than in a region of the state, or vice versa.

Within a place, some segments of the population might have global social networks, while other segments might have social networks limited mainly to the local area. One example is New York City, which is greatly connected to the rest of the world but has a substantial population that has rarely ventured beyond the local area. Consistent with Massey, such variability in people's connections helps define a place. The expansion and contraction of social networks could affect the openness of places to Others in ways that cannot be seen easily on a map. Meanwhile, places become a complicated patchwork of contexts, mechanisms, and events that cannot be simplified necessarily into precise lines of inclusions and exclusions.

GEOGRAPHIES OF EXCLUSION

This study on the event of acceptability is, in more academic terms, a study on geographies of exclusion. A geographic exclusion occurs when an area is closed to one or more groups or individuals. Lack of acceptability for an individual or group in a particular place is a geographic exclusion. Exclusion can be extreme, as when people are literally forbidden from entering a particular country or building. Exclusion can also be less concrete, as when a person feels unwelcome or unsafe in a particular area. Some people feel a greater sense of belonging in some spaces than do others (e.g., an actor on stage, a resident in a neighborhood). Anyone who is different in a particular place is the Other. Arguably, everybody is the Other in some way (e.g., a driver passing through a different neighborhood; a person with different color skin; a person with unique mannerisms or verbal expressions).

Geographic exclusions take place along a continuum, from being welcomed with open arms to being forbidden from entry. This study takes place within that continuum from acceptance to nonacceptance. Geographic exclusions can be considered simply as the event of (non)acceptance in a place, but the explanations behind geographic exclusions also cut across contexts (e.g., race) and mechanisms (e.g., the role of a church). For example, religion and race can serve as contexts for people's feelings toward their own acceptance (events) in one church or another. Similarly, some churches have a more racially diverse congregation, and individual churches can serve as mechanisms for or against geographic exclusions based on race.

Geographic exclusions are often not obvious. Some places may be relatively closed or open to outsiders without being obvious to all sides. Complicating matters, each place has an intangible backcloth of networks and interconnections that can hinder or further a person or group's exclusion. For example, social networks in a place can ease a newcomer's entry into a community. Similarly, making an insensitive remark in some places could have no consequences, but in other places it could stop a person's entry indefinitely. The impact of social networks and connections on each place is different. Moreover, interconnections are not equal on both sides of a social interaction. Power is uneven (Massey, 1995, 1996). For example, power is not evenly distributed between employers in the United States and waiver physicians who do not want to return to their home country. Nor is power distributed evenly when any two people are talking or working together. Individuals can exercise disproportionate abilities to make a place more closed or open. Such conflicts and differences in power occur in every place. It would be impossible to have a place without conflict. Places have multiple identities to the players involved in any conflict (Massey, 1997).

Building on Sibley (1995), geographic exclusion is part of place-oriented conflict. Extreme and pernicious examples include apartheid and Jim Crow, in which people were forcibly separated along racial lines from the rest of an area. Less extreme examples take place practically anywhere, any day. For example, a person might choose not to drive across a particular street, or might avoid a particular part of town altogether. Even a room within a house could be part of a geographic exclusion, if for whatever reason people feel the least bit uncomfortable going into it.

We live in a world of unseen exclusions and social separations with geographic consequences. In a shopping mall, security guards might monitor who may enter and who may not; one consequence is the systematic removal and exclusion from some public spaces of people considered disruptive (Sibley, 1995). Similarly, many neighborhoods might be off limits to homeless shelters, drug rehabilitation centers, mental hospitals, and low income housing. Nearly all neighborhood residents might support the creation of such facilities in principle, but "not in my backyard" (Dear and Wolch, 1987). At a finer geographic scale, a group of physicians practicing together might opt only to hire people from identical racial or cultural backgrounds. Such hiring decisions make some places off limits to other M.D.s perceived to be different. A geographic exclusion can be even harder to identify if it is unclear who is in charge of the exclusion. For example, it is often unclear whether a person chose not to move to a neighborhood because it is unwelcoming, or because of an individual, unrelated reason.

Geographic exclusion is often not documentable or even noticed by the majority or by the people being othered. For example, heterosexuals might not recognize that some places are less open to homosexuals; whites might not recognize that some places are closed to blacks; and a corporation's "old boy's network" might not recognize that it is closed to women. People could live for months in a racially separate area without realizing that they are not welcome elsewhere. There are many places in the world that I should not go, but I do not always know where those places are. In some cases, a geographic exclusion may be alleged without actually existing. For example, a political candidate might claim to be excluded from a forum when in fact he was not. In short, geographic exclusion is often abstract and unseen. It cannot always be confirmed on all sides.

So many ideas, from place to space to specific examples of geographic exclusions and inclusions, will emerge in this study through consideration of contexts, mechanisms, and events.

PROBLEMS IN APPLYING THE THEORETICAL FRAMEWORK

During this study, my own growth as a researcher took place alongside others' expectations that this research should adhere to positivist criteria. I tried to find common ground, for example, by expanding the study to 125 participants while facing the larger than life task of analyzing the interviews in depth for a nonpositivist study.

Advice from other researchers about how to conduct good research surfaced in all stages of the project. For example, while data collection was ongoing, a few health services researchers strongly advised me not to focus so much on contexts, such as gender or race. Instead, I should keep it simple and focus more narrowly on the doctor-patient interaction. Their advice was certainly well-intentioned and based on the need in statistical research to keep a study manageable and focused. However, I could not abandon context, since that was an essential part of the theoretical framework.

Another objection that surfaced focused on the role of narratives. The use of narratives was seen by some geographers to be inappropriate for geographic research, and more akin to reporting. Yet the use of narratives is particularly instructive for physicians who must solve problems by interpreting and reconstructing ideas learned from patient contact (Hunter,

1991). Furthermore, Gesler (1999, 2000) has shown that narratives can be extraordinarily important in gaining rich information and learning from stories about health care. Researchers from a variety of disciplines, including geography, have relied on stories, thoughts, and direct quotations in presenting research findings (Skultans, 2000; Mohammad, 1999; Cutchin, 1999; Laws and Radford, 1998; Atkinson, 1995; Radley, 1994; Kleinman, 1988; Williams, 1984). Simply to do something as commonly accepted as writing a narrative, there needs to be a recognition that geography does not have to focus on generalizations.

A nonpositivist focus was new not only to me, but to most of the researchers around me, who often went out of their way to tell me how to conduct a good (positivist) study. Usually, the advice that I received contradicted this study's theoretical framework. It was a particular challenge to know when to listen to such advice, but I eventually learned to use my theoretical framework as a filter; that is, if the advice contradicted my framework, then such advice simply was not applicable.

Based on most of the advice that I received, a good qualitative study is defensible to researchers concerned about issues such as representativeness (e.g., sampling exact numbers of participants), standardization (e.g., identical questions in each interview), and numerical checks on veracity (e.g., intercoder reliability). Complicating matters, I was studying physicians, a highly educated workforce, and several of them gave me advice, too. Like researchers, physicians typically gave me advice that reflected a traditional conceptualization of science as the quest for repeatable truths. For example, when I asked an early study participant if he would refer me to other physicians who might agree or disagree with his views, he advised me instead to conduct a random sample in order to avoid statistical bias. Similarly, a rural physician advised me to ask every study participant the exact same questions or else the study would have too much bias. Such advice never interfered with the actual research process and was at least a sign that participants were interested in this study. From my perspective, the real difficulty came when colleagues from the health services research community tried but could not understand what I was doing. It was particularly hard to convey to them that a nonpositivist focus has merit, particularly while I was still new to social theory and qualitative research.

Sometimes, in my research, I met other professors from other universities. After one talk in the study area, a professor suggested an article by Arcury and Quandt (1999, p. 128) that aimed for "a representative sample" in conducting qualitative research in complex societies. The authors' sampling framework included grids showing "site-based" estimates of a population's race, gender, poverty status, and age. Inherent in such an approach was the attempt to adjust and reformulate sampling techniques used in quantitative research. Before the beginning of fieldwork, researchers following their methods would know how many people would be interviewed in total and within each demographic cohort.

The use of percentages or raw counts can fall short in making decisions on sampling in a nonpositivist study that, for example, is based on in-depth interviews. I did not choose to rely on "representativeness" in this situation because no two interviews were alike. Moreover, some interviews might go exceedingly well, and some might go poorly, a distinction that precludes easy measurement. One study participant could be as useful as ten others in breadth of insight even though representative sampling would have assumed equal weight. Such differences in the usefulness of interviews made it hard to attach a number value to them. It would also be hard to defend the implicit view that a small number of a race or cohort represented a whole; indeed, to view a young black man as representative of all young black men would be misleading. Such generalizations are not the intention of sampling based on numbers, but still it is a difficult issue to avoid in small sample sizes common in qualitative research. To conduct good qualitative research, should researchers seek to *measure* the representativeness of samples with respect to the general population and, if so, to what end? If the purpose is generalization, then sampling should be based on law-seeking or "positivist" criteria (e.g., Arcury and Quandt, 1999). However, if the aim is to achieve greater depths of understanding and learn about complexity, such sampling criteria are misplaced. So many other pieces of advice could equally make this point about the need for a match between theory and methods—e.g., advice about coding, number of towns to include in the study, and standardization of interview questions.

Whereas my research study built on a critical realist framework, many qualitative researchers adhere to a positivist approach that seems more consistent with generating laws about human behavior. An article by Devers (1999) was especially striking in the author's call to evaluate qualitative methods within the context of each researcher's theoretical paradigm. In her view, researchers should apply positivist (i.e., law-generating) methods to evaluate positivist research, and nonpositivist methods to evaluate nonpositivist research. Put a different way, researchers need to think about theory in designing their methods. If the aim is measurements and regularity, the methods will likely reflect that; if the aim is otherwise, the methods will be different. However, it can be hard to rethink commonly used approaches when, for years, researchers have paid increasing respect to sophisticated quantitative techniques. As Rohrer (2000, p. 1304) recently lamented, "We tend to believe that the answers we get are more accurate because the statistical methods are more sophisticated."

Existing approaches in qualitative research often mimic methods used in the search for laws and generalizations—e.g., counting codes, sampling based on numbers, or predetermining all possible interview questions (Devers, 1999). Using statistics in qualitative research can be an asset except when the methods and the theory are mismatched. In my case, it would have been a mistake to use law-generating criteria in a nonpositivist study.

Finally, one more piece of questionable advice comes from commercials for Nike shoes, "Just do it." Unfortunately, this slogan is also a common piece of advice in qualitative research. For example, in his acclaimed book, *Qualitative Evaluation and Research Methods*, Michael Quinn Patton (1990, p. 89) wrote that "one need not even be concerned about theory." The underlying idea behind this assertion is conceptually simple: *Just do it*, rather than letting theory interfere with your work. He went on to say, "In short, *in real-world practice, methods can be separated from the epistemology out of which they have emerged*" (Patton, 1990, p. 90, italics in original). In other words, Patton stated the polar opposite of my view that social theory cannot be entirely divorced from methods. At the very least, social theory can be useful as a shield against statistical dogma about the "right" way to do good research. Much more importantly, theory can unmask new insights that would remain unseen in a world gone Nike.

Part Two

CASE STUDY ON QUINCY

Chapter Three

Background on Quincy: Across the Unclear Boundaries

I recall waiting in the hospital lobby for a participant to meet me for an interview. The receptionist and I made brief small talk, and she asked me about my research. I explained briefly that I was studying people's perceptions toward physicians from other countries. She said, "Oh, you're here to study—" and then her voice turned to a whisper, "—the foreign doctors." The sensitivity of the topic was in itself a finding, possibly reflecting people's reactions to having international medical graduates (IMGs) constitute over half of the local physician workforce.

In Quincy, I needed to look beneath the surface to find out about people's thoughts toward IMGs. Fortunately, I tapped into the ideas of many people who shared with me their ideas about life in Quincy. I learned from interviews, observations, informal discussions, key contacts, and my time in Quincy. However, sometimes the sensitivity of issues (e.g., referral patterns, political tensions between IMGs and U.S. medical graduates) interfered with open discussion.

Within the broader overview of IMG acceptability, this discussion on occasion turns its lens into sharper focus on IMGs from India. Nonetheless, for the sake of confidentiality, I often blur the line between different countries of origin.

STATISTICAL BACKGROUND ABOUT THE QUINCY AREA

Quincy has approximately 17,000 residents, depending on how its borders are defined (U.S. Census Bureau, 2000). When nearby areas only a few miles beyond town limits are included, the population grows to nearly 20,000. Although not the county seat, Quincy is by far the largest town in Knox County, which has a total population of nearly 60,000.

Quincy is a predominantly white town in a predominantly black county. According to the 2000 U.S. Census, the town's population was 72 percent white and 25 percent black. By contrast, Knox County's population was 46.8 percent white, and 53 percent black. Quincy borders a county that also has a predominantly black (60 percent) population and no town of comparable size. Both counties are classified by the Office of Management and Budget as nonmetropolitan (Area Resource File, 1998).

The U.S. Census Bureau (2000) reported that in 1999, 24 percent of the Knox County population lived in poverty, including 35 percent of all families with related children under five years of age. As of 2000, 68 percent of county residents had graduated from high school, and 11 percent had graduated from college.

According to the State Department of Commerce, government accounted for 25 percent of all jobs in the county in the third quarter of 1999, compared with 22 percent for retail trade, 21 percent for manufacturing, and 16 percent in the service sector. Major manufacturing in Quincy included woven fabric (1,500 jobs), paper (700 jobs), and tires and inner tubes (200 jobs). In a neighboring small town, manufacturing jobs also included work on plastic products (250 jobs), machine tools (237 jobs), and lumber (200 jobs). The hospital accounts for approximately 800 jobs in Quincy, according to the town's Web page.

Looking beyond this preliminary statistical snapshot, the town was, for me as a newcomer, a place with its own identities. My sense as an outsider traveling through the area might help add more of a human face to this discussion, even without being as comprehensive as one would expect from a local resident.

A BRIEF TOUR OF THE AREA

Like many rural towns in the United States, religion has a marked impact on the human landscape. The ride through town leads past many Baptist churches. On the main street, several signs on storefronts tell about bible meetings, revivals, and faith in God. Religion, or more specifically Christianity, is tightly woven into the town's fabric.

It is also easy to spot empty storefronts and pawn shops in the central business district. Amid economic hardship, there is a newly opened restaurant replacing the one that went out of business, a drug store that no longer has a pharmacist, and, among other businesses, a few stores selling various merchandise for gifts or trinkets. A few clothes shops, a grocery store, several florists, and a Christian bookstore also dot the landscape in the few blocks comprising the main drag of town. Now and then, a large truck transporting lumber makes turns with obvious difficulty, at once part of the current landscape and, at the same time, not quite fitting in along roads designed for automobiles.

Being a "mill town," it is not always straightforward to know who is or is not an outsider in Quincy. There are people with family histories and last names that can easily be connected to the town's century-long history. Yet mills have attracted employees from outside of the local area, too, and a nearby lake also attracts migrants from other states looking for a place to retire. The area is thus a composite of people with longstanding, local connections, and people who are either relatively new, or perceived to be new, to the area. Added to such different external connections are IMGs, now constituting approximately half of the physician workforce in the town.

The town has a shopping mall and one movie theater. Near the state highway that bypasses downtown is a Wal-Mart, chain restaurants, chain motels, gas stations, and a number of other externally based stores that are vital to the local economy. One turn off of this road is the hospital, which has importance far beyond being a major employer for the immediate town. The hospital has a geographic pull that extends beyond the local area to the "region," a loosely defined area in the vernacular that has no clearly delimited boundaries or geographic extent. Satellite clinics in nearby areas add to the drawing power and reach of the hospital into the broader region.

Driving past the hospital and onto a road along the edge of town, there is a predominantly black community. This area on the edge of town has several churches, too, as well as homes, a small shop selling sundry items, and farms. There are other sections of town that are predominantly black, by no means limited to agriculture, but you might not notice any racial separateness simply by driving through Quincy. Blacks and whites shop in many of the same stores and walk many of the same streets, and many residents speak highly of the progress that the town has made in race relations over the past few decades. Nonetheless, race relations remain at the heart of many local concerns, especially the controversial issue of school districting.

The Quincy school district is predominantly white. Knox County schools are predominantly black, and so are the schools in an adjacent town. The borders of the school districts do not coincide with the borders of the town. It is common for people to want their children to be in the predominantly white school district because it is thought by many in the local area to be better. Issues such as quality of schools, school districting, and racial separateness by school district are deeply controversial in the area. Such issues are important in laying the groundwork for thinking about the sense of belonging for IMGs in a town divided to some extent by race, particularly considering the importance of the quality of their children's education.

Another small town lies just past the highway overpass and has a predominantly black population of only a few thousand people. Past the community college, the main street in this small town bears even more than Quincy the signs of hard times faced by so many small towns in the United States, such as only a few open businesses. Not far is the county line, which extends from this eastern edge to the north of Quincy.

CONSTRUCTING OTHERS AND IDENTITY

International Medical Graduates' Sense of Quincy as Hometown

If you simply imagine for a moment, you could think of highly skilled immigrants, doctors in particular, calling this area "home." A majority of IMG participants referred to Quincy as their hometown. At the same time, they sometimes mentioned that they had more than one town that they identified as "hometown," including a town in another country.

The term "hometown" had a particular meaning to many participants and perhaps has a special meaning to most people reading this work. In many interviews and informal conversations, I asked people to explain the meaning of the word "hometown." Despite the myriad subtleties in its definition, "hometown" often had to do with either where you were raised or born. Where people consider "home" is a complicated issue that has many nuances and interpretations. For example, one IMG described a hometown as "the place where you feel better" and a few others described a hometown in terms of rootedness in a place, based on having lived in a town longer than elsewhere.

Geographic connections to other areas can be important in shaping attachment to Quincy. For example, one IMG of Asian Indian origin referred to the town as a base from which he can visit other places. Having grown up accustomed to life in a big city, he could travel from Quincy to several larger cities for various social activities. Such connections made him feel more a part of Quincy. "I'm attached to this town," he said.

Just as I found it difficult to tell people where I am from, it can be difficult for some IMGs to name a hometown. For example, another IMG of Asian Indian origin told me that Quincy is his hometown but patients often do not believe him: "Sometime they think that I'm not telling them the truth or that I am trying to act smart—But it really is my hometown."

Discussion and personal observation frequently brought out more complexity than was apparent with a short answer about which town is a hometown. For example, an IMG mentioned Quincy as his hometown, based on the strength of his ties to friends and work in the area. A few minutes later, he showed me pictures on the Internet of the state where he was originally from in India. Throughout much of the interview, he appeared distracted by images on his computer screen, and pointed out the beautiful natural landscapes, architecture, the airport, and, among other places, the front of the building of the medical school where he studied. He clearly had a strong sentimental attachment to the place, or at least to the images on his computer screen, so I wondered again what was his hometown.

"I think I should rephrase that this is my adopted home, and that's my old hometown," he said, laughing, and referring to the computer screen. "That was my motherland."

I wondered what would happen if he were back in his home state in India now, whether he would be looking at images of Quincy with the same sentimentality. He responded that he surely would and then, toward the end of the interview, I asked if he would still be here in ten or fifteen years. "I don't know. I don't think I want to answer that," he said, clearly guarded in his response. In contrast, one IMG who is Hispanic discussed his diminishing attachments to his country of origin, saying that his family and friends are here, and when he goes back, he feels "strange." The word "strange" is an interesting choice because when translated from Spanish it can mean foreign.

The issue of a physician's commitment to the local area and attachments to India or other countries can be controversial. Despite IMGs' strong retention in the area, their commitment to other places and cultures often differs from that of other people in the area. Many IMGs travel every few years to their country of origin, often to see family, friends, and places that remain important to them. One U.S. medical graduate remarked that such attachments and the ability to make money in the area are priorities for many IMGs. Speaking as if he were an IMG, he said:

> And the other things are not really a concern, I usually go to India once every three to four years for at least three weeks. I can afford to send my kids to the best private schools and vacation at the most exclusive hotels and frequent the most expensive restaurants. America is not my home, so it doesn't make any difference to me where I live.

This comment raises two key issues. First, it is difficult to disentangle the issues in this study into discrete entities. The issue of geographic attachments gets interspersed with the importance of children, the role of schools, and the potential for greed (a common accusation against physicians in general), among other issues. Secondly, geographic attachments in and of themselves may be important for acceptability, but so are people's *perceptions* of geographic attachments. Thus, a physician can be perceived to be unattached to Quincy, despite a personal sense of rootedness in the local area. Such rootedeness takes place against a backdrop in which residents have their own ideas about who is or is not the Other. A question is whether geographic boundaries influence such perceptions.

The Problem of Confining a Study to Geographic Boundaries

I had begun fieldwork thinking that I could just focus on the jurisdiction of Quincy. However, I quickly learned that people's conceptualizations of the town did not start and stop at town limits; moreover, social networks transcended the official boundaries of the town. As was evident from informal conversation, formal interviews, and suggested contacts, not everyone had the same ideas about who was from the local area, or even who was a foreigner.

Prior to fieldwork, it had seemed straightforward to consider a clear-cut delineation of a town or country based on political boundaries or other absolute criteria. For example, a foreigner might be someone who is not a U.S. citizen. Similarly, someone from outside of the local area might simply be someone who lived most of his or her childhood (i.e., under age 18) in or within a certain distance from the town. However, criteria based on spatially imposed boundaries, such as lines on a map, cannot convey people's *beliefs* about who is or is not a foreigner, or who is from outside of the local area. A closer look at the social construction of "localness" and "Americanness" is required and is important for two main reasons: (1) to help in understanding what it means to be an outsider; and (2) to set the stage for consideration of issues besides geographic boundaries that shape the acceptability of IMGs.

Localness

In an extreme sense, a town that is highly open to newcomers is one in which geographic boundaries are not important to a person's acceptability. However, not everyone in the world can identify—or be identified—with the same localities. In Quincy, most physicians were also newcomers to the community at some point. Indeed, the majority of U.S. medical graduates in Quincy received their medical degrees outside of the state and the South. It is rare for a physician from the "local" area to return to practice medicine. By "local," I simply mean being "from the area" or "from here," however such terms might be defined by residents. In other words, a person who is "local" is considered neither a transplant nor a newcomer to the area.

In interviews and informal conversations, most residents of Quincy had similar ideas about what is or is not the local area, albeit with differences in terms of its spatial extent. Frequently, people defined the local area as the county or as the two-county area, or as a particular region of the state. In several interviews, people referred to a particular region of the country (e.g., the South) as equivalent to being "from here."

It was also common for people to list, among local places, particular towns that are familiar to most people living in Quincy or that are part of people's activity spaces. For example, one participant defined the local area based largely on where people drive from to go shopping in Quincy. Some participants also raised the idea that there can be gradations of being local. A simple illustration is that someone from Quincy might be more "from here" than someone from a city one hour away, who might be more "from here" than someone from outside of the South, who might be more "from here" than someone from outside of the United States. In my experience in the town, I thought that it mattered that I was not originally from the area, whichever way "the area" might be defined. If I had had a Southern accent, especially one particular to this area, my sense is that it would have helped me gain entry into the community. Such considerations are highly subjective, obviously vary from person to person, and are complicated by many factors, such as professional status or race.

Through such different perceptions, it became increasingly evident that precise, jurisdictional boundaries of the town have limited importance in determining who is or is not "from here." Yet if the boundaries delineating the local area from other places are permeable, it becomes difficult to determine whether people moving into the local area are outsiders.

A nurse who moved to the area over ten years ago explained: "Having based on other experiences, Quincy is not as enclosed as some of the other small southern towns. I believe because of the lake, and having transient people, that we really don't have problems."

A nearby lake attracts retirees, and employment in the mills attracts newcomers to the area for jobs. Whether the area has a substantial transient population is itself open to question and depends largely on perspectives and people's social groups. For example, a manager at one of the major industrial employers in town explained that only about 10 to 15 percent of the employees in his company are from outside of the local area. Of that 10 to 15 percent, he said that the majority works in upper management.

Different people painted different pictures of the town in terms of its transience and its openness to outsiders. For example, a community member in a nearby small town who had moved to the area as an adult said:

> Well, Quincy area is a mill town, and so there's been a lot of, oh, what I would call crossbreeding or inbreeding, to be more precise, here in this area, and people who have grown up in the area have tended to have families who went back into mill work and, you know, this has been sort of a closed society in, oh, the last 50 years or so at least. And so I think that most people who do come in from the

> outside and take a local job, let's say in one of the mills or factories or industries, that person may not be looked upon except askance. You may think that this person has kind of encroached upon your territory.

Obviously, the above statement reflects one man's perception rather than a blanket statement that can be applied objectively to the entire community. However, the underlying premise that length of time in the area has at least some correspondence with outsider status warrants closer attention.

Some residents have a longer family history in the area, which in turn strengthens their ties to the town. A U.S. medical graduate who had moved to Quincy had a less than fluid image of who is or is not "from here" in the town: "Well, I mean, when I say from here, you know, you're talking about people that their grandparents have been here, their great grandparents have been here, you know, the mother and father are here, the children have gone to school here—"

"Where is here?" I asked. "Is that Quincy or—"

"Oh well, you're talking about the whole area. We're taking broad, Knox County."

Another U.S. medical graduate who had moved to a nearby small town approximately twenty years ago also noted that longstanding family roots in the area help define who is or is not "from here." As illustrated in the following exchange, the physician added other issues that paint localness in more complex ways, such as population size and social networks.

"And do you think people tend to think of you as somebody who is from the area?" I asked.

"No," the physician replied, "to be from the area in this area, your grandmother has to be buried here. You know, it's—small towns are different. Now, Quincy is not small, doesn't see themselves as small town. And so in Quincy, I think you can kind of be from the town if you've been here twenty years but in the smaller communities, you're not from the town unless you have grandparents because it's not an unfriendly thing. It's just that you aren't rooted in the community in their view. In Quincy, there's more fluid social structure because they have the textile mill and the paper mill so there are people who are upwardly mobile who come in and go out related to the industries in the area. And course state employees, so if you look at Quincy I think there's a lot more fluidity to that social structure, and I think it's a lot more inclusive than, say, a small town."

However localness is defined, residents with family roots in the area can have especially strong pride in Quincy for being their hometown. This became evident to me during a conversation after a health care meeting in a neighboring county. Two contacts who were helpful in my entry to the town told me that many people who live in Quincy have a sense of local patriotism. In other words, in the view of these two contacts, speaking ill about the town could be perceived by some residents in Quincy to be as unwelcome as speaking ill about America. In much simpler terms, people want to cast their hometown in the best possible light. Such pride in being from the area can strengthen ties among people whose families have lived there for generations.

Outsiders who wish to bring about social change might need to cross an unseen boundary separating them from longstanding local networks. A U.S. medical graduate who had moved to Quincy after having lived mainly in urban areas elaborated on this point:

> I still think I'm an outsider though when it comes to decision making. I've been on a lot of boards, but when you start talking about making changes, you know, deep cuts, social changes, they still look at you as an outsider. You didn't, quote, grow up here, you don't really know the structure here. And I really found that on several of the boards that I was on that made you realize that you're still not in the network, per se, you know, you may be a member of the community, but you're not in the network, and that works a little bit differently.

"Could you say a little bit more about that?" I asked.

> Well, it's just, you know, as I said, there are a lot of social changes that need to be changed here, a lot of the racial things that go on that probably need to be changed. When I started speaking out about them a little bit, even the minorities were a little bit upset because of the fact that I didn't grow up in this area, that I didn't really belong to this area, that I had ties to other areas so I get up and leave when they didn't have those ties. Not to rock the boat too much because a lot of them had to live here and they didn't have any other options and things. It just makes you recognize that you're still not, as I say, in the network. You're part of the community but you haven't been in from the grassroots. And so there are still some things going on that I don't really know about, or I don't know well enough to, according to them, start talking out about, speaking out about. So that's been a little difficult for me, because I like to [laughs] speak my mind when I think there's an injustice. And I still do, it's just that I've gotten some repercussions. And from people that you didn't expect to get repercussions from. So it's been a learning experience, it really has, in that respect. You keep going and you try to educate those people that things can change, regardless of whether they've been here grassroots or whatever, things do change, and people can change. And the more and more probably insiders—excuse me—outsiders we get to stay here long enough, we do see some changes.

Such issues are obviously complex because they are contingent upon people's different perceptions. Indeed, the issue of who is "from here" or not "from here" is complicated by family connections to the area, social networks, the arrival of newcomers, and different perspectives on the identities of the town. Jurisdictional boundaries cannot explain all of the reasons for outsider status.

Americanness

If jurisdictional boundaries have only limited relevance in determining whether or not someone is "from here," do they matter in determining whether or not someone is an American or a foreigner? In this discussion, I refer to "Americanness" as a term for someone who is perceived to be American, and "foreignness" for someone who is perceived not to be American. Since perceptions of foreignness often do not correspond with spatial boundaries, some people who are American might be considered foreign, and vice versa. Why one person from another country might be perceived to be foreign, and another person an American, raises questions about differences in acceptability.

My assumption at the outset of this study was that an American is simply someone who has U.S. citizenship; therefore, it was rare for me to ask participants to define who is or is not an American. Since many people referred to IMGs as "foreign doctors," I assumed further that if you come from outside of the United States, you are likely to be perceived as a foreigner. Fortunately, the flow of conversation sometimes challenged my basic assumptions, and led me to wonder what makes someone a foreigner.

At a senior citizens center in Quincy, I asked a retiree: "What makes somebody a foreign doctor as opposed to an American doctor?"

"A person from another country that speaks another language is what I would call a foreign doctor," she replied.

"If the person comes—Let's say a person speaks Italian, it's a foreign doctor?" I asked.

"Yes," she said.

"If a person speaks English but is from Great Britain, would that be a foreign doctor?"

"Well, technically it probably would. But (laughs) I wouldn't consider that as foreign as I would somebody from Italy or British Honduras or wherever."

Perhaps, because she came from a nearby small town that she described as a few houses and a post office, her views were not representative of many people's views in Quincy. Then again, I did not seek representativeness but, rather, ideas that would shed light on townspeople's perceptions of IMGs.

An IMG of Asian Indian origin explained, "See, if people come from Spain or Cuba or Russia, once they start learning English then they are considered as the same as Americans. Okay, there is no distinction."

"Most people from Spain or Cuba?" I asked.

"Or Cuba or, you know, Europe. Say Germany, Russia, you know. Once they learn to speak English, then they're not considered foreigners, you know. At least once their children grow up, I mean, there are no different [sic] between the white kids here and them."

As the above examples illustrate, whether or not you are considered a foreigner can be complicated by language. In and of itself, however, language is not a sufficient criterion to determine whether or not someone is considered a foreigner. Among many other complex issues, race can complicate people's perceptions of Americanness. For example, I found it particularly interesting that several participants referred to a white physician of Italian origin as an American, sometimes even as someone from the local area. The physician received his medical degree in Italy.

A resident of a homeless shelter explained that "I think he was born and raised in America. He's Italian."

An allied health provider said that "he's from Italy, but he's been here so long we count him as being homegrown. But I mean, he is of foreign background."

A nurse also raised the issue in saying, "He was born in Italy but is very Americanized. He attended one of our state universities."

A U.S. medical graduate also referred to the IMG of Italian origin as an American:

> They tried to entice an American-trained physician to the area, but were unsuccessful. Ultimately, they did recruit an Italian, trained in Italy, who has no noticeable accent. If you were unfamiliar with his background, you would assume that he was American through-and-through.

On the one hand, accent can play a role in determining Americanness. On the other hand, I met other IMGs with little or no accent, but no one was referring to them in conversation as Americans.

The allied health provider had another explanation:

> Well, in this area, skin color, the color of your skin makes a lot of difference in where people think you're from. It does. All the rest of the foreign doctors are dark skinned. The psychiatrist is dark skinned. Both the neurologists, the urologist, [name of a physician], the oncologist, I mean, they're all foreign doctors. So probably [name of IMG of Italian origin] because he's white. But he has been here a long time, too.

The issue of the meaning of race extends far beyond a simple dichotomy about who is or is not American (Pulido, 2000; Kobayashi and Peake, 1994; Smith, 1993; Jackson, 1989; Anderson, 1987). However, race is also intricately woven with other topics in constructing identity as an American. The issue of Americanness is shaped, at least in part, by race, language, and familiarity, as well as many tangible and not so tangible issues.

Just as language is not enough in and of itself to constitute Americanness, neither is race. For example, the town has two brothers who work as physicians in the same practice. The allied health provider told me: "They are from

Argentina. Well, they are white, but their accent gives them away. All they have to do is say a few words and everybody knows they're not from here."

According to a nurse:

> Now when people say American doctors, I'm assuming they mean the white doctor, Caucasian or either the ones that are African American. When they say foreign they're considering the ones from India, Pakistan. I think we have some from some of the islands. So they're thinking—When they look in like the Yellow Pages, they see all these names that you can't pronounce, and they think the only thing we have is foreign doctors.

Thus, determining "foreign" status might be linked to some extent with that which is least familiar, or least common, both in terms of language and color of skin. A more general familiarity can also impact a person's foreign status. For example, a receptionist in a clinic staffed mainly by IMGs said, "I work with them so to me they're not foreign." Then she laughed and said, "You know, they're just American, just like American doctors."

As for my initial thought that country of citizenship determines whether or not someone is an American, an IMG who recently became a U.S. citizen said: "But they still regard me as a foreigner whether or not you're a citizen. Ninety-nine percent of them don't know that I'm a citizen. They regard you as a foreigner."

Most of the IMGs interviewed in Quincy told me that they are U.S. citizens or are on an immigration pathway to becoming citizens. No IMGs told me otherwise, although a few said that it had taken some years before deciding to become a citizen, and one U.S. medical graduate originally from abroad told me that he is a Canadian rather than U.S. citizen.

There are also differing opinions on whether or not someone who has always lived in the United States is a foreigner. For example, a few people said with some amusement that Yankees are foreigners. A few U.S. medical graduates referred to Puerto Ricans as foreigners even though Puerto Rico is a U.S. territory. Quincy had had at least one physician originally from Puerto Rico in the past but now had none.

Whether being a foreign *physician* translates into outsider status is yet another complex issue with no easy explanation. For physicians in particular, professional status might override possible concerns about foreignness.

A social worker explained that people coming from other areas, including other countries, are not necessarily outsiders:

> Now you have to remember now, to most of us, and I think I can speak fairly well on that, it depends on what you're bringing. Your services doesn't necessarily make you an outsider, because we're looking at what you're gonna bring

> to help benefit us. Are you bringing something that's going to—we can overall say, you have brought a product, and I'm gonna use medical as a product, but you're bringing a service. And most of the time if we even call ourself little country people, we see that service coming in that's gonna benefit, that we don't have to run out to the larger cities, then no, they're welcomed with warm arms.

A community member offered similar comments, explaining that there are different standards for the acceptability of physicians and people who do not bring a service. According to his explanation, a person who is highly educated, such as an M.D. or a Ph.D., brings a service or skills to the area that otherwise would not be here. As a result, where a person is from might not be as important as what he or she brings to the community.

Conclusion

As indicated by the above discussion, geographic boundaries fall short as a definitive criterion for Americanness or localness. However, if it did not matter whether a person is from outside of the local area or from another country, this study might never have yielded as much depth about perceptions toward "foreign doctors." Words can be problematic. "Foreigner" and "outsider" are socially constructed terms and have loaded meanings that can divert attention from the broader study. By some definitions, an "outsider" might be somebody who does not fit into an area, and a "foreigner" might be somebody who speaks with an accent. Words have meanings that transcend boundaries, while taking shape differently in different places (see Gesler, 1999).

Considering the words and ideas of people in Quincy, the distinction between Americans and foreigners has become blurred. Even geographic scales of analysis (e.g., local, national) have become blurred; "local" perceptions on nationality are not limited to the precise jurisdictional boundaries that typically distinguish different scales of analysis (see Marston, 2000). Instead, race, accent, professional status, and familiarity are among many issues that obscure such boundaries and make the task of delineating Americans from foreigners difficult. Consideration of such issues adds to the extraordinary complexity of Americanness and localness, and makes a focus on geographic boundaries seem naïve in this instance.

NOTES

1. The Web page is not cited to avoid naming the town.

Chapter 4

Mechanisms and Quincy: Tipping Points For and Against Acceptability

Over half of all physicians practicing in Quincy received their medical degrees outside of the United States. According to the 1998 hospital physician directory, the town had sixty-seven physicians, thirty-one of whom received a medical degree outside of the United States and Canada,[1] and five who received their M.D.s in Canada. Recent press releases, hospital news clippings, and conversations with physicians confirm that the influx of international medical graduates (IMGs) has increased in recent years; nearly all physicians who have arrived within the past few years are IMGs. Only a few decades ago, the town did not have any IMGs.

WHY SO MANY INTERNATIONAL MEDICAL GRADUATES?

An obvious question is why the town now has so many IMGs. This question might seem initially to be easily addressed with a quick explanation about the role of IMGs in alleviating physician shortages in rural or underserved areas. However, the strong concentration of IMGs in Quincy has many possible explanations, such as the role of the hospital, the extent of IMG retention, strength in numbers, and difficulty attracting U.S. medical graduates—all examples of mechanisms.[2]

The hospital, which currently has over 200 beds, had placed priority on recruiting subspecialists rather than primary care providers. While this staffing pattern may have many possible explanations, one that surfaced in several interviews is that the reputation of the hospital could have been increased by having a variety of subspecialists. According to the 1998 hospital physician directory, IMGs are well-represented in subspecialty care in Quincy and specialize in gastroenterology, nephrology, oncology, orthopedics, pulmonology, urology, and other specialties. Advertisements in the local newspaper also indicate a growing number of new IMGs in various subspecializations. This tendency toward subspecialization is consistent with a broader tendency among IMGs nationally toward subspecialization (Mick and Pfahler, 1995).

The recruitment of subspecialists has led to increased access to care for services that patients otherwise would only find by leaving town. For example, many patients with cancer can go to an oncologist in Quincy without having to go elsewhere. The oncologist is an IMG, as are the majority of local subspecialists. The fact that IMG practices have an abundance of patients and are expanding in terms of recruitment, staff, and office space indicates the importance of demand for their services in Quincy.

The flip side of the coin is that the IMGs in the area are much less likely to practice as primary care providers, and therefore are limited in the extent to which they alleviate underservice. Of only twenty physicians listed in the hospital directory as having a primary care specialty (e.g., internal medicine without subspecialization, family practice, obstetrics and gynecology, or pediatrics), seven were listed as IMGs. A few additional IMGs had moved to the area by mid-1999 to practice as primary care providers on the J-1 visa waiver. The recruitment of waiver physicians to this area only began approximately four years ago, and the next updates of the hospital physician directory could reflect further recruitment of waiver physicians among primary care providers in or near Quincy. Moreover, the hospital has shifted its priorities in the past few years toward trying to meet the needs of the "region" and has changed its name to a "regional medical center." The new regional emphasis includes satellite clinics in nearby areas and greater attention to the need for primary care providers.

Yet the question remains, why are there so many IMGs in the area? It cannot simply be attributed to the role of the hospital in recruiting subspecialists. After all, there are also U.S. medical graduates who are subspecialists who could have chosen to practice in the area but did not do so.

Why there are so many IMGs in Quincy is not simply a question of why IMGs move to the area but, also, why they stay. Retention is a complex issue worthy of a study in and of itself (see Cutchin, 1997; Conte et al., 1992). Retention of IMGs of Asian Indian origin in Quincy is especially strong, and some discussion of why IMGs stay in the area helps in understanding their geographic concentration.

According to the 1998 hospital directory, Quincy has eighteen physicians who graduated from medical schools in India. In conversations with IMGs, U.S. medical graduates, and key contacts, I learned that only one IMG of Asian Indian origin had moved away in the town's thirty-year history of having IMGs, and he moved back to India. Even among IMGs from other countries, retention is noteworthy. For example, the medical librarian at the hospital showed me her own compilation of the hospital's welcome notices and other press releases for physicians. Although it was an incomplete collection that had not been updated in at least a year, it struck me that the overwhelming majority of physicians who had left were U.S. medical graduates. I even tried to contact IMGs who no longer practice in the town but, even with help from contacts in the medical community, had difficulty coming up with many names because of the strong retention of IMGs. Based on conversations with key contacts, members of hospital administration, and physicians, I saw that IMGs who have moved away from Quincy are the exception rather than the rule.

The strong retention of IMGs cannot be fully explained by the previous example about the role of the hospital. Other issues, such as strength in numbers, must be important in influencing the recruitment and retention of IMGs in Quincy, and hence why there are so many IMGs in the area.

IMGs of Asian Indian origin have a close-knit community in Quincy. Depending on individual estimates, there are approximately twenty-five to twenty-seven Asian Indian families living in town, including motel owners, physicians, and people with other occupations. Most are Hindu, and many of the families gather once a month for a puja, a Hindu prayer gathering. An IMG and a member of the general community cohost a weekly one-hour broadcast of Asian Indian music on the local public radio station.

There are many intangible, cultural, and social issues that bind the Asian Indian community together. For purposes of this discussion, the important point is that family, work ethic, connections to India, and similarities in cultural backgrounds are part of a larger, complex mosaic that contributes to the strength and supportiveness of the Asian Indian community. For example, according to IMGs and others in the medical community, IMGs on several occasions had acted as nodes for the recruitment of family members, friends, or others from their country of origin. This, in turn, further expanded the size and cohesiveness of the Asian Indian community and, by extension, the community's connections to the town itself. The town's relative location is also important in furthering the connections that IMGs have with Quincy, even if the town is somewhat isolated geographically from urban areas. For example, a little over an hour away is a city of over 200,000 people, where some families travel occasionally for entertainment, or to buy clothes, cooking ingredients, or other amenities.

The geographic concentration of IMGs of Asian Indian origin in Quincy helps foster an environment in which many people are accustomed to having physicians from other countries. Besides India, the hospital directory also lists IMGs who received their medical degrees in the Philippines (three), Argentina (two), Honduras (two), and one each from Italy, Jamaica, Japan, Pakistan, and the United Kingdom. At the time of fieldwork, an IMG was chief of staff at the hospital, a rotating position that had been filled by IMGs in the past, too.

According to an IMG originally from Latin America, it has been an advantage to have so many IMGs in the area:

> And I think it's one of the things that people look when they come. When we try to hire another physician, when somebody comes, they say, well, they have so many IMGs here, and for the IMGs it's kind of an incentive to stay, because it's one of the things that people tell in the hospital when they come for an interview, this community accepts the international medical grads.

The strong concentration of IMGs can also be seen in less flattering terms. The following exchange with a nurse helps illustrate some of the concerns that can surface in considering why there are so many IMGs:

> I think, well, from what I understand, there was a nucleus of Indian community here, and then they have a tendency to bring their own. And they recruit. I mean, it's—they do it. They do it amongst themselves and they become very close-knit. And when there's a majority—the staff is majority Indian. They watch out for their own. They do watch out for their own.

"What does that mean, they watch out for their own?" I asked.

"They will see—if two people apply and one is, say, an American and one's an Indian, the Indian is going to make it, not the American."

She then recounted a recent event that would later be mentioned by a physician, in which the Asian Indian community reportedly worked hard to ensure that the hospital hire a physician of Asian Indian origin in a particular specialty. A similar controversy was mentioned in two other interviews, in which the Asian Indian community allegedly favored hiring an Asian Indian physician for a position.

While there are accusations of favoritism for IMGs, several prominent physicians in the area said that the hospital has tried to recruit more U.S. medical graduates. However, I was told by three members of the hospital administration that they want the best person for any opening, regardless of whether the person is an IMG or a U.S. medical graduate.

Whether true or not, allegations of favoritism are sensitive topics that sometimes blur the line between facts and gossip. Such allegations are important background for understanding how strength in numbers may be linked with potential problems in IMG acceptability.

One way of addressing the issue of why there are so many IMGs in the area is to focus simply on IMG recruitment and retention. However, there has also been difficulty attracting U.S. medical graduates at the same time that IMG numbers have been increasing in the area. Members of the medical community volunteered several reasons for problems recruiting U.S. medical graduates, including:

- concerns among U.S. medical graduates about sacrifices in prestige by moving to a rural, underserved community;
- career decisions that spouses are willing to make;
- reluctance of physicians or spouses to move to a relatively small town that lacks the amenities (e.g., shopping, nightlife) of a larger city;
- perceived saturation of the local physician market by IMGs;
- and possible negative responses by U.S. medical graduates to foreign sounding names in advertisements.

As indicated by these and other possible reasons, the recruitment of physicians is a complicated process that leads to many different considerations. Indeed, even without venturing into lengthy asides about these and other issues influencing recruitment and retention, the strong concentration of IMGs in Quincy is complex and multifaceted. Simply by exploring the clustering of IMGs in Quincy, other issues influencing acceptability begin to emerge, such as: the possible relation between size of the IMG workforce and improvements in acceptance, and the size and growth of IMG patient bases as possible indicators of acceptability.

CASE STUDY: CONCENTRATION OF INTERNATIONAL MEDICAL GRADUATES IN A CLINIC

The first IMGs in Quincy, and the private medical clinic that employed them, played valuable roles in introducing the town to IMGs. At the time of fieldwork, the clinic had thirteen physicians, only one of whom was a U.S. medical graduate. The other twelve physicians on staff included eight IMGs from India and one each from Honduras, Italy, Pakistan, and the Philippines. It is by far the largest clinic in Quincy. By contrast, most practices in Quincy have only one or two physicians. One of the larger practices in town has three U.S. medical graduates and no IMGs; there is also a community health center with several clinics dispersed throughout the region, a few of which have an IMG. A nurse at the hospital explained to me that sometimes people referred to the thirteen-physician-clinic as the "United Nations on the Hill" because of the representation from so many different nationalities. A clinic of its size inevitably has an important voice in hospital decision making. Thus, concerns expressed about IMGs could sometimes reflect some corporate distinctions that are misinterpreted or recast as issues specific to IMGs.

Although the town's IMGs are predominantly subspecialists, the clinic's twelve IMGs included five primary care internists without subspecialty training. Among subspecialists, the clinic had two gastroenterologists, an allergy and immunology specialist, a cardiologist, an infectious disease specialist, a hematologist/oncologist, and a pulmonologist. At the time of fieldwork, the clinic's building had recently undergone renovation to accommodate an earlier expansion of the practice; it had also incorporated physicians from another, smaller group practice. In April 2000, eight months after completion of Quincy fieldwork, I visited the town again and noticed three additional physicians listed on a sign in front of the building, a further indication of clinic expansion.

An IMG who works at the clinic explained that such expansion reflects well on IMG acceptability: "The best indicator to me is that we are doing well as a practice. So it's a thriving practice. At this moment we are not hurting for patients. So to me that speaks by itself."

Why the *clinic* has so many IMGs cannot be easily separated from the issue of why the *town* has so many IMGs. Many of the same issues affecting the recruitment and retention of IMGs in Quincy can also apply to the clinic (e.g., social and professional networks, strength in numbers). At the same time, the clinic's growth is not so much a reflection of IMG acceptability as it is a pace-setter. It was here that three of the first four IMGs in the general medical community were hired.

The growth of the clinic, and the growth in numbers of IMGs in Quincy, familiarized people with physicians who otherwise might be perceived as outsiders—physicians with different accents, skin colors, religions, nationalities, and cultures. A corollary to such growth is that IMGs did not all move to Quincy at the same time. Rather, the process of recruitment began about thirty years ago, and over time a community has been built and still continues to grow.

Vignette: The First International Medical Graduates in the Clinic

"I used to say I didn't want to be a minority in my own practice," a retired U.S. medical graduate told me, "but over the years I've changed that, and it never presented any problems. And quite frankly, I don't know what the medical community would have done had it not had the services of these people."

The U.S. medical graduate and I were sitting in an office at the medical clinic that had twelve IMGs on staff. In 1970, he had hired an IMG, a general internist originally from the Philippines. Based on what both men told me, there had already been one other IMG practicing in Quincy at the time—a psychiatrist who had moved to town as medical director of the mental health center a few months earlier, and who has long since moved away.

The general internist from the Philippines was the first IMG to care for patients in the general population; no participants or other contacts recalled any earlier IMGs to me. A number of physicians had mistakenly thought that the first IMG in town was a urologist from India who had passed away only a few years prior to my fieldwork.

The first IMGs in the clinic—a general internist, a urologist, and a gastroenterologist—gained such excellent reputations in the medical and nonmedical communities that it begs the question, what would have happened if the first IMGs had not been so highly regarded? The first IMGs in town were also among the first immigrants to this rural area, and therefore had an extraordinarily important role as pioneers for future IMGs. As the retired physician explained:

> I guess I suffered as much as anybody because I was bringing in probably the first Asian who had ever spent the night in Knox County, much less lived in Knox County, I guess when [the general internist] came. And I had some—I had some concerns. And I must say, back then, back then even in my training time, the perception was that foreign docs were not up to standard. You know, foreign doctors were not as well-trained in their background as U.S.A. doctors. And I remember a phone call, a conversation I had with a friend who—And I was telling him this doctor was coming, I met him, he was real nice, he is—I think his training is good. We've talked. We have ideas alike. And I said, but I am concerned about how an Asian is going to be accepted in this community and how he would get along. And I was more concerned about him. And my friend said, [name], he said, you know, he said, I spent my military time in Asia, in Japan. And he said, if there's one characteristic that Asian people have, it is their flexibility and their adaptability. And I feel like that that—I believe that to be true. And I believe it is a characteristic that helps Asians, whether it be Vietnamese or Koreans or whoever, in whatever they do, that gives them an advantage or helps them to adjust.

The first IMG recruited to the clinic "was very, very Americanized," the retired physician explained further. "He was as American as apple pie and Coca-Cola. And he was married to a girl who was from just over in [a neighboring state], Caucasian, and he fit into things very quickly." Referring to an early IMG from India, the retired physician continued, "I had concerns about [name of IMG], how he would fit in, and I used—After he'd been here a time, I would marvel how he was able to connect, you know, our country people, some people who've never been out of the county hardly in their lifetime, and he was from half a world away. I really used to marvel at how easy it was to connect. There's a little bit more of a language problem with him than it was with [the first IMG]. But anyway, he came and is here and has made a big contribution to the group. So then as time went on, we would need more help and we would advertise through the media. And I don't know this, but I suspect that the people were looking at our advertisement and they would see a name that they recognized as being that of a foreign medical graduate, and particularly Indian, it sort of attracted the attention of others. And so that's just how it happened that we got more foreign medical graduates."

In the same clinic, in talking with the first IMG hired by the retired physician, I asked, "Was it hard for you as the first international medical graduate or was it—"

"No, I think it was easy," he replied. "One, because I joined somebody who was already in practice, and we took calls together, you know, alternate, so when he wasn't around, they needed somebody, they would call me. So it wasn't hard. And there was a shortage of physicians, and I got, you know, consults right away, you know, from the other doctors. It wasn't hard at all. The hard part was, you know, going out in the streets and people double take and who is that, you know. But that soon wore off."

"So was that common, people would stop and—"

"Yeah, even now, you know," he said. "Yesterday I went to the nursing home on my lunch hour and somebody—Who are you! I said, well, I'm Dr. [name], who are you? I always counter with I tell them who I am but I want to know who you are, too. She said, nice to meet you. But it's out of curiosity. Nothing malicious about it. They just . . . they just want to know."

"What was your reaction when people would stop and do a double take?"

"I looked funny," and he laughed. "I mean, I looked different, you know, that's the reason." Later, he added, " Oh, I can remember once or twice coming in the emergency room and seeing one of [a white physician's] patients and little old lady ask me, you know, where is the doctor of her kind. And I said, well, they're out in the big city making lots of money that they don't have to get up at two o'clock in the morning to take care of you. But these are old people. They're probably all dead now. I mean, you know, I'm talking about twenty, twenty-five years ago, I remember that happening once or twice."

He explained that hard work played an important role in the acceptance of IMGs in the town: "You understand though, that most international graduates that leave their country go because, you know, they're a little bit of an overachiever. I mean, otherwise you'd be satisfied where you are and, you know, with the status quo and things like that." In referring to immigrants in general, he said,

> And these people are going to go work harder, twice as hard at two or three jobs, you know, in order to—at least the first and second generation. I don't know

> what happens after the third, they get soft, you know. My son, he says, oh I worked fifteen hours yesterday. I said my God, I worked eighteen hours for two years, you know. But you know, and he's a good boy . . . but he sees somebody working seven or eight hours, and he's working fifteen, he said he thinks he's just done something, and that's once in a while, you know. And that's second generation already. So, immigrants is the way to go.

The first IMGs earned excellent reputations in the medical and nonmedical communities for the quality of their work, which may have led to increasing openness to having IMGs in Quincy. Private practices and a few small group practices have since opened that are staffed by IMGs, and that helped familiarize people further with IMGs. Such familiarity is important in considering the possible need for IMGs to be "pioneers" who gained acceptance for a broader international medical community.

FAMILIARITY WITH INTERNATIONAL MEDICAL GRADUATES

The introduction of IMGs led to the town's increasing familiarity with people of diverse social and cultural backgrounds. As more and more IMGs moved to Quincy, IMGs became less and less different from people's expectations of a physician.

The issue of change in acceptance over time surfaced repeatedly in interviews, even though the first IMGs seem to have fared well, based on their own accounts and the accounts of others. However, it is difficult to reconstruct the past to find out what people actually thought about the first IMGs. Some things appear to have changed for the better, particularly in terms of the treatment of IMGs by the nonmedical community. For example, I asked a person in administration who works in a health center in a nearby small town that has no IMGs whether IMGs are treated any differently by community members than are U.S. medical graduates. The response came:

> No, because we've had so many to come into our area. At first, I would say yes, but not now. Because we've got more and more to come into the area and they're more acceptable now than they were ten years ago. . . . Ten years ago they wouldn't want a foreigner to put their hands on them. [laughs]

The participant then speculated that it may have been longer than ten years ago. What is important is that familiarity with IMGs is a key reason behind improvement in IMG acceptance, according to many participants who talked about being "accustomed" to IMGs. As explained by an IMG who moved to town within the past decade:

> My understanding is that for the people who came to this town twenty, twenty-five years ago, the situation was a little bit harder, compared to myself that came five years ago. But they say initially people in this small town, they were not used to see a foreign doctor. In fact they had the old primary care physicians, GP, general practitioners, they were here for years, and they were mainly Americans.

Familiarity with IMGs in Quincy also has helped make the town look more attractive to IMGs in search of a place to practice medicine. Almost all IMGs expressed the view that the obstacles to acceptability would be greater in a town that has no other IMGs. As one IMG of Asian Indian origin explained: "One of the things we looked at when we were coming here, that there were other foreign physicians. And I think for us it was easier than for the first person who came here."

Another IMG of Asian Indian origin speculated that to be the only IMG in town, "You gonna get burned out or exhausted by the time you finish."

The strong reputations of the individual pioneer IMGs may have compensated for possible obstacles to acceptability. Also, having other IMGs from the same cultural background can have drawing power. For example, one physician of Asian Indian origin discussed some of the reasons for moving to Quincy:

> Our decision was based on we wanted a little community of our own for our children to be exposed to, and that was the only reason, you know. If it was any other foreigner it would have been fine in terms of breaking down the barrier, but in our eyes we wanted a few Indians because we wanted to have a little bit— You know, you want that community in the place you're going to be settling in.

If familiarity helps in "breaking down the barrier," then is the pertinent issue familiarity with IMGs, with IMGs of Asian Indian origin, or with a more precisely defined group of IMGs? The fact that a physician comes from Pakistan or India or the Philippines is a distinction that does not appear to be noted by many patients, even among patients concerned about seeing a "foreign doctor." I quickly learned that most patients cannot be expected to have a clear idea of a physician's country of origin, or whether the physician received a medical degree in the United States.

On the one hand, IMGs are a diverse group coming from so many different countries of origin. On the other hand, people in the general community frequently confused the different countries of origin. As a result, having a cluster of physicians from a specific country (e.g., India) appears to make people more familiar with IMGs, and therefore to be more open to having IMGs from other countries. At the same time, an important distinction needs to be made between acceptability of the individual physician and acceptability of IMGs in general. For example, according to the president of the hospital, some respondents to a survey reportedly spoke critically of having so many IMGs but commented very positively on the individual IMGs that they see for medical care.[3]

On the one hand, as demonstrated by the above discussion, there may be a tipping point in the size of the IMG community that furthers acceptance. On the other hand, there appeared to be another uncertain tipping point past which familiarity can dampen a town's inclusiveness, which may help explain the sensitive nature of this topic. As more and more IMGs entered the area, some participants expressed unease about whether additional IMGs should be hired. Such unease was underscored by concerns about hiring practices, hospital politics, referral patterns, and the perceived separateness of Asian Indian communities. Some of these concerns have already been discussed (e.g., allegations of favoritism in hiring); others will be explored in depth in the next chapter.

MECHANISMS INFLUENCING TRUST

A patient's trust in a physician is a closely related and highly relevant event to acceptability. A physician who loses the trust of patients will obviously face difficulties being accepted by them, since they would be less likely to see the physician for care again or to follow medical advice. Issues relating to trust are intricately woven with every issue discussed thus far. For example, as explained by a community member who volunteers in a Quincy homeless shelter, familiarity is a key concern:

> Well, you've got to have confidence in your doctor before you can believe that you're gonna get well. Well, if you was a doctor here and I just met you today, I would have to get to know you before I could have confidence in you. So that's what had to happen down through the years. People had to get to know the foreign doctors before they could really believe in them.

Competence

Nearly all participants indicated that IMGs are at least as competent as U.S. medical graduates in terms of their qualifications to practice medicine. Even in interviews in which participants seemed especially candid in relaying sensitive, potentially self-incriminating information, there was rarely any indication of a perception that IMGs are less competent or incompetent as physicians. However, the extent to which participants believed in the competence of IMGs is impossible to capture precisely. At least in the medical community, it is politically wise not to insult an entire group of individuals practicing in the same, relatively small town.

In conversation with a physician who received a medical degree in a U.S. university, I said, "Nobody's saying that international medical graduates are incompetent or less competent here."

He responded:

> It's a very, very touchy subject because, you know, nobody wants to point a finger and say, not to mention, nobody wants to bring a lawsuit on themselves. [laughs] So you know, you're going to find very few people that are going to be terribly forthright with you on these issues.

Yet, just what is meant by "competence" is another complicated issue. For example, in my interview with the above physician, he relayed concerns about the quality of medical schools, concerns about communication, and cultural competence. In those specific terms, he spoke critically of the competence of IMGs on a national level and, despite delving headlong into deeply controversial issues surrounding hospital politics, did not criticize the quality of care provided by IMGs in Quincy. Instead, his view was that the competence of the town's IMGs and U.S. medical graduates varies by individual.

It was also rare for IMGs to suggest that the medical or general community had any difficulty accepting that IMGs are competent physicians. On a few occasions, IMGs told me of incidents in which their competence may have come into question. For example, a few IMGs relayed concerns that some local residents might think that they received their medical training in the equivalent of a community college. In discussing concerns about people's perceptions on competence, one IMG of Asian Indian origin talked about a recent case in which he was sued for malpractice:

> So I said, well you know, see a foreign medical graduate going before a jury probably would not look good, especially when the expert witnesses were, you know, from America. Two of the expert witnesses were from a medical center, you know. So I ran this by the lawyer, you know. . . . He said, well, you know, when we have to represent a doctor from a small town, we get our expert witnesses from a medical center because the plaintiff will get their witnesses from a medical center and it goes over better. In other words, to the jury. So I felt—Well, I said, you know, I think I will not get a fair deal, I mean, in the sense that I'm going before all of these people and I'm a foreign medical graduate, I probably might not get a fair

> deal. So I told him, you know, settle the case. And the insurance company said, no, you know, they don't—they're not going to settle this case because there is no merit in the case. Well, I went through the court system, it went to the—And actually it didn't get to the jury because, you know, halfway through the case the judge threw out the case. He said there was no merit in the case.

He explained further that the process of jury selection was gratifying in making him aware of people's perceptions of him: "The jury may think, well, this guy is an outsider. I wasn't scared of the lawyers or the judge, but I felt that the local people in the jury may think that he's an outsider."

"He, meaning you?" I asked.

"Yes," he said. "But then it was interesting that—You know, in the jury selection—I don't know if you have gone through this process, but they had—You know, they called about sixty people for jury duty and, you know, they interview everyone and ask their questions if they could be biased. In the process—You know, the majority of them had to be eliminated because I took care of them, [laughs] and you know, they all had good impression of me, so they said they would not, you know. So, I mean, that made me feel, well, you know, it seems like the community recognizes what I do."

Another IMG of Asian Indian origin told me that he thinks that most people accept IMGs, but there are some instances in which other medical staff appear to question the competence of IMGs. In his words:

> Yeah, there are some nurses. There are some nurse practitioners and physicians who are angry at us because we know more than what they expected us to know. They're expecting an international medical graduate to be just stuttering and stammering and just coming down with an old status quo, who knows nothing and they thought they were above us and all of the sudden, we came here, we turned around things and our clinical knowledge is better than the average training that they get so I've had that, like, ah, you know more than us.

I asked, "Are they expecting you to provide substandard care then, and then you surprise them by providing better care?"

> That's what I'm talking, yeah, mm-hmm. That's what they think, like I mean, coming from a third world country probably he doesn't know much but they don't realize, you know, that people who come from a third world country, to this country, to have to do that transition, they have to be the cream of the third world country to come here. Otherwise they cannot come here. An average graduate from a third world country cannot make it, cannot get through all these exams, most of them cannot get through all the residencies if he's not smart enough, I mean, he cannot do it.

Most IMGs did not express such concerns. Furthermore, almost all participants in the study spoke highly of the competence of IMGs. However, on two occasions, participants expressed a concern based on a misunderstanding that IMGs do not have to undergo further training once they come to the United States. An elderly participant who commutes from a nearby small town to a senior citizens center in Quincy for activities had some concerns:

> Do they have to adhere to American standards, do they have to pass some sort of board or something before they can practice in the United States, so that we know that they are as qualified as American doctors? They may be more qualified for all I know, but that is my concern, are they as qualified?

A U.S. medical graduate had come across similar concerns that put the above comment in some context:

> Well, a lot of people, like I said, I'd say more of the older population, again, think that—They may think that the foreign medical graduates may not be as competent as the American trained, U.S. born and trained graduates, but once they've learned that they've had to do a certain amount of residency in this country, they feel pretty comfortable with them.

Whether a critical view of IMG qualifications is more predominant among senior citizens cannot be determined definitively from the fieldwork conducted for this study. Several participants posited that senior citizens would likely be a source of concern, but I rarely tapped into such sentiment in direct conversation with seniors.

Critical views toward the competence of IMGs were uncommon even in interviews in which participants appeared to criticize IMGs on other fronts (e.g., communication, assimilation). In several interviews, participants indicated that IMGs are actually more competent than U.S. medical graduates. As explained by a nurse:

> I think some of them are more so because some of them's had I think more education really than the American doctors have, because as I said, some of them's been to school in their country, plus they go to additional school in the U.S.

A pastor in town expressed a similar sentiment: "I actually think that they are more qualified. I think that they are more educated. I think that they're more dedicated. Some Americans would prefer to have a foreign doctor because—for those reasons."

A few participants speculated that there might be differences by country of origin in terms of qualifications. However, no clear dichotomy emerged in terms of which countries would be better and which worse. Instead, the list of qualifications (e.g., degrees, residency training, location of medical school) may have limited usefulness in conveying the qualifications of physicians to a number of people in Quincy. According to a worker in the Emergency Medical Service:

> As far as doctors and physicians coming in, we're seeing a whole lot of physicians coming in that we don't know anything about, and the public doesn't know anything about. I mean, you can list—I've seen them listed in the newspapers, it's kind of funny to me, they'll list in the newspaper all their accreditations and, you know, degrees and stuff. No offense, it doesn't mean a hill of beans to me. I want to know what kind of physician they are. They can have all the school in the world and be a bad physician.

REFERRALS FROM PRIMARY CARE PHYSICIANS

Almost without exception, participants explained that they trust their primary care physician's judgment on referrals. As a result, the competence of the intended subspecialist—IMG or U.S. medical graduate—generally does not surface as a concern. As explained by one patient who said she prefers U.S. medical graduates for primary care but has no preference for or against IMGs in seeking subspecialty care: "Well, if you got to go to a specialist, you want to go to whosever the best in the field that's near you. You don't want to go all over creation. And if you've got good doctors in your hometown, whether they're American or foreigners, that's who you're going to."

"And who decides who is a good doctor?" I asked.

"Your regular doctor," she replied, and laughed.

The names of at least three U.S. medical graduates who are family doctors in the area were mentioned repeatedly by patients for being so trusted, including a physician who has taken care of many patients in Quincy for their entire lives. Still, I wondered why trust in IMG subspecialists might not be as strong an issue as trust in primary care providers. A nurse in the hospital explained:

> Cause you only see a specialty doctor once or twice, you know, you just want him to take care of that one special problem and that's it. You don't use him to take care of your medications, you don't need to see him every so often, you just need him to do that one little thing and that's that one thing that he's supposed to deal with. So I don't care if he was a green little munchkin, as long as he did that one thing and one thing well.

"I'm thinking there must be a lot of trust that you have of Dr. [name] that you would let him refer you to a green little munchkin," I said.

> Yeah! If he do that one thing, if I had a bad heart and all he needed to do was fix my bad heart and he did that one thing and one thing well, well, fix my green heart, little green munchkin, you know what I mean? That's basically what I think about it. I mean, specialists, you don't see them very often. You don't communicate with them, you know what I mean? You just need them to fix whatever problem you have, you know, and that's how they make their money.

A U.S. medical graduate who is a subspecialist in the area expressed a similar sentiment, expanding on the issue of communication:

> Generally speaking, the public has no prejudice when it comes to seeing a foreign-trained subspecialist. If you are there for a procedure, such as endoscopy, colonoscopy, or lung biopsy, you will probably not establish any long-term bond with the physician. However, for a family physician, being able to speak English well is quite important.

Broader contexts, such as communication, cannot be disentangled easily from mechanisms (e.g., competence, referrals) or events (e.g., trust, acceptability). For example, a family physician said that he considered the issue of communication in deciding on his referrals. He explained that "way less than ten percent" of his patients would balk at seeing an IMG for subspecialty care, and he knows his patients well enough to know which patients might have more of a problem with being referred to an IMG:

> You just got a way of talking to that patient and knowing that if they will resent a foreigner, and sometimes I catch myself saying to the patient that I can't quite feel out yet, I say, I'm going to send you to Dr. [name], he's a gastroenterologist, he's board certified, trained in the United States, very good. Now I hardly ever say that about an American. But I find myself saying that sometimes about—And then sometimes I add on, he speaks very good English. There's a few doctors who don't speak good, and I don't refer patients. If I can't understand them, I know my patients can't.

Several community members who told me that they were the above physician's patients were interviewed for this study, and confirmed that he knows best in deciding where they should go for subspecialty care. In the words of one of his patients: "I figure that if Doc doesn't know where to send me, I certainly don't know where to go, so, you know, nobody else does if he doesn't, so that's what I do."

Since most IMGs in the area were subspecialists, questions on competence often did not come to the surface for the general community. Instead, the patient and primary care physician—in most cases, a U.S. medical graduate—had already established a bond and connection, which in turn translated into a trust in providers that the physician says are good. Nonetheless, IMGs often told me that they needed to prove themselves in order to do well in the area.

It may seem puzzling at first that IMGs appeared to be well accepted and yet they also felt a strong need to prove themselves as good physicians. So many explanations surface in considering this paradox. For example, there was a stereotype among many members of the medical community that IMGs of Asian Indian origin were especially hard-working. This work ethic may be attributable in part to the high expectations that immigrants might place on themselves or their families, as discussed in the previous vignette. Possible differences in attitudes toward work in different countries may also play a role in individual IMGs' work ethic.

In the words of a U.S. medical graduate: "Let's face it! The Indians work hard—day and night—harder than the average American-trained physician. They've earned their keep."

This sense that IMGs needed to have "earned their keep" adds another nuance to the work ethic of many IMGs. This work ethic may be one key reason why IMGs have had successful medical practices in the area. In Quincy, it is fair to say that IMGs have built thriving practices and, in general, gained the trust of many people in both the medical and nonmedical communities in the area.

NOTES

1. One IMG had two medical degrees: one from a U.S. medical school, and one from abroad.

2. Beyond such brief examples, the exact delineation of items as mechanisms or nonmechanisms serves no real purpose other than to force items into categories. Still, for organizational purposes, it is important for the reader to at least bear in mind that mechanisms—even though not pointed out specifically—are the driving force behind this discussion.

3. The survey, conducted by the hospital, is confidential and not available to the public.

Chapter Five

Contexts and Quincy: "Breaking that Ice"

"I don't see a problem with the trust issue, other than the fact that it's hard to trust somebody that you don't communicate well with."

Those words, uttered by a community member, add to the already difficult issues of trust and, more generally, acceptability. In interview after interview, no single issue surfaced more frequently, or seemed more important to participants, than problems with communication. On one level, the issue of communication can appear quite simple, as when would-be participants provided mere soundbites like, "I think they are good doctors but I can't understand a word they say," as if there was nothing more that could be said on the topic. On another level, the complexity around international medical graduate (IMG)-patient communication warrants its own separate linguistics studies in order to understand the construction of words, accents, language, and meanings attached to physician-patient encounters.

The issue of language, as complex as it is in its own right, is only one of many abstract contexts that complicate IMG acceptability, and yet no list of subcontexts (e.g., communication, accents, word choice) or other contexts (e.g., race, gender, religion) would do justice to the complicated, nuanced nature of this study.[1] Doctor-patient communication is obviously a crucial issue for all physicians and not simply IMGs (Gesler, 1999; Atkinson, 1995; Good, 1987; Helman, 1984). Communicating ideas in everyday terms, reading subtle cues from patients, knowing how to be persuasive, and understanding local or regional accents and expressions are only a few of the many complex issues raised by both IMGs and U.S. medical graduates in Quincy. IMGs not only faced many of the same issues with communication as U.S. medical graduates but also had the added difficulties of being from another country and, in many cases, learning English as a second (or third or fourth) language.

Obstacles to IMG-patient communication often centered around the difficulty of many patients in understanding the accents, pronunciation, speed in talking, and word choice of IMGs. For example, a common concern expressed about physicians from India was that they talked too quickly. Several participants explained that the pace is slower in Quincy. According to a cancer patient:

> Most of the foreign doctors probably have an accent, or maybe not foreign specifically, but if they're not from this area. They probably talk a lot faster than people in this area. That was my problem with them, they would talk so fast that I didn't comprehend what they were saying most of the time.

Some of the issues faced by IMGs are obviously not exclusive to them, but, rather, part of what it is like to be a doctor in Quincy. Moving to the area from anywhere leads to obvious concerns about finding the best way to talk so that it is most appropriate for this town.

Complicating matters are other difficulties faced by all physicians that inhibit patients from understanding the doctor and from asking questions when something is unclear. For example, a nurse explained about some of the difficulties when doctors ask patients if there are any questions: "I mean, that's just a general consensus around here, you have to say, do you have a question? And some of them will say noooo. Then they ask the family member, because they don't want to bother the doctor, because, you know, and that's how they refer to it, as, well, I didn't want to bother the doctor. You know what I mean? And it's like he's some special human—or she—human being that you can't tell them that because, you know, that's the doctor, you know, that's the doctor."

"Do they ask you?" I asked.

"Yeah, they'll ask us."

"They'll ask you and the family—they can ask the nurse—"

"Yeah, that's—the nurse is just a nurse, but the doctor, he's a doctor, you know what I mean? He's the—the one that you only meet in the case of an emergency, but the nurse, you just can ask them anything."

The nurse went on to say:

> A lot of patients come in and we have foreign doctors on staff and they don't understand what they're saying to them. So this—And the whole while the doctor's talking, oodloodloodloodloodloodl, and they're saying, Mm-hmm, Mm-hmm. And then they say nurse, wait a minute, what did he say? So I think it's more a communication thing than anything else, because they always say, What did he say? And it's always the foreign doctors. They don't never have to ask you to—what they say to the American doctors at all.

Most IMG participants acknowledged the added difficulties that they face with communication. Moreover, the IMG patients who were study participants, and IMGs themselves, agreed that they are often more likely to go out of their way to use the help of nurses and other staff (e.g., assistants working in the office, pharmacists clarifying directions if necessary) in communication. According to a person working in hospital administration:

> I'll tell you an interesting story. One of our physicians who was from India and he passed away about a year and a half ago, but a wonderful doctor, was a surgeon, and just very well liked by the community and his patients because he was so caring. He was real interesting, he was a little guy with a real loud voice. But when he would go in to see patients he'd always take a nurse with him to the room when he was going to describe the surgical procedure that he was going to do. And he'd just talk to the patient and give them the risks and benefits of the operation, and he'd get through and he'd turn to the nurse and he'd say, now you tell them. [laughs] Because he wanted to—he knew that sometimes they might not understand him as well. So he had the nurse then repeat what he had said.

An IMG from South Asia relayed a commonly mentioned approach to ensuring that the patient understands the medical advice:

> Sometimes I have a hard time explaining to people, it is difficult for them to understand foreign accent. But I have my assistant, and if my patient doesn't explain to them—if I can't explain to the patient, my assistant explain to the patient. It's very individual, a lot of people, a lot of my patients, the majority of my patients, they do understand, I will say 95 percent very well. But once in a while I see patients, they really don't want to listen to me or what I have to say, they just turn their face to the assistant, what he said. They're sometimes, they're very nice to me and they come again and again, they bring their family, but they just think in their mind they don't understand.

The issue of whether there even is a communication problem surfaced in only a few interviews with IMGs. For example, another IMG from South Asia said:

> I don't think it is a language barrier. I think it is due to impaired hearing, and they are in a different state of mind. Some people are depressed. Some people are sent here by another physician, referred to me, they don't even want to come, but they will come kind of halfheartedly sent to me and go. But, you know, for example, population, we haven't had much problems. But maybe you ask them, they could say that, you know, we have a little bit of accent problem. That is true. Because I wasn't born here, I wasn't raised here. And it is difficult to have the same accent as the people here.

Later in the interview, he said that some IMGs do need to "improve their language," and discussed some of his efforts to make sure patients understand him. In discussing IMG-patient communication in Quincy, he said:

> I think I have heard some people, some patients say that he's a good doctor, but I don't want to go to see him because I don't understand a word he tells me. I agree with it. And I tend to speak to my patients on a slower pace. I'm talking to you a little faster, because I know you can pick up anything. But to my patients I speak a little bit at a slower pace, you know, I don't go double speed, I go one speed. If I go at my normal speed they understand me reasonably well. If they don't understand, most patients, they know me very well they will ask me, what did you say?

Despite my ease in understanding him and others, a transcriptionist who helped me often remarked about the difficulty in understanding IMGs' accents on tape.

Another IMG, who was one of the first people that I interviewed in Quincy, explained that it is difficult to understand medical terms on top of an accent and differences in pronunciation. He gave a minor example. Having been raised in India, he explained that he pronounced "vomiting" as "womiting." With less familiar medical terminology, he said that it becomes an added concern for patients already trying to understand the physician's speech.

In another early interview, a U.S. medical graduate told me about similar difficulties with language faced by an IMG from Southeast Asia. I asked whether such incidents were isolated examples of problems with communication. The physician replied:

> No, no, the Indians have a real problem with it. The Indian. Now, for example, [name of a physician from Southeast Asia], if you talk to him, doesn't have a trace of an accent. He's totally American and we had a Japanese who had no accent. You'd—on the phone, you could understand him. It's an accent issue. It's not a foreign issue. It depends on how good their English is.

According to several participants, it can be even more difficult to communicate over the telephone rather than face-to-face with some IMGs. An allied health provider said:

> Just as a, kind of an aside, I was sitting at the desk with one of the new pharmacists last week and one of our Indian physicians was behind us talking on the phone and she said, is he speaking English? And I said, yeah, just listen, you have to listen real close. They just talk so fast, and sometimes it is difficult to understand what they're saying. Most of the time if I'm looking at them, I can understand what they're talking about. Now if you get them on

> the phone, sometimes that's a different story. But you know, I don't really feel like my interaction with them is any different than it is with the American therapist—I mean, physicians.

Concerns about communicating with IMGs in Quincy typically focused on speech. However, to limit the issue of doctor-patient communication merely to speech would be a mistake. For example, a U.S. medical graduate talked about unspoken communication, that in any doctor-patient encounter there is much unsaid that has great meaning. He explained that a person from the area can pick up on nonverbal cues more quickly by being more familiar with the local culture. Active involvement in the community adds to his ability to know how to listen to and talk with individual patients.

On the one hand, even the strongest supporters of IMGs viewed communication as a problem. However, there are different nuances to communication that resist easy classification. The extent to which IMGs have difficulty communicating with patients is a multifaceted issue, and patients and physicians alike try to improve the clarity of their own explanations, albeit to varying extent from individual to individual.

Despite myriad ways of considering communication with IMGs, a mitigating issue is that patients can adapt to new situations in which physicians speak differently than originally expected. In discussing a visit to an IMG, a community member explained, "Okay, the more we talked, the more I understood. Maybe I was a little puzzled in the beginning, but as I got to know him I picked up on him more, his words more."

The idea of adjusting over time to different ways of talking was also mentioned in other interviews. For example, another community member said, "But if you, you know, if you be around somebody long enough, you begin to understand what they say."

Even for a first time visit to an IMG, people often said that they adapted without much difficulty to the physician's manner of talking and expression. This point was reiterated by another community member who reflected on the concentration necessary to understand the IMGs that she has seen as a patient:

> And you really have to concentrate and, okay, so we got to really make sure that we on the same level here, are we still talking about the same thing? You know. But it's not one of those things where you got to have an interpreter there or anything, you know. It's not as bad as some people would say that it is, I don't think, you know. For the most part, they understand—We understand each other, for the most part. When they are explaining to you after the examination, you have to actually listen and give your undivided attention to some of them because of

their speech. But it's not a big major thing. I mean, you should be giving your undivided attention anyway, you know. [laughs]

UNDERSTANDING PATIENTS

Until now, the discussion in this section has focused on the difficulty in understanding IMGs. Another important issue is that there are local and regional expressions, accents, and nonverbal means of communicating that might not be readily understood by a new physician. For example, some patients in the area use traditional medicine, such as wearing a penny around the neck or taking herbs. Patients often do not tell physicians about the use of traditional medicine (Eisenberg et al., 1993). Therefore, to be effective communicators, IMGs must not only learn about words but beliefs and mores, which relate further to the idea that communication extends far beyond the spoken language (Gesler, 1999; McPheron-Alex, 1993; Admire, 1993; Good, 1987; Kleinman, 1978, 1980).

It is the spoken language that most people mentioned in considering problems with communication. In addition to accents, words used by people in the local area can present difficulties for IMGs. Most of the words and examples that I came across presented only minor difficulty in communication, often to the point of being amusing. IMGs had several examples from communication with patients and colleagues, including:

- "When I came in, they'd say, how're y'all? I'd sort of say, where's you all? I'm just one. [laughs] You know, where's the all here? And I slowly understand, it's not very difficult. But things like that do happen."
- "We can, like for example, I have a mechanic patient, and sometimes he tells me something that is a word [laughs] that has to do with his job, and maybe for an American born person it would be easier to get that word. And to me, it's something I may never heard. It's a little bit difference."
- "For example, one of the things I always mention is they would say, cut the light off, you know. [laughs] That's a difficult—And, where is he at? You know. But you understand what they say."

Less frequently, participants mentioned words used for explaining health issues. For example, one IMG said, "When I came down to Quincy, sure, there were words that I didn't understand. It took me some years to really understand that. As for number two, number one, I never had a clue what those people meant by that, you know, until someone explained that to me. Pee, what's pee? There are others."

Another IMG discussed the word "budges" [sic]: "Well, it's cramps in the legs and is also described as restless leg. So that's one word that I did not know when I got here, but now when they tell me they have got budges, I know what it means. But in general I don't have problems understanding what patients are trying to tell me."

Many expressions that might pose difficulty for IMGs were mentioned by other health professionals and community members in the area, without specifically referring to the doctor-patient interaction. For example, a community member said that he was so interested in the many local idioms that he was compiling a list of colloquialisms, such as "won't" for "wasn't" (e.g., "it won't me"). In another example, a physician assistant said that he learned the term "kneebaby," which is "the second youngest one because the other one is in the lap. The kneebaby is standing by the knee."

A nurse practitioner who is originally from a nearby state talked about IMGs asking others the meanings of unfamiliar slang terms:

> I've seen them do the same thing, you know, they say, you know, they'll come to you and say I'm having a hard time understanding some of the little slang words, you know, what does so and so mean. Yeah, I've seen them come do that. You know, you explain to them what the little slang words mean, oh, okay, and next time—And it's really funny, cause you may see them with a patient, you know, a month or so later and you'll hear them saying these little slang words, and it's their way of trying to fit in with the community. And it works for them. It really works. They say, oh, it's nonsense, I'm not gonna be saying that kind of crap. But as a general rule most of them who really try to fit into the community sort of pick up those, and you can pick up those little slang things, those little communications that you may not see anywhere else. People just pick them up and then use them naturally. If you're not willing to do that, then you're going to have a hard time fitting in anywhere you go.

To ensure effective communication between doctor and patient, some physicians spend more time with patients, despite having busy schedules. At least four IMG participants speculated that IMGs in general spend more time with patients. One of the IMGs, originally from India, conjectured that concerns about communication might be one reason for longer doctor visits. If English is not your first language, you might need to be a more attentive listener and spend more time with patients.

Another physician, a U.S. medical graduate originally from abroad, also viewed communication concerns in relation to the length of time that doctors spend with patients, as well as other issues such as accents:

> I look at the personalities of certain individuals who are often mentioned. It's not that they have language difficulties. Their command of language is often better than most. It's just that they are either in a hurry or they have an accent

which is difficult for many patients to get used to. And so that's why they say, I didn't understand.

SPECIFIC GROUPS MENTIONED AS HAVING POTENTIAL DIFFICULTY COMMUNICATING WITH IMGs

Several participants mentioned senior citizens as a group that might have particular difficulty understanding IMGs. However, it is difficult to discuss one group (e.g., senior citizens) in isolation from all other groups, since most participants said that there was a problem with communication anyway. I found no evidence that senior citizens tend to have special difficulty communicating with IMGs. However, several physicians and others in the medical community who have worked with senior citizens said that there are often such problems. Particular concerns around IMG–senior citizen communication included many senior citizens' hearing problems; difficult adjustments to new accents after a lifetime without exposure to the accents of many immigrants; concerns about questioning the physician to repeat what was said; and some of the elderly's accents and use of archaic expressions that might be less familiar to newcomers.

The uneducated are another group that might have particular difficulty understanding IMGs, according to several participants. As with virtually all other participants, communication surfaced as an issue among the least educated and poorest members of the Quincy community. Some physicians—including both IMGs and U.S. medical graduates—said that there are many less educated people in the area who are difficult to understand. Difficulties adjusting to the speech patterns of the uneducated add another wrinkle to the issue of doctor-patient communication. However, there appeared to be a mitigating circumstance among the poor—they just wanted a good doctor. They did not have the financial means to be selective, so they were also mentioned as a group that was likely to be particularly accepting of IMGs.

Meanwhile, IMGs, like other physicians, reportedly try to adjust their own ways of explaining ideas to people with different levels of education. For example, an IMG reflected on how he communicated with patients who have less education:

> Well, I think that goes back to some degree to patients' education and home situation. If someone is educated and has some knowledge about medicine and what goes on, then it's a little easier to explain to them in more detail. While somebody who really doesn't have much concept about diseases and, you know, human anatomy and things like that, then it's difficult. Well, it's still not diffi-

cult, you can still convey what you want to, but it's that we communicate at a different level. We try not to give too many details and to confuse the person, but instead try to simplify it as best as we can.

Difficulties communicating with patients who only speak Spanish, such as seasonal migrant workers, present another issue of concern for physicians. Physicians generally estimated that Hispanics who do not speak English constitute only a few percentage points toward their overall patient base. Furthermore, the number of Hispanic patients varies depending on the season, since many are migrant farm workers. A minority of IMGs have an advantage over their U.S. medical graduate counterparts by virtue of speaking fluent Spanish.

Based on personal observation, communication in health care settings with the Hispanic population is an area where there is dire need in Quincy. For example, while I was volunteering at the Free Clinic, two men entered the clinic and wanted to see a doctor, but they did not speak any English and therefore did not know how to fill out the paperwork. I tried to help them fill out a form that had basic questions about name, address, and place of employment, but I was of little use since I did not speak Spanish. When I was able to communicate that something as basic as their names needed to be written down, I handed my pen to one of the two patients. To my surprise, he barely knew how to write. Meanwhile, the two men waited for a translator. After about an hour, a friend of theirs came by to help translate but he could only be of limited usefulness since he was on a break from work and could stay only 15 minutes. Later in the evening, a translator came by to help further with communication.

While IMGs from Latin America can be especially useful with their Spanish language skills, the majority of IMGs in the area did not speak Spanish and had no exposure to Spanish prior to moving to the United States. For example, only five IMGs in Quincy were listed in the physician directory as having received their medical education in a country where Spanish is the principal language. Only two physician participants spoke Spanish as their first language; another IMG participant learned Spanish before moving to the United States; and another married a person who speaks Spanish.

"Do you ever get to use Spanish?" I asked one physician whose first language is Spanish.

All the time. All the time. Whenever there's a woman in labor who speaks only Spanish or whenever we have a patient come into surgery who speaks only Spanish, whether I'm involved in that case or not, I'm asked to get involved and translate, and I'm happy to do so. I'm happy to do so because, you know, I try to put myself in the patient's shoes, that if I were in a foreign country, and I was—You know, surgery or childbirth under the best of circumstances is still a

> very emotionally trying moment in any person's life. So I figure, you know, it's got to be a tremendous relief to then to be able to at least hear, you know, their own language and be able to communicate and express themselves, and ask—You know, if nothing else to just talk to somebody who can understand them and talk back to them, you know, in a language they can understand. So I'm more than happy to do it whenever I can to help out with that.

Another physician—an IMG from Latin America—also reported being called upon to help with translation when there are Spanish-speaking patients who speak little or no English. Based on such accounts and my own observations, there is a need in Quincy to have more physicians or medical staff available who are bilingual.

ADHERENCE AND COMMUNICATION

Alongside difficulties in communication, an obvious concern is whether patients will understand enough from the visit to adhere to the physician's medical advice. "Adherence" (also commonly called "compliance") is a complicated topic that is also a serious concern that is not specific to IMGs, according to many physicians in the area. I questioned participants specifically about the likelihood of patients to take prescriptions, return for follow-up visits, and follow medical advice by IMGs.

All physicians—both U.S. medical graduates and IMGs—reported problems with adherence. A very difficult issue can be determining exactly what caused problems with adherence. Communication can be one possible cause, but participants also mentioned trust, education, transportation, income, belief that the medicine is no longer necessary, different explanatory models behind what caused a specific ailment, and stubbornness among patients as possible explanations for non-adherence. Complicating matters, both IMGs and U.S. medical graduates said that they do not know how closely patients are following medical advice, such as whether the patients are indeed taking the prescribed number of pills on a particular day.

The overwhelming majority of participants stated that IMG problems with communication did not affect adherence. A frequently mentioned explanation was that different people (e.g., family members, nurses, assistants, pharmacists) are available to prevent misunderstandings that would lead to non-adherence. In addition, patients receive written directions with their prescriptions. One IMG shared with me some frustration on the issue of adherence:

> I will explain something to a patient, we have two nurses at the office, these are Americans, they will reinforce what has been explained. So they have no excuse

> whatsoever, except that they're just ignorant. They will understand everything that you say, you have it in writing. How else can you explain the fact that the lady will come to your office, she wants to have [name of procedure][2] for instance. You show her the video, which she can see with her own eyes, you discuss it with her, you answer her questions, you give her the pre-admit slip or form to carry to the lab so that she can have her pre-op workup done, which she does. And then on the day of the procedure, she doesn't show up. Surely that's not communication. Isn't it? No way.

No patients reported that shortcomings in communication with IMGs led to problems with adherence. However, a few patients said that the medical advice would have been misunderstood if they had not been so willing to ask the IMG follow-up questions, or if a family member had not been along to help interpret what the IMG was saying. For example, a woman discussed the difficulty in understanding an IMG of Asian Indian origin: "He just talked too fast and I couldn't catch on to what he was saying. And I'd say, tell me that again please, cause I ain't sure what you said. And then he would slow down usually the second time, if you say something like that."

She went on to explain that the doctor was relaying very important information about her daughter's medical condition, but that she asked questions to make sure that she understood his advice. I began to say: "So if you had not asked—"

She interrupted: "I wouldn't have known what I was doing with the medication, what the medication for, and what her problem was."

Despite the consensus among nearly all participants that communication does not affect adherence, three of the U.S. medical graduates interviewed for this study stated otherwise. For example, one U.S. medical graduate who spoke very highly of many IMGs acknowledged the seriousness of concerns about communication. In the words of the U.S. medical graduate:

> If I look at [name of IMG], for example, the biggest problems that [he] has, I think, is in getting himself understood to the patient what he wants, and I think by the time he gets it understood to them, he doesn't have time to figure out if they understood it really. I mean, he's doing that and he can't talk on the phone to patients because when he's on the phone, his accent is such that then the patients can't understand him. And a one to one basis, he has to work harder at being understood. And I have to work hard at it and I speak the language and I'm from here, but I really spend a lot of time with underserved populations in particular, trying to make sure they understood exactly what it was I told them to do. And that probably, like, one of my patients went to [another IMG who is a subspecialist], and he wrote me back that his nurse had trained her in how to do self-catheterization, and I'm going, there's no way they trained this woman, she's demented. I can't get her to take her pills straight, and I know she's not

> cathing herself, and he's under the belief this woman is going home and catheterizing herself three times a day, and I know she's not so when she comes in, I sit down and say, you know, what's really going on. Well, she's been able to do it once or twice but I don't think he can get that information back from her because I don't think he really—she's not going to tell him that she's not doing it because he's an authority figure and so, I think that part of it's a primary care perspective but I also think part is a communication issue and I think the communication things are the bigger problem.

The participant went on to say:

> When the patients come back to me, I will sit down and say, you know, you saw [the IMG subspecialist]. Did he explain things to you? Yes. Did he answer your questions? Yes. And then I'll have them explain to me what he told them, and it frequently doesn't, there will not be the kind of questioning because they don't understand him. So when he's talking to them, they can't ask a question back because it's that they didn't understand what he said enough to ask a question back but they don't want to tell him and embarrass him by saying, I don't understand what you've said. And so they have to rely more on nurses to do some of the instructing, which is okay, you know, if their nurse is well-trained, I don't have any problem. But my patients struggle more with communication issues, and with [name of a primary care IMG], I know that his nurses have to spend more time communicating for him because the patients won't understand, and [he] will sometimes explain to the nurses and have them explain it to the patient just because his accent is such they don't understand it.

The more common response among participants was that problems with communication presented no problem with adherence. Furthermore, I am not aware of any allegations or legal claims that a patient's illness in Quincy stemmed from an IMG's difficulties communicating with a patient.

UNMASKING COMMUNICATION

I did not have difficulty understanding IMGs, but my conversations were atypical in being nonclinical discussions used toward academic research, rather than firsthand doctor-patient visits. However, I was aware from interviews and other conversations with IMGs that some IMGs had heavier accents, and some had little or no trace of an accent. I recall one interview with an IMG who spoke English with very little foreign accent. Shortly thereafter, I talked with a senior citizen who said that her husband had had so much difficulty understanding this physician's accent that she would come along to help interpret what the physician was saying. This simply did not make sense to me. I wondered whether this participant had a problem with recall or maybe had false expectations that led her or her husband to believe that this physician had difficulty with the English language. I also wondered if it was simply easier to say that communication was the problem when, in fact, it may have been something else.

One IMG raised the idea that concerns about communication may mask discrimination. He said that a patient might change physicians out of stated concerns over communication, when in fact the underlying reason may have more to do with the color of the physician's skin. He said: "I think that's just a camouflage. You know, that's a nice way of putting it because nobody takes offense if you can't understand somebody else. But the real meaning, in my opinion, is very different from that excuse."

The above comment warrants some reflection and rereading because over and over again, participants discussed concerns about IMGs' ability to communicate with patients. Many of the concerns about communication were clearly legitimate, at least based on my own sense of participants' responses. I wonder though if some participants were not telling the truth about communication; in many cases, mentioning communication might simply be easier than admitting to bigotry. I have no way of knowing except to consider that at least on a few occasions, I was concerned that patients discussing problems with communication would not elaborate, or gave an explanation that conflicted with my own knowledge of the physician's accent. Yet even IMGs, and people who spoke very favorably of IMGs, considered communication to be a serious concern. It is difficult to know the real meaning behind all participants' stated concerns about communication, but it is likely that, in at least some cases, some concerns about communication may indeed mask racism and xenophobia.

DISCRIMINATION AND STEREOTYPES

Discrimination obviously does exist in Quincy, as it does virtually everywhere. However, the overwhelming majority of participants, including IMGs, described a town that has very little discrimination against IMGs. Then again, it is difficult to determine exactly what constitutes discrimination (Mohammad, 1999; Holloway, 1998; Sibley, 1995). I have no checklist of discriminatory words or deeds, and do not see any merit in arbitrary delineations of "right" and "wrong" actions. Like virtually everything in this study, discrimination is a complex and multifaceted issue that cannot be encapsulated easily. Potential concerns about racism and mistreatment of women are a few issues that warrant separate discussion. For this section, I want to focus more specifically on stereotypes toward IMGs, with special attention to IMGs of Asian Indian origin since they constitute the greatest percentage of IMGs in the area.

Not all stereotypes are negative. For example, a positive stereotype toward IMGs of Asian Indian origin has already been mentioned, specifically that they are hard workers. Concern for their children, including the importance of education, is another positive attribute mentioned by participants about IMGs from India. In fact, it was commonly mentioned in interviews and informal conversations that the children of IMGs have won a number of awards for academic merit. In one participant's view, the quality of schools in the area has improved because IMGs place so much value on education, which in turn puts pressure on the schools to perform.

In some interviews with community members, participants said that there can be a stereotype that all people from India who are in Quincy must be physicians. However, the person that people think is a doctor may actually turn out to be a motel owner, since not every person of Asian Indian origin in Quincy is a physician.

Some stereotypes can have more negative overtones, albeit to varying degrees. A commonly mentioned concern that surfaced in interviews was that IMGs may have a tendency to be more formal in their professional interactions. As one physician explained:

> The one thing I have noticed is many of the foreign medical graduates I've dealt with here tend to be somewhat more formal and stilted in their dealings with you at first. You know, it takes them a long time to get to the point where you can, you know, just talk to each other on a first name basis. Everything has to be doctor this and doctor that. Which to me is silly. I mean, we're all doctors. I feel silly calling somebody doctor something and having them call me doctor something. But that's just—I guess that just goes in personalities. But most of the American trainees that I know usually it's like go on first name basis, giving the recognition the fact that we all have basically the same letters, or very similar letters beyond our names.

Based on my interviews and conversations with IMGs, I am in no position to confirm whether IMGs tend to be more formal in their interactions with colleagues and patients. I can say that formality in interviews tended to vary by individual more than by any other factor. The age of the IMG might also play a role in formality; most of the IMGs interviewed in Quincy were in their 40s and 50s, and it is possible that a younger generation might be perceived as acting less formally. Some of the perceived differences between IMGs and U.S. medical graduates in formality could also be related to changes taking place in U.S. health care, in which physicians are increasingly becoming team players alongside patients (Robinson, 1999). Obviously, IMGs experience such changes through training in U.S. residency programs, practicing medicine in the United States, and other experiences. In other countries, such as the United Kingdom, which has influenced health care in India, doctors might act more formally toward their patients than in the United States. The issue of formality can have a sharply negative interpretation, as when a few participants expressed concern that IMGs—particularly of Asian Indian origin—tended to be aloof. According to a community member:

> But I would say that on a whole, people coming from other countries really need to be careful about not being aloof when they're coming to practice medicine here, to try to be a little more personable with people to kind of break the barrier. You know, that's one barrier they don't need.

A related concern about IMGs of Asian Indian origin is that they may appear to have a more hierarchical social order. In several interviews, participants reasoned that the hierarchy is related to the caste system in India, except transferred to health care situations in the United States. For example, a nurse expressed concern about her ability to offer medical advice about patients to IMGs from India, while two other nurses voiced particular concern that the social hierarchy can impede some IMGs from functioning in a team approach with female nurses. Meanwhile, participants said that the extent to which IMGs from India have a hierarchical social order varies by individual.

The potential for a hierarchical social order becomes exceedingly complex, in part because of anthropological and sociological overtones about human behavior and social interaction that are beyond the scope of this study (Robinson, 1999; Atkinson, 1995; Kleinman, 1980). Also, physicians must work with nurses, receptionists, X-ray technicians, operating room technicians, and countless other medical staff that are technically beneath a physician in terms of authority and stature in a medical setting. No one suggested that IMGs are deficient in such interactions, although some of the nurses mentioned that there is room for improvement with individual IMGs in particular. Still other nurses said that there was no problem whatsoever with the interactions between nurses and IMGs.

The issue of the role of nurse practitioners (NPs) and physician assistants (PAs) adds another layer of complexity to the social order, since they often perform the same duties as physicians (e.g., performing medical examinations, writing prescriptions, making referrals). Most IMGs, including IMGs from India, came from countries that did not have any NPs or PAs. One IMG of Asian Indian origin was particularly concerned about granting more authority to NPs, PAs, or other health professionals who do not have nearly as much training as a physician:

> For us, it's difficult for us to accept that concept. It's not easy. Cause I'm not used to dealing with—I'm used to dealing with people who are my peers, my colleagues and my peers. But it's difficult for me to deal with somebody who thinks or pretends, or at least thinks that he's as good as I am or I'm better. Maybe! I'm not saying he's not.

Only in one other interview did an IMG have any critical words about NPs or PAs. Furthermore, a few IMGs have employed NPs or PAs in the past, and the NP and PA interviewed for this study spoke favorably of their interactions with IMGs.

Some concerns that surfaced about IMGs in Quincy overlap somewhat with more general concerns that physicians are greedy people. For example, some participants expressed a concern that physicians in general charge too much or otherwise place too much emphasis on money. The same allegation about limited concern for the poor can be looked at with a different spin, focused on IMGs in particular. For example, a few community members alleged that IMGs show little concern for the poor. A related concern was the allegation that IMGs do not put money back in the community, where it is needed, but instead send money back to their countries of origin. A few participants alleged that IMGs are not actively involved in civic activities, and that IMGs receive at least some tax-exempt status. In the words of one community member:

> And there is no money put back into the towns that they occupy, basically the tax base, I mean. What happens that, whether it's true or false, people are under the assumption from the ones that I've talked to that they receive five years tax free, without paying any tax.

Concerns about greediness contradicted my own observations. One of the first IMGs that I met in the area started a Free Clinic to help the poor. Other physicians—including both IMGs and U.S. medical graduates—have volunteered at the Free Clinic. A few participants stated that IMGs do not give to charitable organizations, but the only list of charitable contributions that I saw did include the names of IMGs. It was as if I had two ways of considering the charitableness of IMGs—one with my own eyes, and one based on allegations that are important for this study insofar as they reflect perception. Based on my own observations and conversations with IMGs, there might be complex, abstract cultural and personality differences that are misinterpreted, which help lead a small minority of participants to allege greed as a cultural or professional trait for IMGs.

The few overt incidents of discrimination that I learned about in Quincy took place mostly in relation to medical settings. Even there, the instances of intolerance appeared to be infrequent, according to participants.

An IMG originally from India recounted an incident in which a nurse had a negative attitude toward him: "In fact, I asked one person, I said, why do you do this? She said, you've betrayed your country. You've left your country. I said, but I'm doing good for your country. I mean, why don't you accept us? You're still a foreigner for us."

Another physician told me of repeated instances in which patients, when faced with a choice between a physician with a "very American sounding name" and a last name that "is very obviously foreign," will choose the physician with an American sounding name.

According to an IMG who is originally from sub-Saharan Africa, there are advantages and disadvantages to having a foreign-sounding last name:

> First thing, if you're looking for a physician to take care of your family, and you're looking at the telephone directory, which is a good source of reference, would you rather go to someone with a funny name or would you rather go to someone with a name like Johnson or Jackson or Phillips? It stands to reason that you'd rather go to somebody whose name you can pronounce. It's a different thing if someone is telling you about this person from personal experience. Well, like people have said to me, they say if you can look beyond his color, if you can look beyond his accent, he's really a damn good doctor. Well, unfortunately people have difficulty sometimes looking beyond those things. And so pick up a telephone directory, they see a Johnson, they go to Johnson. So in that respect, it's not an advantage. On the other hand, if they will pay you the compliment of finding out from personal experience what you are, who you are, what makes you tick, they will leave with a better impression of other foreign medical graduates, international medical graduates, because that breaks the ice. It's no longer, gee, he's got a different name. Judge him on the content of his head—what is that?

"Content of his character," I said.

"Content of his character. That's what I find. A lot of them feel pleasantly surprised after they've had some interaction. But it's breaking that ice. And if they could break that ice, things—a new world will open, so to speak. That has been my experience."

"Breaking that ice" can be likened to the removal of a boundary separating patients from providers. From personal contact, patients who had excluded IMGs might then have a more expansive, open view of other IMGs.

Before the ice can be broken, however, a patient's choice of physician can be based simply on looking in a telephone directory. Most patients do not have to rely on managed care gatekeepers for referrals, since managed care has only a small presence in the area. However, IMGs constitute such a large percentage of the local physician workforce that some patients might perceive only a very limited choice or none at all, if they want to see a physician locally. Not often, but sometimes in casual conversation or interviews, a person would say that IMGs are good doctors but we go to them because we do not have a choice.

Even though I found little explicit evidence of discrimination against IMGs, scratching beneath the surface can reveal tensions (e.g., hospital politics, concerns about choice, questions on money) that may have many possible explanations including discrimination. Beneath the surface, beyond the spoken word, beyond what I can observe with my own eyes, a town that is dependent on IMGs has its own instances of intolerance.

THE SOCIAL CONSTRUCTION OF RACE

Race has been an important component throughout the preceding discussion, even while not mentioned explicitly. For example, it is difficult if not impossible to divorce the issue of race from many of the concerns expressed by participants about communication or foreignness. There are other, perhaps innumerable, ways that race can have a marked impact on the acceptability of IMGs. Indeed, the acceptability of black physicians warrants its own separate study, and a detailed analysis of racial preferences in doctor-patient interactions or in the general community is beyond the scope of this study.

The task of delineating differences in acceptability in relation to race is complicated immeasurably by the fact that race is a socially constructed term (Pulido, 2000; Kobayashi and Peake, 1994; Smith, 1993; Jackson, 1989; Anderson, 1987). Pinning down "race" to mean just one thing to all people would be an impossible task, since conceptualizations of race in Quincy borrowed to varying degrees from so many other contexts, including skin color, language, and nationality. What is clear is that race has meaning that fosters separateness (e.g., separateness by church, school, funeral home, residence), but it is less clear from the findings how IMGs fit into racial divisions.

Based on study findings, there is no clear delineation that IMGs who have a darker skin color (e.g., different skin colors among physicians of Asian Indian origin) are necessarily considered "white" or "black" in Quincy. However, some participants raised the idea that IMGs from India are "non-white," but I did not find an absolute gradation as to the social status of "non-whites" in relation to whites or blacks. From my interviews and observations, I also could not predict that "white" or "black" participants would hold certain views of IMGs. Even with such uncertainty, it appears that race can sometimes play a role in a person's judgment about IMGs in particular.

One interview in particular stands out that helped me see a unique role for IMGs in providing health care in needy areas. I had been interviewing a black community member, and I thought that the interview was done. Very little new information had emerged from the interview, and the participant appeared to steer clear of anything controversial. Then I turned off the tape recorder and our casual conversation became more important than the recorded one.

The participant spoke very highly of the clinic that was staffed mainly by IMGs. He also explained that if the clinic were not there, he would probably leave town for health care. He said that there had been white physicians in Quincy who had not taken good care of his family members in the past. He was careful not to say that all white physicians were to blame for their treatment, and said that on an individual basis, physicians can win his trust regardless of race. However, he said that he was skeptical of the quality of care that would be provided to black patients by white physicians in general. He said that IMGs do not have the same history of discrimination against blacks as do white physicians, and therefore he has a strong preference for IMGs over white physicians.

I raised the idea of preference for IMGs to a receptionist who works in the clinic staffed mainly by IMGs. In thinking about her own experiences in the black community, she said: "I think it's easier for them to go to the white foreign physician. It seems to be, yeah. I guess because they don't have that back past record with them as they do."

Meanwhile, participants also indicated that there are some black patients who would prefer to see a white physician rather than a black physician. An added issue is a sense of community pride that surfaced in some interviews with black participants toward the hiring of the few black physicians in the area. To say the least, such issues are deeply complicated, delving into self-perceptions in the black community, the history of medicine in the United States, and economic and social discrimination toward blacks. At the same time, white patients sometimes openly expressed a preference for seeing white physicians but generally, such perceptions appeared to vary on an individual basis, with most participants (white or black) revealing no preference. Based on so much racial complexity and varying meanings of race to different people, it is clear that IMGs walk into a racial history that is not their own, which can be both an asset and a source of concern.

Twelve of sixty-five physicians pictured in the hospital physician directory were "black," or at least had black skin, including an IMG and a U.S. medical graduate who were both born in sub-Saharan Africa. Beyond the specialty of obstetrics and gynecology, it was uncommon to encounter problems in perceptions that were explicitly linked by participants to an IMG's race. Racially tainted perceptions toward IMGs were generally relayed in the third person, in which participants made generalizations about others' perceptions. A community member who sometimes helped find physicians for parents of preschool children mentioned some of the specific concerns that parents had expressed toward individual physicians. She said:

> Well, I've had a parent say to me, I want a black doctor, but not one of those from another country where I don't understand them. I've had that said. So they even discriminate, if you will, between black and foreign. So if it's a black doctor but he's foreign, so I don't want him.

Nonetheless, the receptionist who works at the medical clinic that is primarily staffed by IMGs said that it is rare for her to encounter any concerns relating to the race of the physician: "I have had a couple of callers—Since I been with [the clinic] now for about three years, I've had one caller out of the whole three years that wanted to know what race was the physician. I've had one caller. So I'm sure that there are some people that have some concern about that."

I asked, "The caller wanted to know if the physician is white or black or international?"

"They wanted all three," she said, and laughed, and then said that "the caller wanted a white."

There is no way of knowing how many people with similar concerns did not call the clinic. However, her recollection is consistent with the fact that explicitly stated concerns about the race of IMGs appear to be uncommon in most specialties in Quincy, at least based on my interviews, conversations with key contacts, observations, and the potential hidden meaning behind "communication" discussed earlier.

The issue of race is obviously sensitive, as explained by a physician who was born outside of the United States:

> Cause I mean, in the United States today, you will sooner be forgiven for killing somebody than you will for calling him a nigger. For the latter you'll probably, you know, be crucified. For the former I'm sure somebody will find an excuse as to why you were temporarily imbalanced and felt the ultimate need to kill this other person. But God forbid that you call somebody an ethnic name or a slur or, you know, something like that. So, you know, people are real careful. But in more subtle ways you see it. If you know what you're looking for it's there.

Complicating the hidden interpretations behind race is the heterogeneity of IMGs. With multiple countries of origin, and variations in skin tone within a country, the IMGs in Quincy could not possibly be grouped easily into precise racial categories (e.g., "white," "black") based on skin color. However, race should not be discounted as an issue for IMGs either. For example, some of the quotations discussed earlier about foreignness touched on the issue of race, similar to the following comment from a participant in the medical community: "I think it's still difficult for people to accept others or other cultures, and skin tones, all that. It's just an initial—not altogether fear, but just uneasiness, until you get to know someone."

Again, there is this idea of overcoming unseen boundaries, in this case through crossing racial and cultural differences.

The issue of race can get complicated further if the IMG has black skin. For example, an IMG who is originally from sub-Saharan Africa said that if people see a black physician, they expect that affirmative action helped him get where he is today. In his words: "The general perception is that if you're not white, then you probably have less education. That's the general perception, until you start to deal with the physicians on an individual basis. But that perception will always remain."

Some IMGs expressed puzzlement at racial distinctions that are common in the United States. For example, I asked an IMG who was originally from Latin America to estimate the percentage of his patient base that was white and black. Similar to most of the physicians that I interviewed, he estimated the percentage to be around 50/50, and also noted from another day's schedule that it was about 60 percent white and 40 percent black. He prefaced his estimates by saying that in his country of origin, race is not such an explicit consideration, so he has to try to be aware of racial difference in order to come up with such percentages.

Sometimes, it can be hard to avoid the fact that perceptions on race can be important in Quincy. For example, in an incident recounted by an IMG of Asian Indian origin, a patient preferred to have his appointments around the same time of day. The patient would resist rescheduling appointments for another time. The IMG told me that he learned from the nurse about the patient's reasoning:

> And I told her, I'm going to be kind of busy this morning, I won't be able to see him this morning. Let him come in the afternoon. Then she turned around and she told me, she said, he doesn't want to come in the afternoon because there are other people who are sitting here, and definitely he wants to come in the mornings.

After some questioning, I learned that the "other people" in the waiting room included blacks, and that was why the patient did not want to be there. The IMG went on to say, "I was a little surprised, but then I thought to myself, I said, this is the South, I guess, it's more deeply entrenched in here than elsewhere."

Another IMG of Asian Indian origin had this to say when asked if there were differences by race in perceptions toward IMGs:

> Yes, certain communities like, they treat us better, certain communities they treat us worse. They discriminate a little bit more. Because we fit into certain colors so the black community might treat us a little bit better because we look like them and they don't feel threatened. The white community might, I mean, that's been the difference all the time between the black and white so we kind of tend or steer towards the black side so that difference is still there even though we do not belong to either one of them they look at us and try to push us.

It surfaced only in one other interview with another member of the medical community that IMGs might "steer towards the black side." The only clear rule appears to be that there is no clear rule about how IMGs fit into the racial divide.

Only in obstetrics and gynecology did I find any indication that an IMG's race or ethnicity helped motivate patients to leave town for health care. I often came across the view that there are many white patients who do not want to see a "black" obstetrician/gynecologist (OB/GYN). Of five OB/GYNs in Quincy, one was white and four were black, including one IMG from Africa. While outmigration of patients can have many possible explanations (e.g., perceptions toward the hospital, views that the quality of care is better in a larger town), there appears to be a common perception in the medical community that for many patients, racial preference is a cause for outmigration for OB/GYN services. Indeed, according to several participants in the medical community, one of the reasons for recruiting a white, Canadian-trained physician was to fill a perceived need in the community for a white OB/GYN.

Participants also reported that patients often request the white OB/GYN but the physicians share call schedules. As a result, a patient who chose the white obstetrician may end up with a black obstetrician at the time of delivery. I discussed such issues with an OB/GYN. He was originally from sub-Saharan Africa, received his medical degree in the United Kingdom, and did his residency training in a prestigious U.S. university. He has been practicing in the area since the late 1970s, the third IMG to practice in Quincy.

"Do some leave town for care here?" I asked.

"Yes," he said. "That has been the pattern in this community and will probably remain so. They have two large OB/GYN groups in [a nearby town about 30–40 minutes away]. Predominantly white. And so they troop to that place. Of course now that we have a white obstetrician on the staff, they are coming to him. But primarily they still continue to go to [the nearby town]."

"He gets more patients then than—"

"Yeah," he said. "Because he has the advantage that none of the others have. All the others are black. And he has the advantage that most of them will go to him. That's just the way that things work."

He explained further:

> It seems to me that the men folk are kind of reticent to let their women folk be seen by a foreign medical graduate. . . I don't think they'll be just as reticent to let a foreign medical graduate look into their eyes, for instance, and listen to their heart or their lungs or things like that. So obstetrics is kind of the—very, very private type of pain. I think that that is probably more to do with the color prejudice, you know, because if you have a foreign medical graduate who happens to be white and comes from England, you know, I don't think they'll be just as reticent. I think it's color thing. Which will always be with us, I suppose. You always have a subset of people who will not be able to see beyond the pigmentation of your skin.

The above quotation is rich with the idea of crossing surface boundaries. The human anatomy can be seen through a geographic perspective, in which some parts of the body are more open to examination than others (Nast and Pile, 1998; Dorn and Laws, 1994; Bastien, 1985). Skin colors and physician specialty can complicate such openness, serving as another threshold on the body.

OB/GYN stands out as a case in which race can play a unique role in an IMG's practice. Whether an IMG with different skin color (e.g., a physician of Asian Indian origin) would have similar experiences is merely a hypothetical. The issues are not clear-cut, and no blanket statements can be made about IMG acceptability based solely on skin color or, for that matter, on the broader, more nebulous issue of "race."

THE ROLE OF WOMEN

The issue of the role of women, especially the spouses of male IMGs, was discussed in virtually every interview. I interviewed two female IMGs, one who was practicing in the area and one by telephone who had moved away, and two female U.S. medical graduates. In addition, I had the opportunity to interview two physicians' wives, one the wife of a U.S. medical graduate and the other the wife of an IMG, and to talk informally with other spouses and IMGs. All of these discussions, as well as conversations with other members of the medical community, helped confirm in my mind that the issue of the happiness of the spouse, and more generally the role of women, should not be underplayed.

Amid so many nuances behind IMG acceptability and their retention in rural areas, the spouse can play a major role in the physician's decision to move to the area, to stay or leave, or even to gain a strong attachment to the town (Cutchin, 1997; Conte et al., 1992; Ernst and Yett, 1985; Parker and Tuxill, 1967). These points were driven home forcefully in several different interviews, without being limited to IMGs in particular. For example, a U.S. medical graduate with longstanding ties to the area said:

> I remember in my last year of residency in [a town in this state], one of the fellow residents talking to a local physician about where to practice, what town should I go to, what city? And afterwards he says, you get a map out and he said, you show it to your wife and let her tell you where she wants to live, and he said, that's where you go.

While the happiness of the spouse is certainly an issue that applies to both husbands and wives, most of the physicians in the area are male. According to the hospital directory, there were only five female IMGs practicing in the town; two were not involved in direct patient care because their specialties were in pathology or radiology. All of the IMGs that I interviewed in Quincy were married. I did not come across any perceptions from participants that are specific to problems being female and an IMG. Then again, I only had one interview each with two female IMGs for this town, and a female interviewer might have gained different insights.

Through interviews with IMGs in the local area, I kept hearing that many of the wives of IMGs were highly educated. For example, I knew of at least two IMGs in Quincy whose wives were medical doctors in their countries of origin but who had not gone through the residency program to practice medicine in the United States. I met IMGs whose wives had master's degrees, or whose wives were nurses or had other advanced degrees or specialized training. Usually, I was told that helping out part- or full-time around the office had become the wife's career, and in two cases I learned that the wife was an M.D. who had become a housewife. There are exceptions, such as an IMG whose wife works in interior decorating; or an IMG whose wife practices as a nurse in the same clinic. Among female IMGs, I met husbands who were health providers in the area. For example, the husband of one IMG works as a dentist in the area; two other husbands of IMGs are themselves physicians practicing in the area, too.

In fairness, I also met U.S. medical graduates whose wives had made sacrifices in their professional careers for the sake of their husbands' practices. However, it was far more common in interviews to encounter firsthand or secondhand accounts that IMGs' spouses in particular had made such sacrifices. One IMG was telling me that his wife was a physician who no longer practices medicine:

> She is a housewife. Well, I know that it's been a sacrifice for her, but . . . at the same time, it has been good for the family, for the kids. They enjoy her. And she—we try to stay together and we understand that she's the person who had the biggest loss, sacrifice, because she's been always quite smart. But sometimes it's hard to—You see the way that we have to, in order to be here today, it's a long way. So it's not—it hasn't been easy.

Another IMG talked about the importance of his wife in helping with his practice. He described her in glowing terms as someone he can trust:

> Someone that can mollify everybody. Because people tell me that my wife is one of my biggest assets there. Maybe they're just saying that to be nice. But before someone leaves the office, she asks them how did it go, this and that. And if she sense that there is some conflict or friction, she's probably the first person to intervene, talk to the patient before she leaves the office, as soon as she leaves, those kind of things, keeps track of what is going on, all that.

Living in Quincy can present particular difficulty for some people because there is not as much to do as in an urban area. Therefore, several participants posited that it could be quite difficult for a highly educated spouse who sits at home or helps part-time at the husband's office. Based on my own observation, I was impressed by the sense of community among IMGs' spouses whom I met while attending a dinner preceding a Continuing Medical Education lecture. When the physicians left to attend the lecture, I stayed behind with the spouses, all but one of whom were female. The spouses were good friends with one another. In one of our conversations, one of the spouses was explaining to others at her table about her love of fishing; the spouses who were originally from India were not familiar with fishing and expressed so much interest in learning more about it. Fishing is popular locally, but not familiar to many of the IMGs of Asian Indian origin. Beyond the simple idea of hobbies, a few participants raised the idea that there are cultural differences between the spouses of IMGs and the spouses of U.S. medical graduates, which they say hamper social activity.

It is a tricky issue that the happiness of the spouse is a key consideration for all physicians, but the wives of IMGs often set their planned careers aside for the sake of their husbands' careers. If retention serves as any guide, the strong retention of IMGs in the area could be a reflection, at least in part, of the happiness of spouses. For example, a U.S. medical graduate who has been practicing and recruiting in the area for many years said, "I think retention has more to do with spouse satisfaction than anything else that we deal with."

I did not make any effort to peer into the psyches of the spouses to learn if they really are happy. However, an unanswered question that emerges is whether the happiness of the spouse really is as decisive an issue for many of the IMGs as it is for many of the U.S. medical graduates. Without question, the happiness of the spouse is a key issue that cuts across nationality for physicians in the area.

There are extraordinarily complex cultural issues behind the role of women that affect IMGs in Quincy. At the very least, people have different conceptualizations about the role of women in different parts of the world, and even from one household to another (Mohammad, 1999; Gilbert, 1998; Rose, 1993). Within Quincy, there is an introduction of ideas from other countries about the role of women as interpreted by people within the local area; locally, people might not have the same views as one another about the role of women.

Cultural differences and interpretations were hard for me to overlook when I attended a puja, a Hindu prayer gathering, in Quincy. It was impressive to see the richness of cultures from India taking shape locally, with Hindi songs, children's presentations, speeches about faith and India, and food brought for eating after the service. I was especially impressed by the sense of community among the group of families who attended these monthly services in Quincy. One of the short speeches in particular focused on the diversity of India and yet how it still is one country with so much meaning for people of Asian Indian origin.

Alongside such external connections to India that bind people together locally, I also noticed that women were sitting separately from men during the puja. It looked to me as though there had been a purposeful separation, since there appeared to be an invisible border that separated the seating of males and females in the room. Certainly, there are social gatherings among whites in the United States with separateness by gender, too, so it can be difficult to determine whether such separateness is out of place. After the service, I was eating Asian Indian food at one of several tables that had been set up in the same room as the service, but there were no women at my table. I asked a man—a health professional originally from India and who happened to be sitting near me—why the men sat separately from the women.

He explained to me that it was not a purposeful separation, and people are free to sit wherever they wish to sit. By his explanation, men simply have different interests than women. He said that the men talk about topics like finances, whereas the women are more interested in other topics like shopping or recipes, so it is a natural separation because of people's different interests. He explained further that although people are free to sit at any table, it would be unexpected for a woman to join us at our table. He said that he would wonder if she has a problem with her social group that led her to come to this table. I did not ask other men at the puja to answer the same question about why women sit separately from men. Other informal contacts (e.g., participants in the next town; friends of Asian Indian origin) confirmed that there is such separateness at many Asian Indian gatherings in the United States that can be linked to the belief that men and women simply have different interests.

Different gender roles were also evidenced to some extent by the different style of clothes worn by men and women attending the puja. Most men dressed in shirts and slacks that could probably be found in virtually any U.S. department store. However, for the occasion, most of the women wore clothing that was often more colorful and reflected Asian Indian dress, such as saris. If only symbolically, it appeared as though the men dressed in such a way that they could negotiate external space whereas the women dressed for negotiation of specific internal space (e.g., the room where the puja was held or, more generally, contacts with others in the Asian Indian community).

A female IMG shared with me her thoughts on wearing clothes that reflect her Asian Indian heritage:

> Like now among Indians, you know, we tend to dress differently when we socialize, we don't—I don't always wear a, you know, when I go out to an Indian gathering I wouldn't wear a dress, I would wear one of my Indian outfits. But I—Now if I'm on call, I will always wear a dress, cause I hate to go to the emergency room, you know, wearing the thing that I wear. So in that way, yes, you know, we mold ourselves to the way of life here because you sort of want to be part. I don't want to walk into the emergency room wearing a sari, which is an Indian outfit, because I know that the patients are going to look at me and be saying, you know, what—Now if it were something I used every day and the patient got used to me like that, you know, I think there wouldn't be a problem, but it's not something I do on a daily basis. So I tend to—Well, you know, I dress the way I know that the patients will be more comfortable seeing me [laughs] the way I am rather than, you know, putting on something else that I might use for a social occasion.

As with IMGs in general, familiarity over time has made people more accustomed to seeing people who wear clothes that reflect another culture. For example, when the first IMG from India moved to the area, his wife wore a sari in public, and people would stare at her. That still can happen, albeit to a lesser extent. Although I did not see many people wearing saris outside of the puja, it is simply not as uncommon as it was before the first immigrants from India arrived in the area. Some participants spoke favorably of people wearing clothes that reflect another culture, although usually the issue was broached because it reflected outsider status. In a few interviews, participants spoke critically of immigrants wearing clothes that reflect another culture. For example, I asked a U.S. medical graduate about the involvement of physicians' spouses in community activity:

"Do the wives take part in things that, sort of the auxiliary—" I asked.

"Not a whole lot," he said. "Some of them go to the meetings, but they still wear—a lot of them still wear their Indian habitat."

"And that's—what do you think about that?" I asked.

"I don't like it."

"You don't like it?"

"No. I think if I go to another country—of course the United States is different. The United States is a melting pot, let's say, and we're supposed to accept all immigrants and let them live just like they want to live here. I'm a little bit different. I feel like that if I go to another country, because I love that country, that I should fit in with them and not be a sore thumb sticking out. And I think if I went to India that I would try to fit in with them, language and all, and their customs." At this point he gave a specific example of an individual who dresses differently and said, "And you say, well, why do they come to the United States if they wanted to keep their own identity? If they love their country that much, why didn't they stay there?"

Culturally influenced behavior that may make sense in one setting can sometimes seem out of place when transferred to another setting. Clothes and makeup are examples, but certain practices can also seem out of place to some residents of Quincy. To take an extreme example, a few participants told me about a physician from India whose wife walked behind him on at least one occasion. In the words of a nurse:

> If somebody is Indian, because of their skin coloration and language and all, they're not going to ever think they're from here. Just like the Indian doctor that we had that, you know, he would walk his dog and make his wife walk behind him. And he would put the dog in the car and make the wife sit in the backseat. Now people don't—They remember things like that if they see you walking down the street and the wife is behind you, or you're walking the dog and the dog's beside you and your wife is behind you. They remember, they're not gonna ever think you're from here. [laughs]

The nurse went on to say:

> The nurses are usually women and they're a nurse so they expect them to do whatever they tell them to do. They might look at it a little bit different if the nurse were a man, but they would still think that that person is below them because they're a doctor and the other person's a nurse. And it comes through sometimes, you know. You do it cause I'm the doctor. And people around town have seen some of the doctors—Now all of them don't treat their wives that way. But you know, sometimes the women, they wear the regular costumes with the little stones and the turbans and whatnot, so anybody from around here is not going to think that person is ever from here, I mean, they're just not. I mean, it

> doesn't mean they're good, bad or indifferent, but they look different and their culture's different. I mean, their food's different, everything is.

Thus, concerns about the treatment of women can also tie into some considerations about social hierarchies, the outsider status of some IMGs, and even issues that seem minor in comparison, such as cuisine. As with many other issues relating to IMG acceptability, the issue of the role of women touches on many other extraordinarily complex issues, such as assimilation and religion.

THE ROLE OF RELIGION

Most of the IMGs of Asian Indian origin are Hindu; I also met an IMG from South Asia who is a Muslim; and I know of several Christian IMGs, including two who are originally from the state of Kerala, where Christianity is practiced more widely than in other parts of India. IMGs who move to the area as non-Christians may have a diminished opportunity in using religion as a social springboard, but I see no indication that being non-Christian poses a serious obstacle for IMGs in Quincy.

Based on my observations, informal conversations, and interviews, I came away with the strong impression that religion plays a great role in forming a sense of community in Quincy. For me, this was particularly obvious because I am a non-Christian who is not used to being asked questions about religion; there were several occasions when I needed to respond to such questions. For example, a community member wanted to know my religion before referring me to other contacts; and a member of the medical community wanted to know my religion before agreeing to be interviewed, explaining to me that people in this part of the state want to know something about a person before they can trust him. Such questions were not common, and seemed to be part of a longer litany of questions designed to get a quick sense of a stranger.

On one occasion, I was invited to be the guest speaker at the weekly meeting of a senior citizens' center, which to my knowledge did not have an official religious affiliation. The Baptist Hymnal was passed out to all attendees. As reported later in the minutes on the back page of the local newspaper, the meeting began with a reading of Psalm 133, Verse 1, "Behold, how good and how pleasant it is for brethren to dwell together in unity!" This was followed by the pledge of allegiance and members singing, "Amazing Grace." A member read Ephesians, and as written in the minutes, explained that "Everyone has a gift or talent from the Lord that can be used for others." Then I was introduced to give my presentation, in which I talked for about fifteen minutes about my research study on IMGs. Subsequently, according to the minutes, the meeting also included prayer concerns and, at the end, the members sang "Blessed Assurance," before the meeting ended with a prayer. If this example serves as any guide, being able to participate in gatherings that have a public expression of faith can be an asset for newcomers to the area.

Churches are an extraordinarily valuable entry point into the town, as I found from my own observation. I felt that there was an especially strong sense of community in a black church when the pastor introduced two new members to the congregation. Parishioners rose from their seats and lined up to welcome the new members and embrace them. There was clearly a strong sense of friendship based on fellowship in the same church. Yet, as noted earlier, the issues of religion and race cannot be disentangled easily. For example, the senior citizens' center meeting that was discussed above had only white participants; when I asked about black members, I was told that they meet on a separate day. Furthermore, with few exceptions, whites and blacks generally attended different churches. A deacon put it this way:

"On Sunday morning, if you go to worship, odds are you're going to be segregated, very segregated. More so than anywhere else, any other time of the week. It's sad, but that's the way it is. [laughs]"

A community member in a nearby small town referred to religion to defend the idea of separateness in general, explaining why he did not socialize with an IMG from India:

> And, you know, the Bible says that God divided the nations, and it was a deliberate act of God to separate people out so that they would populate the earth and scatter, and these various differences that I've mentioned, social, cultural, linguistic differences, all of these things, geographical differences, racial kinds of things, they all seem to tend toward separating people. Now, I would then say that I believe in that kind of thing and I certainly do without being a racist. I think racism is a form of hate, and I don't hate anybody, and so I'm not a racist, but I have to recognize that these differences exist. They exist for His purpose, not mine. But the fact is that they do exist. And they divide people.

Nonetheless, religion can play a valuable role in bringing diverse communities together, as explained by another community member:

> If you're involved in the church, regardless to what it is, that's your backbone. You could be the worst person ever, but if you come to church—You know, even the drug dealers, if they come to church—I'm not, you know, going along with what they do, but they're going to be looked at differently once something bad happens to them, you know, because, hey, well, he has tried to do, and he was trying to do right and just couldn't get it right. But if—the Bap-

> tist Church—well, basically the church itself, I won't just say Baptist, but the church itself is the backbone to the community. And if maybe the foreigners would get more involved in, whether it's the black, the white or whoever it is, maybe if they got more involved in what was going on, you know, in the churches, then we would be more open to want to go visit that particular physician. Oh, he was at my church child, you can't tell me nothing, that's my doctor, you know.

In interviews, I learned that some IMGs have reached out to different communities by attending churches or other religious services. For example, a Hindu IMG who recently passed away had been actively involved in a church in the local area. I asked another IMG who is a Muslim originally from South Asia whether he has attended church in the area: "Yeah, my wife is a Catholic and I go with her. And sometimes my patients invite me to their church, then I go with them. So I have been to the Baptist church and all these other churches in many denominations."

He also attends the monthly puja in Quincy even though he is not Hindu and not of Asian Indian origin. He said: "I have good relations with the Indian community and also Filipino community and Nigerian community. I also know American doctors. We are very friendly to each other in every respect. I respect their feelings about religions."

As this IMG has shown by attending different services, religion can play at least some role in bringing people of diverse backgrounds together. Meanwhile, people also have close bonds within their own religious communities, including IMGs who are Hindu or Catholic.

Although I do not know of any IMGs who are Baptists—the predominant branch of Christianity in Quincy—I did meet IMGs who are Catholic. One talked about "Catholic culture": "Well, the Catholic church, or the culture that I meant, is really the fact that you can go to Catholic church in any part of the world and feel at home, because the liturgy is the same, there's no improvisation, for the most part, it's the same."

The sense that adherents to a particular religion might "feel at home" within a specific religious culture also applies to Hindus in Quincy who attend the monthly prayer meetings. In addition to the monthly puja, some of the Hindus in Quincy gather once a week in someone's home, or travel to nearby towns—one a little over a half hour away and another about an hour away—for religious gatherings. One IMG explained about some of the similarities in social networks for the Hindu and Baptist communities in Quincy:

"The community has been nice. We have our own community here, there are enough physicians from our own community and people of other professions from our community here in town."

"What is 'our' community?" I asked.

"That's the Indian community. And so, you know, the people have been accepting, they have been wonderful to us. I just have no—You know, we really are happy here."

"That's great," I said. "Tell me more about the Indian community. Is the community a part of the larger community, or does it tend to be separate?"

"Um, I guess it's—I tend to say we—Our social activities tend to be separate. We participate in the larger community for other things, but it's sort of like—I guess in the South here people are more church oriented and things like that, so people do things according to their church group. And our Indian community have, I guess because of our religion that has brought us together, and so we do things, you know, with our group. So it fits in very well in the way things flow in this area."

While religion plays a role in bringing many people of Asian Indian origin together, my understanding from interviews was that there are many other factors that also influence the sense of community among Asian Indians, such as shared connections to places far beyond Quincy, similarities in background as immigrants, and various intangible social and cultural similarities.

I interviewed most of the IMGs in their offices, which looked no different from any other physicians' offices; I did not notice any visual indication of personal attachments to a place far beyond Quincy, or with Hinduism in particular. However, in an interview in an IMG's home, I saw a number of crafts and paintings reflecting his strong faith as a Hindu, and he had a separate room used for praying. In Quincy, I did not see any public displays of devotion to Hinduism beyond attendance at the puja. The puja itself took place in a building near the senior center; I suspect that, except for the sound of songs in another language, anyone walking by the building would have had no idea that it was being used for a Hindu service. There could still be some public displays of Hinduism that gain little or no notice from neighbors, such as pouring water on a plant as part of a religious observance. For example, an IMG of Asian Indian origin said that a relative visited frequently and they took part in the following activity:

"Certain things, like we do a lot of offering of water and this and that, and you do it on a plant or something. So it's not something done necessarily out on the street, but it's done outside your home, so people would witness it, you know."

The IMG mentioned further that neighbors had said how impressed they were with the devoutness of the relative. In fact, in all of the interviews, informal contacts, and observations, I never encountered any negative reaction toward the Hindu religion in Quincy. Rather, I met people of strong Christian faith who spoke positively of others whose religion is important to their lives.

On a few occasions, participants told me that it helps to have a physician who shares the same religion or belief in God. For example, a community member discussed being referred to a Christian IMG: "And in one case, the Indian doctor was a Christian, a very active Christian doctor. Well, that, I found that that was, well, a good bridge. I thought that the fact that the man had a faith similar to mine made a difference. Not a big difference, but it did make a difference. I felt comfortable."

Another community member talked about the importance of having a physician who shares the same beliefs in God:

> The personal thing with foreign doctors as a rule is I don't like people treating me that doesn't believe in God. That would be my major hang up. I have had some surgery done by a couple of physicians here, minor surgery, that were foreign, and well pleased with the results. A little bit of a problem with communication, but as a general rule, my only hang up would be with religion. I know that a lot of them are not Christians, and it's okay, you know. We all believe what we want to believe, but I prefer to deal with somebody that understands where I'm coming from, particularly that understands my feelings.

Underlying some concerns about the faith of IMGs are misunderstandings or lack of familiarity with the Hindu religion. For example, a participant who spoke critically of doctors who do not believe in God confused Hinduism and Islam, and assumed that neither religion included a belief in God.

Some IMGs who are Hindu told me about their response to a common question about church: "You know, everybody says, what church do you go to? And you say, well, we have our own church, you know, and they accept it."

In the words of another IMG who is Hindu:

> They know that we practice differently, and we don't go to church. Some of them ask, why can't you go to church? I tell them we go to a place and it's like a church, but we just have different—That's how we are brought up. I guess a different belief doesn't mean that one is superior to other ones. But they accept the fact, but they're just curious to know why. They ask, but it's not in offensive way, they're just curious to know what's the reason.

Another IMG of Asian Indian origin remarked the following:

> I have more people ask me about my religion. And honestly, I'm not a very religious person. We gather once a month, not to teach any religion, but religion and culture go hand in hand, and we try to preserve our culture and let our children know where their roots are.

Differences within religions did not come up in conversation as a potential influence on IMG acceptability. However, some health providers raised the idea that there are different health beliefs (e.g., use of folk remedies) among some patients that may or may not be consistent with religious beliefs. In the words of one U.S. medical graduate:

> Well, you've got religion, science, superstition. And those three areas is what we have to face with when somebody comes in to see us. How much faith do they have, how much factual knowledge do they have, how superstitious are they? And you just have got to feel your patient out. And if I was from India and I came here, I wouldn't know beans about how a patient felt, if he was a strong Baptist, about how compliant—about how more compliant that would make him or more superstitious that would make him about wearing a copper bracelet or something like that. And when I have one of my patients come in and I see he's wearing a copper bracelet, I don't mind laughing at him and say, why in the world are you wearing that thing for? He wouldn't have any idea, but I would be particularly careful about it knowing the patient's faith and religion versus his factual knowledge about this as opposed to his superstitious nature.

THE QUESTION OF SEPARATENESS

Toward the end of one interview, I asked an IMG if there was anything that I missed in discussing IMG acceptability. He paused and then replied that this study could be amplifying minor differences between IMGs and U.S. medical graduates:

> I know what your focus is, but I'm not really quite sure that one should make a distinction [between] international medical graduate or an American medical graduate. I think we all compete—should compete at the same level in that . . . the best marketing tool is to provide a better product . . . I understand what you're trying to do, but I wonder though whether you're just making the distinction much more because of the fact that you're writing a book and you're writing a thesis, when hey, we all went to the same school, we may not—the caliber of our medical school may not be of the same level, but when we go for postgraduate training, we all compete for the same places.

I came across absolutely no hint or clue that IMGs practice medicine any differently than do U.S. medical graduates in terms of medical diagnoses, procedures, explanatory models, or the purview of physician specialties. To be sure, there were differences in people's perceptions about communication, formality, amount of time spent with patients, or the issues of race or gender or religion. However, the practice of medicine was where the greatest similarities existed. Many of the IMGs had learned from the same textbooks as did U.S. medical graduates while pursuing medical degrees. Significantly,

IMGs are trained in U.S. residency programs, under U.S. standards, with U.S. conceptualizations of the scope, content, and practice of medicine and of specific medical specialties.

Furthermore, the extent to which IMGs are separate from other physicians or from the nonmedical community varies from one individual to another. The same could be said about U.S. medical graduates. For example, I met both IMGs and U.S. medical graduates who told me that they are members of the Lion's Club, the Rotary Club, or the Kiwanis Club. Simply put, some individuals are more outgoing and sociable than others. For those IMGs who are not part of a cluster of people who come from a particular ethnic group, it might take more effort to meet people initially in the town—not that it would be inherently difficult, but the strong sense of community among Asian Indians in the area helps lead to friendships.

If the distinction between IMGs and U.S. medical graduates is a social construction, a complicated issue is that there might be further social separateness within the IMG community. An IMG originally from Latin America talked about the sense of community among Asian Indians:

> There are some more conservative, and there are some others who are more open. And I think it's—one of the things, since—we have talked about that, since they have several people from the same culture, they have more people to relate with. Like they are able to organize an Indian party, and they would have plenty of people there. Actually you can say this guy's not going to go, we are not going to invite some, who likes this guy. And the other countries—for us, for Hispanic, we have only a few, so that we, I think that we have to reach out to other people to establish more relationships.

An IMG of Asian Indian origin described himself as actively involved in the general community while also acknowledging some social separateness:

> So we are still trying to feel each other out, and that sometimes makes you withdraw. You don't want to go to somebody else and then start all fresh. All—If I say something to you, you'll ask me, well, is that what you did in India? Is that how things were in India? And then it sounds like you're trying to ask me about my things. And which I may want to divulge to you, and I may not want to divulge to you. It becomes a little difficult sometimes to make you understand some things, some traditions, some customs, which are totally foreign to you.

As we talked further, he explained that "you" was in a general sense, and that there are underlying differences in the way that Christians and non-Christians think. Issues relating to separateness and assimilation also became difficult to disentangle from religion, foreignness, or, for that matter, any other issues discussed earlier.

Another IMG originally from India raised similar issues about cultural differences in social settings:

> Well, I think, you know, the interests of the international like and our interests would be different than the people in the local area, what we like, in a social situation. So because of that, we try to integrate with the people in a common interest. So—But still, I think people like to experiment, so that's when we try to interact. But most interactions are in big social functions related to work, rather than unrelated to work. Most of the relationships are related to work. And if you meet the local people, it's mainly as part of the work. Like in hospital parties or medical society parties.

Thus, just as it can be difficult to consider IMGs and U.S. medical graduates as completely separate, it can also be difficult to consider IMGs as one cohesive group. Even within the Asian Indian community, an IMG told me that people in his age group felt less comfortable in large physician gatherings than did younger IMGs. In addition, social and cultural backgrounds can help create bonds between some people more so than among others. However, rural physicians might not have as much responsibility as in the past to be involved in social activities in their adopted towns.

Changes in the Role of the Rural Physician

The concept of the rural physician as an integral part of community activities has undergone substantial change in Quincy and elsewhere. Whether or not a physician is separate from the general community might not matter as much as in the past, or at least might not matter as much in a community this size. A U.S. medical graduate explained:

> I try to go to a different church than my patients do. [laughs] I mean, just so they won't bother you at church or ask you a question and stuff, so you can listen to the minister. But it's just, I think just the rural town physician has changed a little bit. You've changed to the international physician and probably African American physician too, we're not going to be that person that lives next door to you, per se, okay? Or we're not going to be that person that necessarily goes to your church or we're not going to necessarily be that person that you can stop, you know, or call to come over to my house and blah, blah, blah, you know, and I'll go to your house. So it's not so much that we've changed. I think number one, the wave of medicine has changed a little bit, we're not doing that quite as much, you know, practices have changed a little bit, and you know, probably the faces of medicine have changed a little bit. There are a little bit, you know, you have your foreign students, you have your African Americans, it's not just your white males anymore in the rural communities.

A nurse took a critical view of the separateness of some IMGs of Asian Indian origin from the general community:

> And I think it's good always to have somebody that you feel comfortable with and that you can share things with. But if there are too many and you only stay with the Indians or the whoever, then you don't meld into the society as well, and I question whether you understand your patients as well if you don't really get into things in the community that you are serving. So I personally think that to some degree it is a responsibility, if it is not your personal inclination, to become involved somewhat so that you have a better understanding of the people you are trying to serve. That's my opinion. [laughs][3]

Whether or not IMGs—regardless of country of origin—are less involved in the general community might be a moot point, since rural doctors in general might not be as actively involved in communities anymore. The major exception appears to be in the specialty of family medicine. Based on interviews in Quincy and conversations in the next town, I kept coming across the idea that active involvement in the community is key in family medicine. As one family physician in Quincy explained to me in discussing length of office visits:

> And if you were from this town, I probably would've delivered you, raised you, given you all your shots, followed you up through school, college, and you come in and you say, you know, I've got bronchitis and I've got a bad cold and, you know, I've looked at your record and I say, you know, nothing in your record that would make me think that I needed to talk to you about anything else, and so I give you penicillin or whatever, and you'll go, it's a five minute office visit. But if you come in and you sort of hint that you may have a problem, relationship with your wife or relationship to alcohol and I hear the talk in the community that you're slipping and word gets back in different ways that so and so hadn't been seen at church in two months and his wife is coming in asking for tranquilizers and all these kind of, and so then that's when I sit down and have a talk. Whereas this may go on with the foreign doctors, but I don't think they can pick up on stuff like this. See, I go to the Baptist church and 400, 500 people, I know everybody in the town. The foreign doctors coming in know nobody. And they don't get in the cultural, in the community culturally and associate with the people. And so they don't know how to do things like that.

"Fascinating to think of the importance of being a part of the community for being a physician," I said.

"It used to be really like that. Now it's drifting away a little bit, and the people know that when I go to a doctor, that he doesn't know all the nuts and bolts about them. And so they just go in and say, give me my heart pills and give me my blood pressure pills, let me go."

None of the IMGs in town is a family physician. In fact, the overwhelming majority of Quincy IMGs specialize in internal medicine. Quite possibly, any separateness between physicians (IMGs or U.S. medical graduates) and the general community could at least partially reflect medical specialty. Still, the individual physician's personal interests and inclinations can easily override ideas stemming from a specialty about the need for involvement in the community. For example, the above family physician told me his comments to another family physician—a U.S. medical graduate—who had had trouble attracting patients:

> I says, you're not accommodating. You don't fit in the community. You leave this office and you go home and you lock your door and you listen to your music and drink your liquor and there you stay until the next day. What I do, I go home, I go jogging with the high school kids, I play tennis with the high school kids, I go to church with those kids, I teach Sunday school, I'm a deacon in the church, I belong to the Lion's Club, I'm the president of the Lion's Club. And he said, I don't want to be busy all the time. I said, well, it's fun, fitting in with people, talking to them, and enjoying the functions.

The issue of social separateness between physicians and the general community is part of a larger dynamic within medical culture. Some townspeople sensed a division in terms of their social interactions with doctors, pointing out class-based differences in social status. For example, a community member shared with me her recommendations for IMGs moving to Quincy: "I guess the only thing I could recommend would be to try to intermingle with the local community more. But then again, I guess it doesn't matter what nationality or what faith they are, doctors' families tend to put themselves on a pedestal above the average community anyway."

Amid concerns about separateness and changes in medical culture, it would also be unfair to overlook the importance of physicians' time commitments, which can impact their ability to be active in the community. The physicians whom I met worked long hours, with most dividing their time between working in a clinic, working in the local hospital, and trying to find time for family. As one IMG explained, "You get nights and every other night call and all that kind of stuff. It gets old after a while. You know. And missed birthdays and . . . dances, I mean, dance recitals, soccer games. It's part of being a doc, you know, I'm sorry, [laughs] but that's the name of the game."

A paradox appears to be that IMGs have thriving practices with large patient bases even though there was some concern mentioned that they are not more actively involved in the community. Then again, it may not be a paradox but, rather, a reflection of the changing role of the rural physician.

Separateness in the Medical Community: A Focus on Referrals

Although there is no apparent difference between the practice of medicine by IMGs and U.S. medical graduates, social differences such as differing cultural backgrounds cannot be entirely separated from professional practice. For example, the issue of hospital politics includes its own set of complicated turf issues that are far too particular for discussion here; yet there is a sense that the Asian Indian community—or IMGs in general, for that matter—are part of hospital politics. For example, an IMG of Asian Indian origin expressed a concern about possible "competition" and "resistance" from other physicians, but then declined to elaborate when asked because it was a "very political question." Other participants shared with me some of the major concerns in hospital politics that can affect the acceptance of IMGs, such as hiring practices (see chapter 3) and referral patterns.

Referrals can be a deeply contested and sensitive issue, with some members of the medical staff expressing a concern that IMGs primarily refer to other IMGs. Of the twelve IMGs interviewed for this town, only one said that he had any preference for referring to other IMGs over U.S. medical graduates. However, this is not an easy issue to gauge, since I cannot simply ask people about preferences in referral patterns. Virtually all physicians said that the number one priority in making referrals is the well-being of the patient, which must take precedence over any other issue. When asked, physicians were generally understanding when I suggested that social circles, such as people known through residency programs, could influence referral patterns. Having said that, I cannot document whether the social circles of IMGs influence their referral patterns. One U.S. medical graduate did briefly show me his records, claiming that it was uncommon to receive any referrals from an IMG of Asian Indian origin. I did not look at the records for any length of time to support or reject what was said to me. However, the perception certainly was there, at least for this physician, that there is a problem with getting referrals from IMGs of Asian Indian origin.

A person working in hospital administration commented on the issue of the possible separateness of Asian Indian IMGs from others in the medical community:

> I see them more as separate, and I think the other members of the medical staff see them acting, for the most part, together. If another Indian physician comes in, say a surgeon, then the other medical staff members think well, they're going to get all the referrals from all the Indians, other Indian physicians, because they're Indian.

I did not come across any claims that U.S. medical graduates avoided referring to IMGs. In fact, since IMGs constitute a majority of the subspecialists in the area, it can be difficult not to refer patients in need to them. An added consideration is that like other rural areas, there is a mindset in Quincy that the next larger town will provide better care, with the best care being provided by a teaching hospital a few hours away. Some participants told me that IMGs at the major teaching hospital were regarded very favorably by patients from Quincy since they have the university's "stamp of approval." Physicians also told me that referrals are based on many individual factors as well, such as previous patients' experiences with the referred physician, thoughts about who might provide the best care, and finding a good match in personality between patient and physician.

Integrating into the Community: The Role of Children

As mentioned earlier, the children of IMGs are often perceived to be among the best and brightest of all students in the area. Most IMGs have children, and the children help their parents become involved in the community through public school functions and activities. A U.S. medical graduate who has worked closely with IMGs was telling me about the involvement of IMGs in community activities: "But the thing that draws them into the real community, the participation, is when their children go to school. It's when their children go to school. And they get involved with things and that kind of pulls the parents into it too."

Similarly, a pharmacist also said that children can play an especially important part in IMG involvement in the community:

> They're gonna have children, their children will be going to school with mine, they'll be of the same age, they'll be in class plays, they'll be in sporting events, as you mentioned, or social events, and you get to know people and they integrate themselves into the society like that. And once again, I think you've got just the normal, what I would call normal distribution or bell curve. You've got some people that like more social activities and will integrate themselves into the community, just because that's their personality more than it would be whether or not they were from India or Pakistan or where, you know, or [a nearby U.S. state] for that matter. Some people just, their personalities lend that.

Nonetheless, cultural differences can emerge in people's attitudes toward children. For example, one IMG told me a story about a time when he made small-talk with a woman whom he met while waiting to see the attending physician at a hospital in the United Kingdom. This was before he had moved to the United States. She was a clerk at the nurse's desk, and she showed him pictures of her dogs. She had eight dogs of a breed known as "salukis." He asked her how she was able to afford taking care of so many dogs, and she explained that she had friends who are butchers, and she gives the dogs meat and dog food, and said that "we're able to manage." The IMG continued with the story:

> And I saw him coming through, the attending was coming through, and I said, well, it's time for me to go, but I just sort of wanted to ask her one more question. I said, I'm going to ask you one more question. She said, good. I said, how many children do you have? She said, I can't afford them. [laughs] And that sort of shocked me totally, I couldn't believe my ears.

"It was no joke either," I said.

> Yes. It was not a joke, it was very, very straight, she was very serious about it. For us in India, or for that matter, Asia or certain other parts of the East, children are a big thing. For you to think that you don't want to have children is unknown, that's how I felt. And here I was with a person who was more—who had more interest or whose life was devoted to an animal rather than to another person of her own kind. And that totally shocked me. But since then I have had many experiences and I've slowly got used to how things are thought differently here than we think out there.

The issue of the role of children in creating a sense of community is complicated in part because of the role of school districts in separating whites and blacks in Quincy. Finding the best schools are of extraordinary importance to many people interviewed for this study, including IMGs. IMGs overwhelmingly placed special value on the importance of their children's education. Most—if not all—IMGs live within the predominantly white Quincy school district. The school districts not only reflect racial divisions, but there is a perception among many people in Quincy—rightly or wrongly—that the white school district is better. Thus, simply by being concerned about their children's education, the locational preferences of IMGs may be influenced at least to some extent by others' racially influenced attitudes toward schools.

Many IMGs live within a particular area of Quincy, but not as a separate geographic cluster; many U.S. medical graduates live in the same neighborhood, too. It is a newly developed area that is among the more affluent in Quincy, a town that does not have many wealthy neighborhoods. The role of schools may be one influence on locational preferences within Quincy, but a more targeted study could point to a variety of other reasons why IMGs live where they do (e.g., distance from hospital; education of others in the community; proximity to others of similar cultural background; friendliness of neighbors).

On several occasions, IMGs told me that they especially wanted to practice in a small town. Some IMGs came from small towns originally, albeit in different countries where the conceptualization of "rural" could be completely different (e.g., much less developed; more heavily populated; not necessarily as distant from an urban center). Some IMGs had practiced in small towns in the United States prior to coming to Quincy. New IMGs to the area were at various stages in their medical careers, with some fresh out of U.S. residency programs in large cities (e.g., New York, Chicago) and others having experience practicing medicine in another country and in the United States. A few IMGs told me that they had been practicing or studying in a major city, such as New York or Boston, and people there wondered why anyone would want to move to a rural area in the South.

Separateness Revisited

The separateness of IMGs in Quincy has been put under a microscope for this study, with differences magnified for the sake of observation and analysis. In reality, IMGs are physicians like other physicians, going through many of the same experiences with missing school plays, working long hours, and being the town doctors. Some IMGs told me that they feel a sense of appreciation for their hard work, as was so evident from an IMG who collected letters of thanks sent to him by his patients. The words of a U.S. medical graduate show further a sense of appreciation for the contributions of IMGs, and a sense that IMGs have become an integral part of the town:

> I've been here twenty years, and what I will say about it is I think we are dern glad and should be dern thankful that we have foreign medical graduates here because this community would have nothing. And the problem I have with it is I think it's bad that we're letting other countries train our physicians. I see it as bad to do to these other countries. I don't think it's bad that the foreign medical graduates come here. I'm appreciative of having them. I'm appreciative every time I have a cardiac, myocardial infarction that I've got two cardiologists cause I've been here when we had no cardiologists. I've been here when we had one surgeon. I've been here when we had one OB. So I've been here when the things have been really bad and you had to handle things but I do think it's a problem for this country to not deal with its own medical needs and depend on using, being a sponge to either take up or not take up the excess in, you know, the brightest out of these other countries. We're not getting the dregs of those other countries. We're getting the best they've got.

NOTES

1. Consistent with the previous chapter on mechanisms, contexts will be highlighted in this chapter, albeit without being pointed out specifically as contexts.

2. The name of the procedure is not listed because the specialty is masked to preserve confidentiality.

3. After reviewing the written quotation, the participant suggested the following rewrite for clarity: "But if the IMG's create a subculture that prevents being involved in the community at large, this may prevent melding into the society and developing an understanding of the people who make up your patient population. So I think that to some degree it is a responsibility, even if it is not your personal choice, to become involved so that you have a better understanding of the people you are serving. That's my opinion."

Part Three

CASE STUDY ON HAMILTON

Chapter Six

Background on Hamilton: Tapestry on a Different Fabric

It is especially fortuitous that Quincy was studied first, thereby preparing the reader for further consideration of acceptability in a more complicated place. In the simplest conceptualization, both towns could be viewed merely as empty spaces or canvasses, and acceptability the picture that emerges in this study—but this is not a simple study, and the canvasses are not empty. The canvas for Quincy seems relatively simple in comparison with an intricately woven Hamilton tapestry that has more bumps, notches, and colors on a different fabric. Not only are the two towns unique—with Hamilton being part of a racially diverse county that has no clear majority—but my place in them led to different perspectives and levels of depth. My status as an outsider doing research was different in the two towns, particularly considering the greater openness of Hamilton to me in conducting this research. Thus, not only does a different picture emerge in the two towns, but it is as if the medium has changed, too, like from oil to watercolor.

In doing fieldwork in Hamilton and environs, I had the sense of being able to find useful contacts and interviews with any population in the area. At times, it seemed as though every corner led to another helpful person who was instrumental in my progress. The friendliness of the community toward me as a researcher had obvious advantages, since people were more open in presenting ideas than had been the case in Quincy. A disadvantage was that there was, in some ways, too much information about Hamilton. Many different nuances of the complexity of the area (e.g., local history, racial conflict, personal anecdotes) could be explored as complete books in their own right. Indeed, it can be easy to get lost in byways and tangents about Delano County. As an outsider, my view is limited but then again, I may be able to see things not evident to a person from the area.

My interviews in Hamilton were fuller, richer, more interesting, and longer than in Quincy. The reasons behind such progress with my research could be instructive about acceptability, or might simply be a question of luck. I knew in advance of fieldwork that my entry into one case study town would likely go more smoothly than in another, since each place is different; Hamilton happened to be one that went more smoothly. Then again, for whatever abstract reason, I felt like I fit in better in Hamilton and much of Delano County than I had in Quincy. Perhaps that was because of the diversity of people in Delano County with different educational levels or geographic attachments, or the presence of a nearby university, or my personal interest in being in places that are not easy to figure out. Yet progress in this second case study area might be attributable mainly to my improvements in interviewing people, in introducing myself or explaining the study to strangers, or in simply being more patient and less hurried in conducting fieldwork. According to a key contact, people in the area are also used to being researched, and he suggested that may make them more open to being interviewed. Another useful contact explained that the community is more open to outsiders than it is to insiders. As a result, people who are part of local conflict might have more difficulty gaining access to different communities than someone who has no such history (e.g., a newcomer to the area, or a person from another country).

Having said that, there were some parts of Delano County that presented more difficulties for me than did other parts. Fortunately, my contacts helped me meet the right people, and bridged different places and communities. Such contacts helped me realize even further that Hamilton is just one part of a broader equation of complexity in Delano County. It would be nearsighted to focus exclusively on Hamilton without considering the acceptability of IMGs in Delano County more generally.

STATISTICAL BACKGROUND ABOUT DELANO COUNTY

Delano County's 949 square miles make it the largest county in the state. As of 2000, the U.S. Census reported that the total population for the county exceeded 120,000. The county seat of Hamilton has nearly 21,000 people, easily the largest population of any town in the county. By contrast, the other towns in the county range in population size from a low of 79 to a high of nearly 3,500. Approximately 30 miles away in an adjoining county is Filmore, a city with a large military base and a population of over 120,000 people (U.S. Census Bureau, 2000).

Many of the employment opportunities in Delano County are concentrated in Hamilton, where the majority of manufacturing facilities and service-sector employment are located. According to the State Department of Commerce, manufacturing accounted for 29 percent of all jobs in the county in the third quarter of 1999, including work in a poultry processing plant (1,300 jobs), canned soup company (1,100 jobs), and a number of textile mills, such as manufacturers of knit fabrics (750 jobs), children's wear (600 jobs), and shoes (560 jobs). Twenty-three percent of all jobs in the area are in "service," 17 percent in government, and 20 percent in retail or wholesale trade. The county is undergoing a transition from being an agriculturally dependent area to one that is more industrially based. Agriculture accounted for only 0.9 percent of all jobs during this time period, although, according to a 1994 book of summary information about the county, just over 4 percent of the population works in agriculture. Tobacco is easily the number one crop in terms of production and total sales.

The county is also undergoing transitions in terms of its racial composition. According to the 2000 Census, the county's population was approximately 38 percent Native American, 33 percent white, and 25 percent black. Based on population projections, Native Americans may constitute over 50 percent of the county's population around the year 2010. Different races vary in their geographic distribution in the county. Hamilton, which is in the eastern central part of the county, is 49 percent white, 36 percent black, and 13 percent Native American. Only about a 15 minute drive to the west is Berry, which is 85 percent Native American. Whites tend to have greater percentages in the eastern parts of the county; Native Americans in the west; and blacks are more geographically dispersed, without constituting a majority in any individual township. Racial diversity and community ties vary further within individual towns. For example, south Hamilton is a majority black area in a majority white town. Meanwhile, there is a growing Hispanic population in the county, including many non-English speakers who work long hours for low pay at poultry processing plants. Informal estimates of the number of Hispanics vary, often around two percent of the total population, with apparent growth in their numbers in the last few years.

The U.S. Census Bureau (2000) reported that 26 percent of the total population in the county lives in poverty. This total includes 46.1 percent of all families with related children under five years of age.

IMPRESSIONS OF THE AREA

I first found my way to downtown Hamilton during a preliminary trip prior to fieldwork. It was a Saturday and most of the businesses were closed, except for an ice cream parlor and a comic book shop. In front of the courthouse was a memorial to Confederate soldiers of America killed in battle—standing atop a tall pillar was a Confederate soldier carrying two guns. For whatever abstract reasons, my initial sense was that this could be a violent, explosive area, and I wondered how difficult it would be to do research here. Then again, perhaps I had simply picked up on a feeling that participants would later tell me about, and I would wonder what they meant because the place had seemed so friendly and open to me. On my next trips to the area, I felt comfortable and relaxed walking these same streets, browsing through downtown stores, or meeting people in their offices only a short walk away.

On one of my first days of fieldwork, I was in downtown Hamilton and I walked into the public library. I asked the librarian for assistance in finding a book on the history and culture of Delano County. She responded that there was a book on the history and culture of whites, several books on the history and culture of Native Americans, no book on the history and culture of blacks, and no book that integrates discussion of all three races. Subsequently, I went to a university library in a nearby town and asked the same question. The librarian there also did not know of a book that effectively integrates the history and culture of all three races in Delano County. I have since found a book of short summaries of descriptive information compiled largely from available government statistics about the county. Still, in the literature, there does not appear to be a multiracial cultural history written about the area.

Such racial separateness in reporting the history of the town took me by surprise, but that day in the library also helped prepare me for what I would later find. The town was not always as friendly to others as it had seemed to me. As my fieldwork progressed, it seemed as though the black community was often forgotten or overlooked in important decisions in the area—consistent with the fact that there was no book on the history and culture of blacks in Delano County. For example, at the time of fieldwork, there was not a single health care facility located in south Hamilton, which is a lower-income, predominantly black part of town. Moreover, my early contacts in the general community led primarily to interviews with Native Americans and whites, but not to blacks—again, making me think that blacks might often be forgotten or overlooked in Delano County. Fortunately, when I asked about references to the black community, a contact who was white called a friend of hers who was black. I was invited to a black church, and doors opened easily in the black community.

I met helpful people at the hospital and in the general community who had worked hard at building strong social and professional connections across multiple communities. Their achievements in networking across communities made my research much easier. As one participant explained to me, the networks in the area can take you "anywhere you want to go." The strength of such networks was particularly notable within the medical community. For example, I was referred to the same physicians in Delano County by a number of different people, in contrast to Quincy, where it was uncommon for me to be referred to the same person twice. The extent of referrals to the same people could be another indication that Hamilton was well-networked, since different people had the same ideas about important contacts. If my experience served as any guide, there were plenty of helpful people in Delano County who at least had a working dialogue and friendship with others from different communities.

In working my way into different communities, I also realized that a short distance on a roadway can lead to a seemingly different world altogether. For example, I felt like an outsider in Berry, a nearby town that was predominantly Native American. Participants and contacts there even told me that I looked and sounded very much like an outsider. I was taller than most people, and my hair was red; when I opened my mouth, my accent was different. One contact explained to me that such differences are why people stare at me, but I never noticed people staring at me. My sense of being an outsider was especially strong when, early in my fieldwork, I was having trouble finding the street number for a meeting with a Native American physician. In a neighbor's yard, I asked a couple of children if this was the right address. The mother and a neighbor walked out, both seeming very concerned, and I sensed that they were afraid of me. I was not expecting to be met by fear, particularly in a scenic small town with only a few thousand people. The mother and neighbor assured me that the physician was not working today, but pointed me to the building which was his home and office.

One of the first things that struck me about Hamilton in particular was that it was more difficult to find my way around than it had been in Quincy. In Quincy, it had taken me only five minutes to get from one end of town to another. In Hamilton, there was more traffic. The layout of the area was more complex, with major roads converging at different places in the local area and the county. As in Quincy, an interstate intersected the town, but Delano County also had a number of other major roads that I needed to use to get where I was going. Sometimes, roads had the same name in different towns only a short distance away. For example, I once had to reschedule an interview because I had been driving back and forth on the wrong Martin Luther King Boulevard. Another time, I showed up an hour late for an interview in a nearby town because highway construction had blocked access to the interstate exit, and I tried in vain to follow an alternative route that took me through a no man's land. Although it was not really difficult to navigate the area, the businesses and residences were much more geographically dispersed in Hamilton than had been the case in Quincy.

I only entered Delano County as a visitor, but it left a major impression on me, leaving so many ideas that cannot possibly be summarized in just one work on IMGs. Anyone who has lived in Delano County for any length of time can, no doubt, raise other points that I have not mentioned thus far.

BACKGROUND ON THE HOSPITAL

According to information in the physician directory, the hospital employs over 1,600 people and annually has over 11,000 inpatients and 75,000 outpatients. With 314 licensed beds, the hospital has grown substantially since it was first built in 1953 as the consolidation of two separate hospitals in the area. New wings have since been added, leading to an increasingly complex structure with several adjacent buildings, a winding hallway connecting different parts of the hospital, and multiple points of entry. In entryways to different wings of the hospital, receptionists busily speak into their headphones to answer telephone calls. Sometimes I would wonder, is the receptionist talking to me or to the person on the other end of the telephone line? It was easy to get confused in finding my way around, especially as a newcomer to the area. In some ways, the layout of the hospital seemed like a reflection of the town—confusing to an outsider, with different meeting points at geographically dispersed places. Elsewhere in the hospital, the emergency room has about 70,000 admissions each year, according to the hospital's Web page. The hospital, which changed its name in 1994 from a "general hospital" to a "regional medical center," also has a close working relationship with one of the most prestigious teaching hospitals in the United States (about two hours away) and owns several clinics throughout Delano County. A fitness center, a nursing home, a hospice, and a community health education center are among many affiliated divisions that promote the local hospital's outreach to the broader community. The local hospital also provides financial incentives to attract new physicians, even paying for some students' tuition in medical school in exchange for subsequent practice in Delano County.

The population is also served by the county health department, several clinics independent of the hospital, and a community health center with four sites throughout the county. At the time of fieldwork, the community health center had 152 staff, including eight physicians and nine midlevels.[1] Hospitals in neighboring counties, including one over the state line, also attract patients from the area. Clinics in Delano County range in size from solo practices to a clinic with ten physicians on staff. IMGs are employed in solo and two-person practices, community health centers, group practices with U.S. medical graduates, and, in one case, a facility that has four physicians, all of whom are IMGs of Asian Indian origin. Two IMGs work as hospitalists; i.e., their provision of care is limited to a hospital setting.

Of 105 physicians (i.e., M.D.s or D.O.s) listed in the hospital directory, twenty-three (21.9 percent) are IMGs, including nine who received their medical degrees in India, three from Caribbean medical schools, two from the Philippines, and one each from Argentina, Bulgaria, France, Guatemala, Lebanon, Nigeria, Pakistan, Poland, and Taiwan. The three IMGs who received medical degrees from Caribbean medical schools include a married couple, one a U.S. citizen originally from Haiti, and the other a Canadian citizen originally from India. By my count, based on knowledge of the area and review of the hospital directory, six of the area's twenty-three IMGs have primary practice locations outside of Hamilton. At the time of fieldwork, none of the IMGs had a full-time practice in Berry, the town that is 85 percent Native American, although one IMG split time between there and another small town.

Unlike Quincy, where the majority of IMGs worked in subspecialty care, sixteen of twenty-three (69.6 percent) IMGs in Delano County provide mainly primary care. This includes five in family practice, ten in internal medicine without subspecialization, and one pediatrician. No IMGs work in obstetrics and gynecology. Four of the nine IMGs of Asian Indian origin have subspecialties in cardiology, gastroenterology, neurology, or pulmonology. Although only about one in five physicians in Delano County is an IMG, thirteen of twenty physicians with residency training in internal medicine are IMGs. As I learned earlier in looking for a book on the history and culture of the county, blacks have largely been overlooked in many important decisions in the area. Similarly, the Native American and white communities are often seen as separate. Health services present an avenue for looking at such issues.

Even though blacks constitute 25 percent of the county's population, a much smaller percentage of the physician population has "black" skin, depending on how "blackness" is defined. In an effort to alleviate disparities in access to health care, the hospital has a health clinic under construction in south Hamilton, a lower-income part of town with a predominantly black population. South Hamilton did not previously have any health care clinics. Burdened with layers of local politics and disagreement about what needs to be built and who should build it, the construction of the clinic is evidence of the struggles that are underway so that health services can meet the needs of disparate communities.

Meanwhile, many Native Americans are reluctant to use the hospital or even to visit Hamilton. A deep history of racial conflict remains at the heart of such concerns, including the idea that north and central Hamilton—including the hospital—are part of a "white power structure." As evidence, several people interviewed for this study claimed that there is almost no representation of non-whites in hospital administration. Concerns about inadequate representation lead some Native Americans to look elsewhere for care. Two hospitals in adjoining counties have also opened up clinics in Berry, a predominantly Native American town.

Perhaps another indication of the historical separateness between races, a wall in the hospital has portraits of retired physicians. All of the pictures are of white males except for one of a black male physician, taken down for a dedication to the new clinic in south Hamilton. I asked a member of the hospital administration why there was not a more diverse representation of physicians' pictures in such a racially diverse town. His response was that it was a reflection of the times; there had not been as much opportunity in the past for minorities in general to work as physicians; soon other faces will go on the wall, too, and he named physicians close to retirement who are not white males.

When those next pictures get put on the wall, physicians of completely different backgrounds will effectively be honored alongside one another. Different-sized worlds come together at different places, and new physicians from other countries add to such convergences.

CONVERGENCE OF DIFFERENT WORLDS IN A LOCAL AREA

Discussions of people's views toward the hospital and the town overlapped significantly, since "Hamilton" often meant north and central Hamilton, which includes the hospital. Some of the strongest and most lasting impressions of Hamilton and the hospital came from people in other towns in Delano County. In Berry, a nearby town that is 85 percent Native American ("Indian" in the following quote), I asked one of the leading figures in the Native American community about his thoughts toward Hamilton.

> There's much antipathy. I mean, there is—it's almost a palpable animosity. I mean, it's like it's perceived as the conservative, white capital of the world as far as, you know, within this county. That's the county seat and people are—You just have to look at the social and political history to realize that until most recently, Indians were denied political opportunity. I mean, they were denied the right to—It was difficult for them to win elective office. So for many years, you had this tri-racial population being administered politically by the white community, so there's some built-in animosity from that.

Later in the conversation, I asked him whether he goes to Hamilton for health care.

> I was raised when segregation was in place, so I do have that animosity in my makeup. Not as pronounced, I'm not going to berate anybody about it or bother anybody, but I mean, it's there. And if I have a choice, I'll go someplace else. I do that for everything, shopping, whatever I do, if I can do it somewhere other than Hamilton, I do. Not because I hate anybody in Hamilton, but because I was raised in a segregated society, and that was the bogeyman, so to speak, you know, socially and ethnically speaking. But decent people in all three races obviously, but we're talking about how I respond emotionally.
>
> [The hospital's] reputation is certainly much improved over the years, and it's run much more democratically now. Although, the way I look at things, if we have a hospital in the area, I always want to know who makes up the board of directors that administers that hospital. So when you look at that, we usually still have just one token Indian on the board, so that's crap to me. When I see that, I just tend to shy away. And also the staff, I think, is underrepresented at the hospital. But I have seen much improvement. So many Indians do go there, but as I said, there is that perception that you're treated differently outside the county, more fairly and more decently.

Similarly, a Native American physician said that "there's no minorities in the whole administrative branch of the hospital. And that's a shame. . . And on its board maybe one or two, maybe two or three minorities, but again, the vast majority white."

I asked a black U.S. medical graduate in another nearby town whether there was any truth to the statement that the hospital is run by whites. The reply focused on the quality of care provided at the hospital:

> Well, in the past I think there was some truth to it. Now, you must realize, you only have to have two or three bad outcomes for it to be a perception that the whole hospital's like that. You must understand it's like a couple drops of blood in a toilet bowl, it looks like you're hemorrhaging to death, which is not the case. Right? Which is not the case. But I think particularly you look towards the Native American population, and particularly as it applies to the Berry area, there was that perception.

Talking with a Native American physician in his office in Berry, I asked, "And do you practice in Hamilton also?"

"No, right here," he said.

"Do you have hospital privileges?"

"I do, but I seldom go over there. I seldom have a need to be in Hamilton, so I don't go very often."

I asked him to explain to me the reasons for the divisions between Berry and Hamilton. He said, "It's the fact that at one time Berry was the, and still is, the seat or head of Indian country here. And Hamilton was seen as the seat of non-Indian country. And you couldn't—You know, you couldn't just go to Hamilton as an Indian person and deal socially or commercially. I mean, even—And I'm—I like to think I'm a fairly young man, but I remember going to Hamilton where, you know, you'd have to sit in the balcony. I would have to sit in the balcony or I'd have to go to a different bathroom. So that's not been that long ago. So now people still remember that. So I have patients come in who there's no way under God's green earth they're going to Hamilton, forget it. Child's sick, dying, they're not going to go to Hamilton, they'll go somewhere else."

There was three-way segregation in public spaces: whites only, blacks only, and Native Americans only. Even further segregation in the school systems added to social and geographic exclusions based on race. The end of legally coerced segregation did not erase deep-seated racial conflict in the community. Rather, social and geographic separateness continued in other ways. For example, a health care administrator, who is Native American and works in a small town in Delano County, talked about the importance of boundaries, and their implications for outsiders:

> You know, our kids go to school together and da, da, da, but you still have Indian churches, you got black churches, you got white churches, and there's very little crossing of the lines, you know. And there's still white communities, black communities, and Indian communities, you know. For the most part there's not a lot of intermingling in terms of communities. And this has been going on, you know, forever. And I think with the tension that continues to exist between the groups, probably plays—has a lot to do with how we view other people coming in. Our own mistrust amongst our—the people that live here in the county, amongst the groups, you know, automatically, I think would impact the way we view other people coming in, especially foreign medical graduates. And exactly to what degree I don't know, but I think it would have to have some, play some part in that.

Considering the social and geographic separateness within Delano County, the administrator also described some of the whites' choices to live in Hamilton:

> Because if you're living outside of Hamilton, you're living with the African Americans and the Native Americans because Hamilton is basically a white community. And so you're only going to live in Hamilton, we're not going to live, you know, in the rest of the county, especially unincorporated areas of the county. That's really where the Native Americans and the African Americans

> live, so you have people who don't want to go outside these little walls. I can remember growing up being told that we were not allowed to go to Berry, we were not allowed to go to Wilson, there was certain places in the county that we were not allowed to go to for whatever reason. I never did quite understand, you know, why. But as I've grown up and I've matured, it had a lot to do with the fact of people's attitudes about how people in other communities perceived them. Wilson was perceived as a white community,[2] so you were considered to be discriminated against if you went to Wilson. The same thing with Hamilton, and I live within the Hamilton mailing address. Although I'm out in the country, Hamilton is my mailing address. You know, Hamilton was just always—You only went there if you had to go there, you know, to do your critical shopping needs or whatever. But you just stayed away from it. You just didn't go because it was the white power structure and—I'm Native American, by the way, so I'm coming at it from that perspective.

Newcomers to the area cannot possibly know all of the intricacies of the histories of the area's separateness. I explored this issue in talking with a real estate agent in Hamilton who shows houses to IMGs.

"It's illegal for us to steer people to one neighborhood or the other, you know," she said. "As tactfully as I know how, I try to encourage them to stay in town. The schools are better, number one. Number two, if you're out—In this particular county, we're tri-racial, we have American Indian, black, and whites, and we're about a third, a third, a third." Referring to the Native American population, she said, "Especially the Berry area are more the Indian population, and these people—They're wonderful folks, they really tend to stay to themselves and they—There are still some little Indian schools and it's just—And if you live out—How do I say it? It's just harder for new people to really get incorporated in the community because they're sort of already set themselves apart, you know. And so I try to encourage them, especially if they have children, to be in town because then they're going to get—If that's the lifestyle they want, to be involved. It's harder if you're further out. That's not true in all communities, but we just don't have the kind of country here."

Even within particular racial communities, there is social separateness based on location. For example, when I asked about attending a Native American church, a contact discouraged me from going to Berry. Although the town seems small in size to me, with only a few thousand residents, it was described to me as more upscale, as if less down-to-earth, than smaller towns. As other contacts confirmed, perceptions of class differences can be important in social separateness in the county.

Separateness between towns can narrow people's worlds to exclude some places. For example, a community member interviewed in Hamilton said,

"There are hundreds and hundreds of people in Hamilton that have never been to Berry, in this county, because it's an Indian town." Then, in discussing another town, he said, "The people in Pierce[3] don't want to shop anywhere but Pierce. They're so clannish—They're all Scotch over there, and they're—They're like another breed over there." Even though Hamilton is also often perceived to be in a separate, social world from the rest of Delano County, the town is still difficult to avoid for a variety of reasons, including employment opportunities, access to health care (e.g., the hospital and numerous physicians' offices), and the fact that the town is the county seat.

Another aspect of separateness is that there are people whose worlds do not extend beyond Delano County. In the words of a health care administrator:

> I have been outside the county before, you know, and I've done traveling, I've met people from all walks of life, so I think it has to do more with your experience base. Because you would be surprised how many people in this county have never been outside the county. . . . And that really impacts people's perceptions and their realities, you know, and the way they view the world.

In many ways, Delano County appeared to be a juxtaposition of external geographic linkages transposed against internal separateness. It was common to meet highly educated people who were well-traveled or who came from different parts of the country, or to meet people who had moved away and returned, or who commuted frequently to cities a few hours away. Also, the nearby city of Filmore has a major military base, and several participants told me that their military experience exposed them to people in different countries and from different walks of life. Furthermore, participants often projected a sense of familiarity with parts of Delano County beyond their immediate locations. For example, the apparent separateness of the area did not apply equally to everyone living there and was frequently contradicted when participants gave me good directions from one town in Delano County to another. Put another way, the separateness of the area was often a perception or a feeling, rather than firmly set boundaries between places.

It is as if a shade of gray is cast over local impressions of outsiders, since different communities and individuals have different perspectives. The issue of race in particular complicates immensely any generalization about people's impressions of outsiders in the area. For example, in the Native American community, I learned that often non-Native Americans are outsiders. In the white community, I frequently came across the idea that Yankees, particularly people from New York, were outsiders. Besides social networks, there is a further, underlying unity that arguably cuts across all races, at least in the sense of being a part of Delano County. A community member explained about the idea of unity occurring alongside difference:

> There are areas within the county where people can tell if you're from this part of the county or that part of the county, even Hamilton, this part of Hamilton and that part of Hamilton. But there's also sort of a bigger sense of—I was going to say if you're from Delano County or not Delano County, but I think there's some little pockets near Delano County where people who are from here sort of moved a little, and they sort of would be identified culturally by people here as, you know, fitting in, I guess people from here, they wouldn't be outsiders. But there is a real strong sense of a Delano County native, I'm from Delano County. And then a lot of people who live here don't associate with being a Delano County person or who won't admit to it or who just don't identify and have lived here like decades. [laughs]

"Why won't they identify with it?" I asked.

"I think culturally they still feel alienated or they still feel different."

Another participant raised the idea that there are across-the-board similarities in the behavior of people, even if they do not socialize much with one another:

> But, the thing about it is, people in Delano County are so clannish, they're very clannish. Once you get into a community and they get to know you, and it's very difficult for them to get to know you, then they would take you in as their family. And that's across the board across the county.

Transience is another common characteristic of the area, at least according to several participants in the white community. As explained by an attorney:

> We have a lot of people who come here and stay a few years and move on for one reason or another. So I think we're accustomed to seeing people come who are not natives of this county, let's say, that come into Hamilton.

As explained by a U.S. medical graduate:

> In many small Southern towns, particularly in eastern [name of the state], if you haven't been there several generations, you might as well forget it. That's not—I don't think that's really true here. And I don't know what the reason for this is, but we've had—Before we had a lot of foreign medical graduates, we had a lot of new industry come into this area. And in many cases, the people that they brought in, in their upper levels of management, were from the North. And those people came in, were bright, were well-accepted and are

> part of things. And actually if you look around at who runs things in the community, there are very few natives running things. If you look at the board of the Chamber of Commerce, for example, there's hardly anybody on there that's a native. They're almost all from outside somewhere. And, you know, maybe that's typical everywhere, I don't know. I don't think it is. I spent a little bit of time in other towns of this size where there's kind of a nobility and there's a—I don't know what you call it, but it's the people that have been there several generations and they're the ones that are in charge of everything, and unless your grandma grew up here, you don't have a chance. And that's not the case in this area.

Such comments about family history might not cut equally across all races, particularly considering that family linkages are of extraordinary importance in the Native American community in Delano County. There were also some suggestions that, at least at one time, people with a long family history in the area were more likely to be considered from the area. In the words of a retired, white physician: "Some people would say I still don't belong to this area. I was not a Colbert, I wasn't born here, Colbert's a local name. I wasn't a Johnson, you know, I wasn't born—I'm not a hometown boy so to speak."

As demonstrated by the above comments, Delano County is not a set of fragmented, unlinked cells but, rather, a place with at least some sense of unity. Indeed, having so many internal differences can be considered one more reason to think of Delano County as a whole.

DIFFERENT-SIZED WORLDS FOR INTERNATIONAL MEDICAL GRADUATES

Against the backdrop of the collective qualities and divisions of Delano County, the size of each person's world obviously varies from individual to individual, and from one community to another. Most people that I met had ties to places outside of the area, and IMGs were no exception. In fact, the geographic pull of some IMGs' social worlds outside of Delano County can be considered another part of the internal separateness of the area.

In one interview, I asked an IMG of Asian Indian origin who had been living in Hamilton since the 1980s if he had ever been to some of the areas near Hamilton. He said that he had been to south Hamilton a couple of times. He had been to Berry and Wilson a few times, and had never been to another small town that I mentioned except en route to another town outside of the county. He explained: "Yeah, but you know, it really, it's because you don't know too many people in certain areas. So unless there is a reason to go like shopping, or there is some business related activity, you know, you don't go to certain area. There is no need to go."

Later, I said, "So that means your world is parts of Hamilton, maybe north and northwest—"

"Hospital, around hospital," he replied. "Around where we live. [laughs]"

Even without visiting many of the places inside Delano County, he traveled frequently to urban centers outside of the county. He described going to Filmore for Hindu religious activities every Sunday, and also going to New York City frequently, and traveling once or twice a year to India. His strong faith led to many of his travels beyond the local area, for example caring for an ailing spiritual leader. Meanwhile, he had a thriving medical practice with patients coming from all over Delano County to see him.

It seemed like a strong contradiction, on the one hand a geographic separateness from the rest of the area, while on the other hand having patients from throughout the area. Furthermore, the convergence of different-sized worlds was particularly striking, with people who have never ventured outside of Delano County seeing a physician who has seldom ventured much within Delano County. At the same time, it can seem unrealistic to expect a physician who is so busy with his family, medical practice, and other obligations to find the time to forge additional social worlds within the area.

I saw firsthand that the city of Filmore, approximately thirty miles away, can be an important meeting point for some IMGs. I attended Diwali, a Hindu New Year's Festival in Filmore, after learning about the festival from talking with IMGs in Hamilton. The event attracted hundreds of Asian Indians, filling a high school auditorium. I arrived there as the guest of the head of the state association of Indian Americans. He walked me to some empty seats and said, "You are at home," and walked away. A few people approached me, wondering what I was doing there (was I a reporter?), since I looked like an outsider. I had different skin color, and was not of Asian Indian origin. Through my conversations with people at the festival, and my own observations from being there, I learned that the Asian Indian community has a strong social network across both Hamilton and Filmore. Also, Filmore has a larger population of people from different countries of origin, which could help explain some of the initial pull of IMGs to Hamilton.

The importance of Filmore in furthering people's own comfort with life in Hamilton also extended to IMGs from other countries of origin, too. For example, in Hamilton, I asked an IMG who was born in Nigeria, "How large is the Nigerian community in this area?"

"Here in Hamilton, I don't know any other Nigerian," the IMG replied. "Probably there are but I haven't met them."

"They're in Filmore though?"

"In Filmore, we have, I would say I've met personally like ten families, yeah. . . It does help to know that, you know, there's somebody who comes from the same area, probably speaks the same language as you do. In Chicago, we had a very large Nigerian community there, and I felt a little uneasy leaving there and, you know, to a place where I don't know, you know, I don't know anybody and I kind of miss the, you know, the familiarity, you know. But it did help to know that there are some Nigerians around here and you can always interact and relate to them."

An IMG from South Asia explained that attachments to different parts of the United States are not important in his own happiness in Hamilton:

> What really doesn't matter in terms of me working in rural or cities, or non-rural settings in the U.S. is that I really don't have any close attachment to anywhere in the U.S. I don't have family here. I just have my wife and my kid. And so it doesn't really matter. I'm looking for work, and I can work here or I can work in New York City or Chicago. I don't care.

Thus, a complicated picture emerges of many different social worlds transposed against one another. Some IMGs have strong social connections to different parts of the United States and beyond, while others enter Hamilton seemingly free of such connections. As an IMG of Asian Indian origin explained:

> I know some international medical graduates, not necessarily Indians, are unhappy. One of the major areas, and it really depends on your personal degree of comfort with it, but one of the major areas where people find Hamilton more remote in that it's not as closely connected to a city, you know, away from the city life. And for anybody where that factor is more important than it is to me, I would certainly think twice about coming here, you know.

The IMG talked about traveling to New York about once a month, and feeling a strong sense of connection with different places in the "West," including Hamilton.

> I'll tell you where the divide comes. It's bizarre, but it's convent school, convent educated and non-convent educated people in India. You'll find that the outlook is very different. The convent schools were run by the Jesuit priests and the nuns, so we—I say we, and this sounds terrible, but probably you're exposed more to a Western—more Western ideas than some of the non-convent schools. And I think that's where the difference is. That's why I consider myself more of a hybrid. I'm not like quite Indian, not but quite American, but some amalgamation of both. And I like to think that I have the best of both.

Another IMG of Asian Indian origin expressed a similar sentiment, referring to her own hometown in India:

> I went to convent school there, so I guess my education was a little different having been taught by Irish nuns, you know. So our exposure was a little different, and my parents were different in the sense that, you know, they took us basically all over the world on travels during vacation time, you know. So we were exposed to different cultures at very young ages.

Just considering South Asia, some IMGs grew up more exposed to "Western" ideas than did others. Hence, the migration of physicians from India to the United States is not simply the transplantation of individuals from one location to another. Rather, the convergence of different-sized worlds in India is now juxtaposed against such convergences in Delano County (see Massey, 1997). By virtue of living in Delano County, or even walking from one side of a street to another, people constantly cross unseen social or geographic boundaries. With networking across communities within Delano County, social and geographic separateness, and the introduction of immigrants, everybody is, in some sense, an outsider. This "cosmopolitan" nature of having so many different worlds converge in the same place serves as a complicated backdrop for the acceptability of IMGs in the area.

The convergence of different worlds is also evident by considering IMGs' responses on the issue of whether Hamilton is their hometown. It had seemed relatively easy to determine whether or not IMGs viewed Quincy as their hometown. In Delano County, determining "hometown" status was not nearly as straightforward an issue. Of fourteen IMGs interviewed, plus the wife of an IMG, the answers tended to reveal more ambiguity than simplicity. For example, I said to an IMG, "And if I were to ask you what's your hometown, what would you answer now?"

> Mmm, you know, I always have this question, and I say that I have a little bit of all the cities that I've lived in. I mean, Bombay is still, you know, is still part of me, but I'm part New York City and part Hamiltonian now. I'd be hard pressed to say where I am from right now, honestly. I don't call myself a Bombayite anymore, I don't call myself a New Yorker. Not quite exactly belonging to Hamilton. I guess just an amalgam of all three.

The wife of an IMG also reflected on being a part of more than one place. After she told me where she was from in India, I asked her if she would consider that to be her hometown. She said yes. "More so than Hamilton?" I asked.

"Well, now, now Hamilton's home, we've—He's been here now about twelve years," she replied. "I've been here almost seventeen, eighteen years, in the United States. So, this is more home than back home now. Everything's changed, you know, back home. So this is more home."

Another IMG explained:

> Home when I came was India and then when I was waiting for my residency, I was here. Home—It's never one place to us. I think—When you say home, if I'm say out shopping somewhere in [a city], and if you say I better get home, I mean, I better get back to Hamilton. When I have a big vacation and I think I might as well make the trip home, then I'm talking of India. So it's a relative term for us when we say home.

In another interview, an IMG said that Hamilton was his hometown. "And how long did it take before you started thinking Hamilton is my hometown?" I asked.

> Possibly . . . after my children were born, sort of, the feeling start when my wife, is from Bombay, she's from a big city, she was kind of apprehensive of going to a small town in the beginning. It was almost maybe six months to a year. After that, you know, you could see in her also that, you know, she liked this place more than New York or Bombay. Right now we're part of this community and we have so many friends, I mean, we go to all the soccer games and [laughs] we travel together and we go to different games.

Later, he added, "I think most of my adult life I have been in Hamilton, comparing to any part in India too, I've never been in any town this long."

Another IMG also said that Hamilton was his only hometown: "Well, you see, I left India for good, so I wouldn't say that's my hometown because I haven't been there for the last nine years. [laughs]"

A few IMGs looked to the future in naming a hometown. For example, an IMG who had been in the area for only about a year said, "It's too early in my career in U.S. [laughs] so . . . I would like to pass for now."

Similarly, an IMG who was only a few weeks away from leaving for a job in another part of the United States said, "It depends what you would like to put into the phrase hometown."

I responded, "Well, let's suppose we put into it the place where you have the strongest attachments, where you feel most like it's your home. Does that—"

"Okay, well that's the next place I'm going to," and he named the town where he was recently hired to practice medicine.

Another IMG, who had been living and practicing in the area for about a year, said that a town in Nigeria was her hometown. I asked if Hamilton could be considered her hometown in the sense of having a very strong attachment to the area, more so than almost anywhere else. She replied, "It's getting there."

As some IMGs talked of transitions to a new hometown, it also became clear that some people adjusted more easily than others to life in Delano County. For example, an IMG answered the question about "hometown" by naming a town in India. Then later in the conversation she said, "You know, I have this ability to quickly feel at home in a place. Much to my husband's chagrin. [laughs] I just do."

Repeatedly, I came across the idea that a "hometown" is not a stagnant, fixed point throughout IMGs' lives but, rather, a process. People *become* attached to a town, and may or may not want to stay attached to other places in the past. Meanwhile, people who are originally from Delano County have their own set of attachments to the area, too, which further adds to the idea that the area is a nexus within which different identities are constructed.

DIFFERENT-SIZED WORLDS AT THE MICROSCALE

The meeting of different worlds also takes place at the microscale, particularly considering different conceptualizations of personal space (Hall, 1969). In some places, standing a particular distance away from another individual can be a norm; in another place, it can be an intrusion. Individual differences in behavior and work experience add further to perceptions of personal space. One nurse practitioner told me about an IMG of Eastern European origin who, at first, would stand too close to patients:

> I noticed very early on that he would come too physically close to some of the patients, cause some of the people in the area just do not deal well with that. If you're going to like come up and do something to them or talk to them, you have to like do it gradually or tell them what you're going to do. I actually saw a couple of patients that he would like—I would ask him to come to a consult, and he would come in the room and go up so close to them to talk to them about like this. And they would start doing like this. And he was concentrating so hard on what he was doing, cause he's very intense, that he didn't realize.

In another interview, a real estate agent marveled about the above IMG's perception of how much space is needed to live comfortably:

> I had one gentleman tell me—I think he was one of like four or five children, and they lived in three rooms. And they come over here and—He was a well-off person from Bulgaria, and they come over here, and you know, we live in two or three thousand square feet. You know, that's unheard of in his country. And they're not sure they want two or three thousand square feet, you know, they're happy in a smaller situation. . . And I'll never forget the gentleman

> from Bulgaria. You know, why do you need all this? Do I really—No, you don't need all this, it's just whatever you want. You know, if you want fifteen hundred square feet, we can certainly find that too, you know.

Beyond the introduction of people from one locale to another, there is also an introduction of different perceptions of space, all in one rural area. Furthermore, many IMGs have activity spaces that pull them outside of the local area, while at the same time intersecting with the activity spaces of people whose worlds are limited mainly within a town or county. Self-perceptions of being more "at home" in one place than in another lead to even further convergences of different worlds. Such convergences help give Delano County its identities.

NOTES

1. Terms such as "midlevel" or "nonphysician" include nurse practitioners, physician assistants, and certified nurse midwives.
2. Wilson's population of 2,600 people includes 59 percent blacks, 30 percent whites, and 10 percent Native Americans (U.S. Census Bureau, 2000).
3. Pierce's population of nearly 3,500 people includes 49 percent blacks, 38 percent whites, and 9 percent Native Americans (U.S. Census Bureau, 2000).

Chapter Seven

Mechanisms and Hamilton: Exclusions and Uncertainties

The first international medical graduates (IMGs) in an area can play a crucial role by their example in furthering or inhibiting a town's openness to other IMGs. It is therefore fitting to begin this discussion of mechanisms[1] by recounting an interview that I almost missed with one of Hamilton's first IMGs.

I had been conducting interviews in Delano County for almost two weeks and was still having trouble with my directions. I missed my turn off a highway and, finally, once rerouted, got caught in five o'clock traffic in Filmore, a city about 30 miles from Hamilton. I pulled over from traffic at 5:05, ten minutes before a scheduled interview, to call an IMG's office to say that I would be arriving late. The receptionist put me on hold. Ten minutes later, I called again and was told that he had left for the day but that he would come back to the office to meet me.

It was close to six P.M. when I knocked on the front door of his office building. He let me in the building and walked me into his office. Some interviews are more formal, and some more relaxed; this felt more formal. He sat behind his desk, the tips of his long fingers on one hand pressed against the tips of his long fingers on the other hand.

> I came here December 1981. I trained in New York. My internal medicine and cardiology fellowship at New York Medical College. I actually—I like New York but I just wanted to go to a smaller town, because I am from a small town in India too. I like small town, and thought the opportunity also will be better in smaller towns. I was traveling on [the highway] and came to see another town nearby. On the way back we stopped in Hamilton and just wanted to see the hospital. It happened that they told me that they needed a cardiologist here. Later on I approached some of the doctors around here, some of the local people, you know, just, in the beginning it was kind of a—not a—you know, not everyone

> wanted me to come down here, but it looked like, you know, I thought a few of the people were very—they gave me a lot of warm reception. Pretty much started my solo practice. Later on I—the main thing I stayed here was the patients and the people around here, they were extremely nice to me. Actually maybe I'm the first Indian internist and a cardiologist to come to this place. Beginning I was slightly apprehensive about this area, but soon I realized that people are nice and this is a nice place to live. I think I've done pretty well here. After one year I found a [medical] partner, and he's also here with me even now. And we have one more doctor right now. She's also same way, I mean, she was looking for a smaller town, so she's with us almost two years now."

After further conversation, I asked, "And you said that not everyone wanted you to come down here?"

> See, initially when I came down here, maybe half the doctors, it was really half the doctors strongly supported me that they wanted a doctor here, and after I came here they all liked me. They all thought that I'm hard working and they are getting consultations whenever they wanted, day or night time. Two groups, they thought, you know, we will be competition for them. And, you know, that's the main thing I think, more than anything else. They were not that happy, because they thought one more new doctor coming here. And I don't blame anyone, because you know, I came from somewhere else and I look different and talk different. But right now, all those groups, you know, we are in good terms. Not that we socialize, but professionally we don't have any problems. I am the chief of medicine in this place here.

I sat there, my mind still reeling from the pressing feeling of being late. Several people had suggested that I talk with this physician, but it was common for me to be referred to the same person by several people. I had not realized in advance just how important he had been in paving the way for other IMGs.

"The two groups that thought there would be competition, are they also cardiologists or internists?" I asked.

"Internists," he replied.

"And you mentioned that some of the concern might have been based around the fact that you look different or talk different."

"No," he said. "What I was telling you was that I don't blame them, because when you come from somewhere, they're always, you know, skeptical that, you know, how good you are, you know, what you are. There's something for people to—it's a small town, Southern town, some foreigners are coming from somewhere, they might have thought that, you know, they may be thinking that I may not be that good, or the way I practice may be different. You know, first of all I don't know if they were exposed to any of the international medical graduates in this place."

"So is it the general community or the medical community—"

"Only the medical community. The general community, I never had any—I can only say that I never had any problem."

He explained that he could see positive changes in physicians' perceptions toward him in the first six months to a year of practice. He said that he had faced strong objections in trying to bring a partner to his medical practice:

"When I want to take a partner, they opposed. I took it as, you know, if I can't take a partner, there's no way I'm going to stay here without working almost twenty hours a day, you know, I worked like that almost one year. It was getting to a point that I was—I mean, I still thought I had enough energy to do that, but I didn't think I could continue that pace. I didn't have coverage from anyone when I first came here." Referring to a medical staff meeting in which the pending partnership was discussed, he said, "The majority of people in the medical staff meeting, without me not knowing them, they supported me. They told that these things are not going to happen, this is a free country."

"That these things are not going to happen?" I asked.

"No, opposing me, for taking partnership," he said. "They—Actually most of the people who opposed on that meeting, I didn't even know them. You know, I knew them a little bit, but not—they were not my friends or something." Further in the conversation, he said, "Right now it has changed. Possibly, you know, they have seen us for a long time. You know, newer doctors who are coming here in town, I'm sure they were much better acceptance, because they look at all other doctors who are here, and they think that, oh, you should be like—some of the people here now, they think that India is a small country."

My immediate understanding was that people became more accepting of IMGs by having been exposed to the quality work of pioneer IMGs. Familiarity with the work of the first few Asian Indian IMGs may have made it easier when other physicians from India moved to the area.

Trying to put myself in the shoes of a new IMG, I asked him for advice that he might give me if I were an IMG who was about to move to the area. He responded:

> Don't feel that people won't like you before it happens to you. Even if it happens, you have to think that always there's something—if human beings are animals, then something else comes to the field, it looks different, you are taken as like, in a suspicious eye. So if you do your job the best you can do, you'll be fine.

Thinking later about the interview, I was impressed by the IMG's willingness to cast even negative experiences in a more positive light. He did not seem to hold grudges against anyone who had mistreated him but, instead, said that he was now friends with people who had expressed early objections to IMGs. He did not dwell on past problems. However, the fact that he mentioned some of his early negative experiences was telling. I reasoned that the objections that he and his medical partner had faced must have been so strong that it would have been untruthful to say that the medical community had been more open.

I had not known about such objections prior to talking with him, and indeed had only a limited understanding of the early exclusion of IMGs based on my interview with him. Subsequent interviews with other participants confirmed how important he and his medical partner had been in overcoming obstacles for future IMGs.

COMMENTS FROM A RETIRED PHYSICIAN

In one interview, I was sitting in the home of a retired white physician in Hamilton who had been a leader of the medical community around the time that the first IMGs came to the area.

He said, "I haven't had any experience, you know, trying to recruit a foreign medical doctor. I'll be very frankly, I've been in the recruitment phase almost all the time I was in practice, and I would not have considered a foreign medical trained doctor."

"You would not have considered one?" I asked.

"No," he said. "Not as an associate, no, because they don't know the mores and the social, you know, ways of going on with women in this area, and I just never did. And while early in practice we had residents in training from [a university town] here, and I remember a guy who went to medical school in Switzerland, a nice guy, I really liked him and liked his wife. He was born in the United States, his father is an American trained doctor, he just couldn't get into medical school. But his knowledge of medicine was not what I would have expected. We had another guy who—This first guy happened to be Jewish, the one that followed him up was an Arabian, they came through the same program, but not adequately trained, as far as I was concerned. And this influenced my thinking."

Later, when asked about IMGs from India, he said, "They have to prove themselves. I mean, I would think that [the IMG cardiologist] and [the IMG's first medical partner] would tell you it took them a while. They had—their practice for a long time was the economically lower levels and it's gradually picked up. They have a good level of people."

"Would there have been resistance from the medical community?" I asked.

"Oh no. Nn nnh."

"No? From the nonmedical community?"

"From the nonmedical community, yeah, yeah. The medical community would try these people and would take them on—And this is how they made their reputation, they did a good job when you asked for a consultation. That was the way it was."

His account of a lack of resistance from the medical community was not consistent with the previous interview in which I learned that there had been resistance to the first IMGs. It puzzled me further that the retired physician said that there was no resistance while also saying that he never wanted to hire an IMG. I wondered whether some of his concerns about IMGs might be minimized if the doctor were to come from a western European country, as opposed to India.

"I wouldn't consider either one of them," he said. "I mean, I went through lots of resumes. And at one time I was in charge of physician recruitment here, and we had resumes for everybody here. And because of nondiscrimination clauses, we had to interview and get these people here. But, you know, you just—you don't—If you really want to recruit someone, you go all out, if you don't, you sort of let it go. And I remember there was an otolaryngologist that—he was Lebanon . . . his wife's a concert pianist, had two lovely kids, but he had been trained in Detroit, been to medical school in Lebanon. He came to town here but he never fulfilled the position that we needed filled. He actually ended up leaving to do that. But we really didn't recruit him. I mean, we gave him an interview and then he called up and said he wanted to come. Well, it's an open staff, he met the criteria of the credentials committee, but that's not someone I would recruit."

"Now how long were you in charge of physician recruitment?" I asked.

"A couple of years. I don't remember exactly, it was back in the 60s, late 60s."

"So there weren't that many international medical graduates applying at the time, right?"

"Oh, there were a lot."

"There were?"

"Oh yes, there were a lot. There really were. There were a lot."

"But there weren't that many coming here?"

"Oh no. Nn nnh."

"And why not?"

"Well, our criteria was that most of them had to be American graduates. Unless they pushed it, we didn't really, you know, push to get them here."

Even after IMGs entered practice in the area, he was slow to accept them as equal to U.S. medical graduates in the practice of medicine. By his account:

> I think the international medical graduates' medical decisions were scrutinized by the nursing personnel much more in-depth than the American graduates'. To be frank to tell you right off that if a patient asked me who to send them to, until [the

IMG cardiologist] and [the IMG's first medical partner] had been here for a long time I would not refer a patient to them. They had to prove themselves whereas a young American trained internal medicine guy, I would refer to immediately.

Despite his concerns about IMGs in general, he has shown an ability to accept individual IMGs who have proved themselves. Regarding the IMG cardiologist, the retired physician said, "He's very smart, he's kept up, he takes good care of his patients, and he's been an asset to the medical staff."

COMMENTS FROM A MEMBER OF THE NURSING STAFF

A participant who works in the nursing profession also recalled some of the difficulty faced by the IMG cardiologist and his partner. Her words helped me understand some of the personal aspects of the early exclusion of IMGs:

> I worked in the hospital in other jobs that—My last job was director of critical care there for right many years before I went into this job, and even in that setting was some excellent doctors, cardiologist is one that I was thinking of right then. And he probably was the first non-American to get on staff there, and there was a great deal of, I don't know if it's stigmatism—I don't have the right word in my mind right now. But he was shunned and sort of held at a distance by the other members of the medical staff. And there was open discussions about it initially, and he was such an excellent doctor. Now, he's like probably one of the top respected doctors in the hospital, chairman of multiple committees, and blah, blah, blah, very well respected. And he sort of like broke the barrier. But there's just—in this area—I don't know if it's in this area or if it's everywhere, but totally from what I've heard from other people and from myself, you know, I would have thought—I would have rather seen an American doctor, you know. And now that I've worked with [an IMG] for three years, I wouldn't feel like that.

Reflecting further, she said, "The thing that I remember is when [the IMG cardiologist] came to Hamilton, cause I was working there then, that the medical staff, in the halls of the hospital, actively talked about it wasn't going to be easy for him, they weren't going to make it easy for him. And he really did have a difficult time, but he was such an excellent doctor, that he overcame all that. It was a very painful thing, because everybody—all the nurses knew how well—how smart he was."

I asked her, "What were they saying they were going to do?"

> They didn't say what they were going to do, they were just going to say—You know, he could—Well, it's just going to be difficult. They weren't going to make it for him. And it felt like, and everybody understood that he was not welcome,

> and it was because he was an outsider. But he certainly transcended all that. He probably is the person that paved the way, if you want my personal opinion, because he really was a—He was nice despite whatever. He was nice and he was extremely smart, and it's a 360 degree turnaround now. He's like the person they would all ask advice from, you know.

She said that opposition to the first IMGs came entirely from white physicians. The medical staff was almost entirely white at the time. Referring to physicians from India as "Indians," I asked about the views of the white physicians who had opposed having IMGs on the medical staff.

"Where do these physicians stand now in terms of interacting with the Indian physicians in the area?" I asked.

"They're working in their offices with them," she replied. "It's like the people at that time when they were giving [the IMG cardiologist] such a hard time were the biggest office in town, and still is probably, is the [clinic], was all white, and now, they have Indian physicians employed in their offices. I mean, so that's the transition. And they refer people to [the IMG cardiologist] or get him on consult. Before, they wouldn't have given him a consult or helped him with anything probably. So, it was actually very mean."

COMMENT FROM ANOTHER INTERNATIONAL MEDICAL GRADUATE

An IMG of Asian Indian origin who had moved to the area only a few years ago said:

> Well, you know, we have heard in days past when this was more a homogeneous community, physician wise anyway, that a foreign grad or just a doctor of different origins was just not—They were just not welcomed here as readily as we were. I mean, we were given the red carpet treatment. And of course, we didn't hear about that before we got here. Had we known about it then we might have been more skeptical about even coming here. But we heard it after we'd been part of the community for a while, and you know, talked to these folks. So I guess in retrospect it's good we didn't hear about it originally coming here. [laughs]

VIGNETTE: INTERVIEW WITH ANOTHER PIONEER INTERNATIONAL MEDICAL GRADUATE

My greatest insight into the early experiences of pioneer IMGs came from a two-part interview with a pulmonologist who had moved to the area in the early

1980s to join the IMG cardiologist's medical practice. Our first meeting was in his office, and we had to reschedule because he was on call and needed to return to the hospital. Our second meeting was held in his home in one of the more affluent areas of Hamilton. His account of his early experiences effectively filled out the story of the early exclusion of IMGs. This extended excerpt from the transcript is provided to let his words lead the story, rather than mine.

"I am a pulmonologist. I also do internal medicine. I have been in Hamilton since October of 1982. . . . I think when I came here, they were kind of suspicious about quality of care we would give or whether we would fit into the medical community here. In fact, I personally had opposition to come here. The hospital didn't give me privileges for almost three months. And then they approved privileges after a lot of discussion in the medical staff. And the response was very slow from the doctors to accept in the beginning. And some doctors wouldn't talk to you, wouldn't look at you."

"Wouldn't talk?" I asked.

"Uh huh. They would just pass by, wouldn't say hello to you. And since, over the period of time, the same doctors are very friendly now. Very nice. So we had to prove ourselves that we're as competent as anybody else around to be accepted."

"Tell me more about the denial of hospital privileges," I said. "Was that a resolution that was passed or was it just something that was de facto and not written down?"

"Well, what hospital did, they hired [name of firm], this [name of firm], this accounting firm to investigate if we needed any pulmonologist to this area. So they give them report that there is no need for a pulmonologist in this area. And that was not well accepted by some of the doctors which favored for me to be here. And they fought against that and then they reversed their decision that there did need for a pulmonologist. I think after that they approved my privileges. They thought I was too qualified to come to this area. [laughs] I had done some research in all these things and they thought they didn't need somebody with that background and subspecializing in pulmonary diseases. There was no pulmonologist between [two cities a few hours apart in driving distance] when I came here, so this hospital is very fortunate that there was somebody here who was trained in pulmonary diseases. There were none even in Filmore when I came here."

I asked, "Did other early physicians, early IMGs in this area, have similar experiences?"

"There's only one here as I told you," he said, and he spelled the name of an IMG who had come to the area prior to the cardiologist. "He was also pretty good guy. He was actually a friend of Governor [name] and all of that, so he was well accepted. Then came [the IMG cardiologist]. Actually [the IMG cardiologist] came to join two other IMGs. They were practicing in [other counties]. And one was internist and one was gastroenterologist and they were having some part time offices here so [the IMG cardiologist] came, he settled the practice. They were planning to move here too. But they were not allowed to come here. I don't actually know the details but their privileges are denied here so they couldn't come. And then [the IMG cardiologist] was by himself. And by that time it was for almost eight months and he was very busy being the only cardiologist, was getting a lot of critical care. And because I had a background of critical care, he asked me to join him. We knew each other from residency. We did in same place. And I decided to come here. I liked the area, peaceful, quiet. I was born in rural area in India and I always like the peaceful quiet place. I did my residency in New York and I did my medical college in Bombay, so I didn't really like the big cities. I wanted to be in quiet small places."

I said, "I'm wondering was there an institutional objection to having international medical graduates on staff?"

"I think both side," he said. "From the hospital and from the staff. Some of the staff was very opposed I think probably for foreign residents to come here. So this from both sides. But some staff were very supportive, very open-minded. I think because of them, I could come. They were very supportive. They did not like the objection for coming here."

"There was an objection to your having hospital staff privileges that lasted three months?" I said.

"Yeah," he replied, "it shouldn't have lasted, because I was going to join [the IMG cardiologist]. I was not coming here primarily to do my own practice, so there should not be that much hassle, and all the paperwork, everything in order before I came here. In fact, I moved here. I had rented apartment so, they wouldn't give privileges, I had to go back to New York and find a job in VA [Veterans Administration]. I stayed there for three months. And then I came back. [laughs]"

"Came back once you had the privileges approved?" I asked.

"Approved. Yeah. But I had moved here anticipating that there was no problem because [the IMG cardiologist] told me everything looks in order, move in here. So after fellowship I moved here directly."

He continued, "I think, I don't know, I don't know, I think it's just, you know, just, maybe the people are like this here. They're not supposed to see other world people here. They didn't like to have other world people to come here. So it's a close community. Things have changed tremendously here. I think this area is opened up now, more open-minded, even hospital. Because when I came here, a lot of local Indians, they didn't want to come to this hospital. They would like to go to [a neighboring] county. Said they are better treated there. Once we had good rapport with them and had good relations and said, well, I'm going to take care of you, you come here, I'll give good care, and they started coming. Things are changed now. No more have that kind of feeling anymore. People will come here without any hesitation, reservations."

I asked him what brought about the change in people's attitudes toward IMGs.

"I think this is what happened with the people migrating here. [laughs] Different people. Lot of ethnic groups now here which we didn't have before. But I think hospital has been open. They're very progressive, and very forward-going. So I think—I don't blame the hospital. I think they go with the hospital staff wishes that time. I don't think administrative itself had any problem with anybody coming here. They had to go slowly with the staff, they were very powerful at that time. So I think they didn't want to make that their doctors unhappy. So I think these people very nice to me after that. I didn't see any problem. I didn't have any problems with the administration actually. Except the first, you know, kind of administrative hassle, which may be technical. But nobody gave me any hard time here. Hospital has been very nice to me and very supportive and very helpful about what do I want to do here. It's a very progressive hospital."

When we met later in his home to continue our interview, he said, "Last time we talked about the difficulty I had about being accepted in society, especially—not especially, only—by medical community. But I think the patient population accepted me very, very easily. So it was the physician population have difficulty accepting somebody else. But it has changed, gradually it changed. The relations have become very cordial, very friendly. No problems anymore. But initially, it was some problems. Definite problems. [laughs]"

I said, "I was invited to a church by [name of a mutual contact] and I was talking with her later. And I didn't tell her which physicians I had interviewed. And she said to me that she used to have lunch with you, and that when you first came, you would be upset—"

"Well, I guess—"

"—about how you were treated, I guess."

"I think when you're young, you're more sensitive," he said. "More aggressive. As you get older, you mature, then you don't care about those things. . . . If somebody have doubt about you, it's natural, you have to prove yourself to those people who have doubt about you."

I asked, "What do you do to prove yourself? Just work extra hard?"

"I think they see how I treat my patients and I take care of the patients and, you know, eventually they felt comfortable enough to call me on consult for their patients. That's the level of their confidence level. I think it's a natural process. I don't blame anybody because we are dealing with a whole different world. [laughs] They're not exposed to foreigners. And you know, they might have some kind of suspicion about our medical training and all kind of stuff."

I asked him what would happen if I were a physician moving here.

"No problem," he replied. "I think they would like it too. Especially foreign origin. So I think that gate is opened up now. That's past."

Today, praise for the IMG cardiologist and pulmonologist is widespread. Without even being asked, participants in the medical and nonmedical communities spoke of them in glowing terms. This happened so often that if a participant was speaking highly of a physician, I became accustomed to hearing that the physician was either the IMG cardiologist or pulmonologist.

OTHER PIONEER INTERNATIONAL MEDICAL GRADUATES

The first IMG to practice in Delano County received his medical degree in Taiwan and actually did not practice at the hospital or in Hamilton. He had located in nearby Pierce about thirty years ago, and practices family medicine there still. The pioneer IMGs in Hamilton did not refer to him in discussing their early experiences in the area. He was rarely mentioned in participants' recollections about the first IMGs in Hamilton, and therefore was probably not as central in IMGs' acceptance in Hamilton. It seemed as though his experience had a different geographic center than encountered by the other IMGs, and therefore might pull the study in a new direction. We talked only briefly by telephone near the end of my fieldwork, and I never did manage to schedule a formal interview with him. Consequently, his experiences will not be explored in this discussion.

I saw no evidence in the historical record that IMGs practiced in Delano County any earlier than thirty years ago. A book published by the county medical auxiliary in 1959 listed biographical information about physicians in the county from the 1700s forward; no IMGs were listed. In 1985, the medical staff directory included four IMGs out of seventy-two physicians; two years later, with a total of sixty-seven physicians listed in the directory, only one more IMG had been added. At the time of my fieldwork, there were twenty-three IMGs in Delano County, constituting over 20 percent of the physician workforce.

In talking about the first IMGs to come to the area, participants often recalled an Asian Indian physician who had moved to Hamilton in the mid-1970s. The physician, an orthopedist, lost his hospital privileges in the early to mid-1990s and subsequently left his Hamilton clinic about five years ago. He appears to have been the first IMG to have a medical practice in

Hamilton. The orthopedist was referred to earlier as someone who was initially well accepted because of his connections with the governor.

Comments about the orthopedist were sometimes positive but often circumspect or critical, possibly reflecting the fact that he left fairly recently under less than ideal circumstances. Some of the comments about him matched negative stereotypes encountered in Quincy about Asian Indians. For example, several participants said that he did not treat women fairly and would make his wife or nurses walk behind him. Several participants said that he became too interested in money; as evidence, they referred to a business venture that had consumed much of his energy. Other concerns expressed by participants included questions about his accommodation of patients (e.g., alleging that he scheduled too many appointments at the same time) and about his personality, particularly in his final years of practice.

Whether or not the IMG orthopedist was an obstacle or asset to IMG acceptance is a question that has no easy answer. In being first, he had been the lone example of an IMG for many people at the hospital. In the late 1970s and early 1980s, people in the area simply were not familiar with what to expect from an IMG. When the physician staff had the opportunity to oppose the introduction of other IMGs, they did so.

The question of why acceptance is greater now is not easy to answer either. Certainly, the IMG cardiologist and pulmonologist played valuable roles in opening up opportunities for acceptance. The internationalization of the local area could be another contribution to acceptance, i.e., that which had been unfamiliar or exotic is now part of the local landscape. About twenty years ago, a question relevant to this study was why the IMGs faced such strong resistance to practicing at the hospital. Today, a relevant question is why IMGs are moving to Hamilton to the point that there are now international communities in the local area.

GEOGRAPHIC CONCENTRATIONS OF INTERNATIONAL MEDICAL GRADUATES

After the initial struggles of the pioneer IMGs, the immigrant community has grown in Delano County. Among participants, estimates varied as to the size of the Asian Indian community. There may be around twenty to thirty families of Asian Indian origin who live in Delano County, with even more who live in the nearby city of Filmore. Besides health providers, the Asian Indian community also includes motel owners and other small business owners. There is also a Filipino community that, by one participant's estimates, has around thirty to forty people in Delano County, and much fewer in Hamilton.

A geographic concentration of immigrants in or near a rural town can have advantages, according to participants. Discussing the reasons why Asian Indians move to the area, one of the pioneer IMGs told me:

> Their reason is there are enough Indian people so they have some social interactions. Plus, you know, good days, bad days you need some support from your friends because basically I think in every ethnic community, you feel more close to your ethnic background people, for, you know, hard days and bad days, so I think all people probably go to any other people of their kind. So that probably is the determining factor where people go for practice. When I came here it wasn't that thing, I just went for opportunity. I was young. I thought I could do anything I wanted to do and I could be strong to face anything. As you get older, I feel that it is essential, that you have your own community around you. I think it's for kids also to know their heritage and background.

Some IMGs have recruited other IMGs to come practice in the area. The pioneer IMG quoted above mentioned the names of three other IMGs of Asian Indian origin that he helped recruit into the area. Family connections also furthered recruitment of IMGs of Asian Indian origin. For example, an IMG told me that she had joined a group practice with her brother-in-law, also a pioneer IMG. In another example, the wife of an IMG told me that her aunt introduced them to an IMG in Hamilton, which led to future practice in a Hamilton clinic. The wife of the IMG who had been recruited to practice in the area said to me:

> If we already knew that there's a good opportunity in, let's say, Wyoming, some town in Wyoming, at that time, if we had known, you know, that there's not much competition, there's a lot of underserved area, it's a good town. And if somebody had given us the confidence to go there, then we would have probably chosen that town as opposed to this one. It's just information, the feedback you get from the physicians who are in that area. In that sense we feel comfortable coming to somebody who's already in this area and who's given you the correct information, that if you settle here, you're not—your practice is going to, you know, get established basically. These are the problems, but these are the opportunities too. You know, in that sense, it's good to know somebody who's already in that area. And it could be an American doctor too, I mean, it doesn't have to be, you know, an Indian, a foreign doctor. You just have to have, probably trust for the person who's providing you that information. You want it—If you are looking to establish yourself, you want it to be like on the up and up so that you get there and you're established and you don't have any pitfalls.

In her case, it was a pioneer IMG who was trusted, further adding to the status of the pioneer IMGs as people who are held in high regard.

Most of Delano County's IMGs live in Hamilton, regardless of where they practice, and the same could be said for physicians in general. Several of the more affluent neighborhoods in Hamilton have attracted IMGs, and I saw new construction and expansion for their homes. The reason for living in or near Hamilton often had to do with requirements by the hospital that physicians need to respond to calls within a certain time frame. Thus, proximity to the hospital can be a deciding factor in terms of choosing a home in Delano County, at least for physicians who work on the hospital staff.

A Geographic Concentration of Asian Indian Physicians in a Clinic

Specific reasons could be posited as to why IMGs move to individual clinics. For example, the clinic that has two pioneer IMGs has now expanded to four physicians, all of whom are of Asian Indian origin. I wondered why there was a small concentration of physicians from the same country of origin practicing in the same clinic.

At the time of the interviews, an IMG was about to leave his current practice to become the fourth physician in the clinic. I asked him if it was just a coincidence that the clinic was going to have four physicians from the same country of origin. His reply:

> Well, I don't know, maybe the senior most person there brought in a friend of his, and then two of them practiced for a long time. And then one of them is a relative of—The third doctor who joined them is a relative of the senior doctor, and it's my joining them is kind of coincidence or—They were looking for doctors and then they saw me and I was coming up. There was another doctor, not from India coming up, and I don't know what criteria they used to ask me to join them. We do get along better. I don't know if I should say better, or I should say we get along well. And in fact, we do have a very friendly relationship. Maybe it might have played a part, but I'm sure if that equally competent person, they could have probably chosen him too at the right time.

I said, "It's just interesting to consider how it comes about, and it could just be friendship and nothing—"

"Right. And once you start—When I came here and met with more doctors, some of them were from India, then you sit down and talk and then you can, you know, learn about their roots back home, and you might find certain things common amongst you. It's interesting, it kind of does create a certain bond, yes."

In talking with another partner in the clinic, I said, "That's interesting that there might be this cluster of physicians originally from the same country."

The physician replied:

> Ah, that's not necessarily true actually. This was just incidental. It was just because . . . we did have a PA [physician assistant] who was working for us who was not Indian, who was American, and she worked out great with us. In fact, that was one of the things I was talking about, because we worked for almost six months together til we discovered that we had, you know, quite a lot of stuff in common. So I think this was just incidental and I don't think his being Indian was specifically the reason why he was picked up. Given the situation, actually it was just opportunity. We were looking for a physician and he was—the physician who is joining us was one of those people who was just finishing his contract at this particular time. Rather than go through all the hassles of finding somebody we didn't know, it seemed easier to take on someone who is already in the community, who knew the community well. He was—the physician we're taking on was also working right here for the hospital and was under some contractual obligations which ended and was looking for a job. So it was just incidental that he happened to come in here. And I don't think his being Indian had anything specifically to do with it.

Such comments lend credence to the notion that sometimes, geographic clusters do not have deep explanations. It was also interesting to me that all four physicians had a strong social connection through personal experience, family, or training in the same city in India. This similarity could conceivably have added to a sense of inclusiveness for the newly hired IMGs.

Primary Care Recruitment and Waiver Physicians

In Quincy, many IMGs came in response to the hospital's earlier emphasis on the recruitment of subspecialists. In Delano County, the reverse appears to be the case. In other words, the movement of IMGs to the area could be a reflection, at least in part, of the hospital's recruitment of primary care providers. Furthermore, the IMG influx could also be a reflection of national and state emphases on primary care. Even though such a shift in emphasis took place nationally approximately twenty years ago, different hospitals and places adopted a more primary care–centered approach at different times. Most of Delano county's IMGs moved to the area within the past decade, and added more primary care. Recruitment of physicians seeking J-1 visa waivers is a further reflection of the Hamilton hospital's emphasis on primary care. By comparison, the shift to primary care in Quincy has been much slower and is reflected by the subspecialization of many IMGs who practice there.

According to the hospital recruiter in Hamilton:

> We have for this upcoming year, the need for four family practice physicians, two internal medicine physicians, one pediatrician, one OB/GYN, general surgeon, a dermatologist, and an otolaryngologist. And also we have need for one

> half, point five gastroenterology. People, I'm sure, have a puzzled mind when I say that, but we would be looking for someone who has done a fellowship, subspecialty training in gastro, and also anticipate doing some internal medicine, maybe a 50/50 mix.

A U.S. medical graduate involved in physician recruitment also emphasized the need for primary care:

> The big emphasis now is on, you know, primary care. And that's where the big influx of the international doctors are coming from, because of primary care needs. Cause, you know, American docs want to go into cardiology, cardiothoracic surgery, ENT, derm, all the, you know, specialty and subspecialty and subsubspecialties, and family practice kind of got away from that. And now you see the resurgence of primary care. A lot of foreign international doctors have come back and try to do family practice residencies so they can get a place in America.

J-1 VISA WAIVERS

One approach to the recruitment of primary care providers is to hire IMGs on a J-1 visa waiver. As explained in Chapter 1, waivers allow IMGs to stay in the United States in exchange for service in an underserved area. Six of the fourteen IMGs interviewed for this study area were on or had recently completed a J-1 visa waiver, compared with only one in Quincy. According to Hamilton's hospital recruiter during an interview in late 1999, Delano County's first waiver physicians had been recruited only three and a half years earlier.

A major problem with J-1 visa waivers is that applying for them is a long, drawn out process. Through bureaucracy and paperwork, employers may have no choice but to have delays when hiring waiver physicians. According to a waiver physician of Asian Indian origin:

> Whatever the process it takes to get these people into rural communities or underserved communities has to be much faster. It shouldn't be going around, beating around the bush, and take a year to just get in there. You're wasting valuable time. So if that's what the physician really wants to do, to serve the community, and integrate into the community, then it has to be much faster rather than beating around the bush and delaying the process. What I have lately seen is that with each year there is some changes that delays the process. There may be several reasons why that's happening, but if the goal is to serve the community and if there is a physician, in this age and time it should not be difficult to match.

In other conversations, I also learned about the long, drawn out process of requesting J-1 visa waivers. The CEO of a multisite community health center remarked:

> It's tough. It is tough. I mean, you got to get all these lawyers involved. You're on the phone with your senator and your congressional representative trying to get the paperwork because it will get stuck in the process. And this one particular person that we were recruiting, and I don't remember who it was at this point in time, if it had not been for our senator, I don't think we would ever have gotten the paperwork processed. . . . And plus, the physician had a lawyer that was working with him, and then we had the senator's office working with us, and we had our own lawyer that was working with us. I mean, it's a tortuous process. And I'm not sure if that's good or bad or what the reason, you know, what the politics are behind that. You know, I don't know. But when you've got communities, and especially at that time when we were down—You know, we had all the medical centers and all these patients and we were down to trying to contract out for services, and Dr. [name] was running himself ragged, and we had midlevels, and we had to have—You know, the midlevels, you have to have signers, you have to have primary physicians signing off for them. It was horrendous. I mean, we thought we were going to have to close the place down because we had no providers. Or at least, you know, close everything down except maybe the one across the street. And it was awful. And the hospital was working with us, trying to help us find someone. It was a real, you know, community effort in terms of trying to find somebody to get in here. So the powers that be really worked with us on that one.

In a conversation with the hospital recruiter, I asked about mistakes that might be made by waiver physicians who want to move to the area. He replied:

> So often the biggest mistake, I guess, is when I get calls or faxes, they appear too desperate. They call and say, my husband—you've got to help us, my husband or my wife is finishing up her training and we must have a position. And oftentimes they call way too late. If they know they're going to finish in June, and I have a pretty good understanding it's going to take a year to go through this—Obviously if they call in January or February or March—There are all kinds of snarls and tangles, so they need to start very, very early in their process, and they need not appear as desperate. They need to have a focused agenda as to what they're looking for and how they can best serve that opportunity, and then let their skills compete with the other people in the market.

Immigration pathways are exceedingly complex, and people who are not immediately involved in a physician's employment can misperceive whether or not he or she is on a waiver. The line between being on a waiver and moving closer toward a green card is obviously not differentiated in everybody's eyes. From a legal standpoint, there can be distinctions in immigration status, and indeed such distinctions can be very important to individual IMGs or their employers. In terms of work environment, the distinction often appeared to be only a technical one, since there can be good and bad employers regardless of the waiver. When there is a bad employer, the waiver or other early immigration status can make the physician vulnerable to mistreatment. Waiver physicians in Delano County already had to work for a year or more through the difficult process of *obtaining* a J-1 visa waiver. Then they have to be careful to keep the waiver, which adds pressure to anyone in an uncomfortable working relationship.

The vulnerability of waiver physicians to mistreatment was an awkward topic. Most people obviously do not want to speak ill of their employers; nor do people want to be quoted as saying anything negative about others with whom they have close working relationships. Mistreatment of waiver physicians was typically discussed in the third person, often in reference to acquaintances in other parts of the country.

Here is how an IMG of Asian Indian origin explained what it was like to be on a waiver:

"Well, waiver kind of is like a—kind of a chain. It kind of keeps you like whether—What's going to happen next? Once you get the waiver off then you know at least one thing is taken care of, now you can concentrate on the job of looking after your patients. But waiver was only kind of a legal or a formality to go through in the entire process of moving from like Bombay to this place and then coming to serve the rural community here." He went on to say, "I had to make some compromises because of my J-1 with respect to compensation. An equally trained American graduate would have made much more compared to what I took in when I came here."

Waiver physicians are paid on salary, and therefore cannot be expected to be compensated as well as most other physicians for working long hours. Beyond the issue of compensation looms a more complicated issue of IMGs' vulnerability to employers' work demands.

The Experience of One Waiver Physician

Exactly what constitutes mistreatment is a difficult issue. For example, waiver physicians take jobs that are often less desirable, a point that came out in conversation with an IMG working in a clinic in a nearby small town. We were talking in the hospital only a few weeks before his last day of work. He would soon move to New England.

"Well, see, it doesn't make sense to say to someone that the job is busy and it's very difficult, because there are levels of difficulty," he said. "And probably it more would make sense that it's unattractive because it requires substantial time commitment that most physicians are not capable. I am not also capable. You have to have some time to regenerate from dealing with patients' problems. Most people are not capable of committing that much time for others. So that's one of the difficulties that make the position here unattractive."

I found it interesting that waiver physicians might take jobs that would be seen as less attractive for other physicians.

"Well," he responded, "I would think that that's the purpose of the whole system that was placed at that time. Nothing bad in such a system, but that's what it is. I think that this job is less attractive because of the time commitment that it requires."

A month later, his work experience in Delano County surfaced in an interview with a nurse practitioner who had worked closely with him. In her words:

> The thing that has surfaced is that the pay, from what I understand—I don't know what [his] pay was. You know, we talked about various things and ballpark figures, so I don't know what it was. But he perceived that his pay was less than people who weren't working in the clinics doing the same job, that if he were out working in a private office he'd be making much more money. The other thing, the other side of that, the administrative person I told you about, he was never satisfied with anything, he was always looking for the numbers. And he perceived that [name of IMG] was not, and he made it plain, was not earning his money, because he needed to generate a certain amount of things. Well, you know, we got reports, and we knew that we all generated a heck of a lot more than we got paid, you know, like bunches and bunches more. But, you know, of course there's overhead and stuff that goes with clinics too. But it never—It always seemed to be the opposite way, that [the IMG] was working very hard and taking very unfavorable call, and probably not getting rewarded what he would have had he been in a private setting, even in Hamilton.

"Do you think part of that is related to being on a J-1 waiver and simply having to make more sacrifices because of that?" I asked.

"Uh huh!" she replied. "The fact that he signed a contract to help get his green card—Well, he always told me from the beginning he would be out of here when he got his green card. He got his green card and he's out of here. [laughs] Of course part of—I think that that wasn't all of it, but that was—You know, he felt like he had to like walk a chalk line until he got his green card, which is, you know, the permanent visa. And he felt very much more at ease once he got that, that nothing could be held over his head cause they were, you're not doing your job here, you know, go back to [country of origin] or something."

I commented that the issue of call schedules can be an important issue for physicians, and she said, "It was terrible for [this IMG]. And I think this was one of the times that he got burned from not knowing how things worked. And I always tried to tell him, this is how it works. But he was very meek in the beginning, so nice. And he still—He just had that—He leans towards not making a fuss, you know. I'm not sure why that was. He didn't want to be seen as somebody who rocked the boat too much, he just wasn't sure how things went. But he would—He probably took up the job of doing the scheduling for his call group, and several people in the call group were extremely uncooperative. And what he would do was he would always take up the slack. He would like work the inconvenient times, work the times nobody else wanted. Remember, they didn't get any more money for taking call. They would have this horrific weekend call schedule, they would be on call twenty-four hours a day, Friday, Saturday, and Sunday. And then he was expected to show up in the office on Monday. And I used to say, [name of IMG], the docs out in the clinics, I mean, in their office, they don't do what you do. They're on call the night before, they either work a half-day and they're gone, or they don't work. They got to get some time back. And you guys need to talk about that. Cause he was like dead on his feet. And he'd say, well, no, I don't seem to be able to do anything about it. But he would like not rock the boat. Their call schedule was extremely demanding. He would often work and come all day and work, and it was like—It was a killer, I don't how he did it, to tell you the truth. And he would always work the holidays cause nobody else wanted to work, and so he would like work the holidays, he did it all. So I guess he learned—I'm sure that he has learned things from his bad experiences to take to his new job, and he won't be dealing with the same kind of stuff there."

She explained further, "You know, he would typically have eight to ten internal medicine patients, probably on an average, in the hospital unless he'd been on vacation or something. And that's a pretty heavy load. And they are very sick, of course. Internal medicine patients who have migrated to the hospital are like big train wrecks. And so he would go start to make rounds about—probably about eight, eight-thirty, and to do the rounds and the kind of stuff that he did, and sometimes he did stress tests too, he could never be at the office before noon time, and he would start working then. But the guy that I was telling you about, he wanted him to be there by nine-thirty or ten, and he didn't care if it meant that he had to go to the hospital at six-thirty or seven o'clock, that's what private people did. But private people were making a lot more bucks than he was. And he gave him grief about that all the time, all the time. And he would be making remarks to the office about it, and it was a continuing problem. And [name of IMG] probably could have stood up for it a little bit better, you know. He just—He wasn't assertive enough I think out of just not wanting to cause a fuss. He would just let it roll over, you know."

As indicated in the above example, waiver physicians do face some of the same constraints as other physicians, such as pressure to generate productivity. However, waiver physicians can be more vulnerable to the demands of administrators, simply because it can be a precarious situation to be on a J-1 visa waiver. Even if the IMG has the ability to resist excessive demands on his time, there can be a sense that causing trouble can lead to revocation of the waiver. Adding to such difficulty, some individuals might simply be more passive in dealing with confrontation; there might also be cultural differences that impact whether or not one person stands up to another.

A blatant example of mistreatment was mentioned in other interviews. This time, however, the physician was not on a waiver while facing even stronger pressures from his employer.

ALLEGATIONS OF MISTREATMENT

Allegations of the mistreatment of an IMG surfaced in multiple interviews with members of the medical community. In discussing this sensitive issue, I want to reemphasize that my interest is in perceptions, rather than investigative journalism. Perceptions toward an allegation of mistreatment are important in understanding further the acceptance of the individual IMG, and IMGs in general. An IMG of Asian Indian origin who used to be on a waiver told me that he has heard about the mistreatment of waiver physicians. However, the discussion led to consideration of the experiences of a non-waiver physician in Hamilton:

> I have seen it happen to people. Mostly I couldn't say I faced it much. I might have had kind of certain, you know, assessments where they thought that maybe he would really not ask for more maybe, you know, but I've seen people really being almost like a bonded person. I've seen a doctor who was not even a J-1, he was an H-1 [which allows for application for a green card], and he had—It was almost like as if he was being traded by one doctor to the other for a price, and this one wouldn't know what he—what the compensatory, you know, actions were. But there is a fellow Indian colleague who has been through this. He is still with us in the area. Luckily for him, he was rescued by a group, which I would say is essentially a group of white doctors. They helped him out of that situation. Although, the other doctors who were dealing with him were also white guys. [laughs]

The precise accusations that surfaced in these interviews focused on contractual obligations that led to an unfair workload and unfair pay. In the words of another IMG in Hamilton, "It is well known, everybody knows about it."

The IMG may have signed an unfavorable contract without any understanding that he might be mistreated. As explained by a social worker: "Well, the one incident I'm talking about is where a doctor came and did not know the other doctor well enough, his reputation here was not that great anyway."

"The other doctor?" I asked.

"The other doctor. Okay? So then he came into a situation where the other doctor probably wanted him to do most of the work, but yet he got the pay because he owned the office and already had established the business. And this foreign doctor ended up—In a way, it's sort of like a slave to him."

The conversation continued, and I asked, "Do you think the way he was treated had anything to do with the fact that he was a foreign physician?"

"I think maybe because [he's] a little naïve when he came here I don't—from that particular doctor that was treating [name of IMG] the way he was, he would treat me and you that way too probably. Okay? So I don't think it's a—I think if you're naïve—I'm naïve, he'd certainly have taken advantage of me probably before I realized what was happening."

Certainly, anyone in virtually any profession can have employers who make unfair demands. The naïveté of an employee, combined with uneven power relations, can be key issues affecting a new IMG's experience. Being unfamiliar with some of the ways that employers might mistreat their workers can be a major problem for IMGs who are relatively new to working in the United States. Then again, anyone who mistreats an employee has to contend with word of mouth that, in a rural area, can be damaging professionally and personally. The social worker continued:

> I think our town will embrace—our community will embrace [the IMG] against this other doctor. He's more the outsider cause he's from probably up in another state, like up North somewhere. And they will embrace [the IMG], they will not embrace this other guy.

I did not mention these accusations of mistreatment to the IMG when he was interviewed. Instead, I was much more interested in knowing simply his perceptions about what it was like to practice in Hamilton. He told me that he has practiced or studied medicine in three different continents. Prior to leaving his first Hamilton job, his wife had a premature baby. His words about uncertainty stayed in my thoughts long after the interview:

"It is tough, being professionally—being professionally satisfied and to do the best we can itself is a challenge. On top of the other issues which we have no control of. . . . Particularly in my case, I mean, because I moved from another country to here, so it's kind of a second migration to me." He continued, "I hate the word *uncertainty*. [laughs] You know, unfortunately I have to live with it. And I really sincerely want to get that out of my head. It's bugging me now."

"The uncertainty?" I asked.

"The uncertainty."

"What is uncertain?"

"About this visas and, you know, what if this doesn't work, or what if— You know, to find another place and to go through the square one. So I was in fact joking to my wife, perhaps we haven't seen a couple of other continents. [laughs] Wherever there is a continent with an entrance exam, perhaps we should go."

RETENTION

In its simplest conceptualization, retention could be considered a bellwether for acceptability. Simply put, people might stay longer in a place if they feel like they belong there. Of course, people also move for many reasons besides acceptance. As with any job, people might move because of better opportunities elsewhere, family situations, personal conflicts, or any number of explanations that were mentioned by participants in Delano County.

Retention as a Justification for Exclusion

Consider a conversation that I had in the hospital with a physician who did not want to hire an IMG for an opening in his practice. He told me:

"In my group one of my partners categorically just doesn't want to hear about foreign medical graduates, or international medical graduates, because there's enough out there who have regional ties to the area, better chance of retention, without considering the international. Of the three of us I'm probably more open than they are to screening internationals." As we talked, he explained further, "Well, we only see those that [the hospital recruiter] has sifted through. And I think he knows one of my partner's views on international graduates and simply, you know, doesn't pass forward those at all. The other part of that was we've had a fourth doctor a couple of times, right out of school. They stay a couple of years and their spouse drags them away. So, the match we're looking for begins with somebody who's got ties to the area, either by spouse or by training, or by themselves some roots in the area or their parents or some way of nailing down their foot to the floor and more likely to keep them for the rest of their career here. And that pretty much—That alone, pretty much closes the door on international graduates."

When asked to define who would have a strong enough attachment to the area to be recruited to his practice, the physician said that he means people who already have strong ties to the state or to a neighboring state.

In essence, the physician has constructed a boundary. On one side stand people who *belong* to the area. On another side stand people who do not have any strong connection with the state or local area, and hence who are perceived to be more likely to leave. Through his group's decision not to hire IMGs, the boundary is now impossible to cross, at least in his practice.

Several other participants also raised the idea that IMGs might be less committed than U.S. medical graduates to long-term practice in Delano County. For example, a nurse practitioner told me that he also thinks it is best to recruit health providers who have an attachment to the local area or to rural areas:

> In an ideal situation, you get your best outcome as far as recruiting and retaining health care providers if they are indigenous to the area, if they're from that local area. And I—Just in the seven years that I've been here, I've seen the revolving door where health care providers, and not just internationally trained health care providers, but people who are just not from rural areas, come in and they do their time and they're gone.

Hence, a fuller picture emerges in which the boundary between newcomers and outsiders is also drawn through rural life. People who grew up in areas similar to where they are practicing might stay longer; people who grew up in urban areas might prefer practicing in urban areas. However, such a demarcation says little about IMGs who grew up or lived in rural areas in other countries. "Rural" in one country might not necessarily be considered "rural" in another. Furthermore, urban areas in many less developed countries may actually have a rural feel in some places, so it becomes difficult to make categorical statements about the rural backgrounds of IMGs. In addition, concerns about the spouse's happiness, employment opportunities, leisure activities, shopping, and quality of schools are among other possible influences on physician retention in this and other places in the rural United States (Crandall et al., 1990).

Perceptions on the Retention of Waiver Physicians

Legal obligations form another concern for retention, according to an IMG:

> You want people who are committed to stay. They get their loan fixed, they spend two or three years and then somebody else comes in. There's no con-

> tinuation of care. Where is that feeling that my physician knows me? Okay, this guy is going to stop for few days and leave. There isn't that commitment from the physician cause they know they're leaving. And I'm just here for my J-1, I'm just here for whatever. You need people that are willing to stay in this community, that are willing to commit themselves in this community.

It is not clear that, simply by having a J-1 visa waiver, a physician will establish only short-term ties to the area. In fact, there are examples already in Delano County of former waiver physicians who appear to be staying over the long-term. Of course, there are also examples of IMGs who have left their jobs. Because of individual and cultural differences in behavior, IMGs who come from different countries and cultures will probably not respond identically to the J-1 visa waiver by leaving or staying en masse. Furthermore, it is not simply the physicians or their families who are responsible for mobility, but their *employers* as well.

A waiver physician reflected on problems with retention, not necessarily limited to Delano County:

> I don't think it's the people, the physicians who are making the mistakes. I think it's the institutions who have hired them are making the mistakes. If they would make more attractive to them to stay, I think people will stay. But if you're rigid and you think that you've got to stay for three years, pay them two thirds of what you would pay an American graduate, and keep them, and you can hope that you'll find another one, you can let that person go. You can work somewhere else and you find somebody else. And that's what happens. That's what I think the philosophy is unfortunately. And they're strapped for cash too, you can—a federally funded clinic can't pay a doctor similar to private practice because their populations are restricted to other—to less monetary gain and more—insurance is different and whatnot. There's just too many things going on. So obviously they have a unit that they're trying to run on limited resources, so maybe they can't afford to pay as much. So then when the choice comes for the physician, they kept their promise for three years, now they can make a choice of going somewhere else, they leave and they go somewhere else.

Explaining further, he said that there are IMGs "who come into the community with probably initially one goal in mind, to get that green card, and then after that goal is met, they have that choice, so they go up probably to the hospital administrator or their job provider and say hey, I have a choice now. [laughs]" The IMG, who is on a waiver, told me about how fond he was of the area, and that physicians who moved there by choice might stay longer than others:

"I like it. I love it, up til now. Because—the problem is that initially people don't want to make that first step and first move. They'll come here, they'll look around, and they'll say, hey, the biggest store is WalMart, and the only grocery store is Food Lion, and there's no private schools. And I look at San Diego, there's everything, I have a job there, I have a job here, which should I take? I didn't have a choice initially, so I came down here, but I like it. Maybe if I had the choice, I wouldn't have come. You understand that?"

I told him yes.

"Give any human a choice, they'll try to see what's best for them and they will take that," he said. "And unfortunately places like this will keep on suffering because they just don't provide that attractive influence for people. So that's the main reason that's stopping people from coming here and staying here. People who've made the choice, have stayed here, but they've kept it for two or three years, you've got people working here for fifteen, twenty years, without a problem. And they're from Canada and whatnot, and they like it, because they took the choice, they lived here, and now they like it to an extent that this is their home."

Whether or not IMGs tend to be less rooted than other physicians in Delano County is a matter of perspective. Among other possibilities, retention could be studied in relation to the J-1 visa waiver, or on an individual or collective basis, or through differences by institution. In addition, retention can be influenced by call schedules, peer contact, financial incentives, affinity with rural practice sites, or requirements to practice for a certain timeframe in an underserved area (Crandall et al., 1990).

A Few Contradictory Perceptions on Retention

A plethora of cultural and social issues makes the task of understanding retention even more complicated. For example, an IMG of Asian Indian origin explained about the lack of mobility among people from India:

> At least I speak for graduates from India, I can't speak for the rest of the world. But most Indians form roots really fast, and we're not a transient kind of population. If you find most of us will be in one area for a really long time. We build roots really quickly, and once we build those, they kind of remain, you know, you remain rooted to that area for a really long time. You won't find a lot of Indians moving house very frequently. It's just . . . you know, it's just that once you enter into a community, you by and large stay there. And I think that's one of the biggest advantages which international medical graduates offer, at least as far as Indians are concerned. I'd say some of the other Asian groups too, that wherever you go, you tend to set roots really quickly and . . . that's one of the major problems, is providing continuity of care to patients. I like to think that fifteen years from now I can see the next generation of the patients I'm seeing and we'll be following them up too, you

know, and just . . . give them more one-on-one kind of approach. And I think that's something which doesn't get quite there with people who are forced to form, you know, who are trying to pay off their debts and they're in that area because of that reason.

Another IMG of Asian Indian origin viewed mobility differently through his own family's experiences:

"So basically, my great-grandfather moved from one place to other in India. My father moved, he didn't stay in his hometown, he moved to a bigger city. And then I didn't stay where I was born, I moved too, so it's pattern. It's kind of a constant trend."

This was a different view of retention than I had just heard in the previous interview so I asked if people from India might be less mobile.

"No, in fact I would expect more mobility there. It may be more from a case to case basis. . . . But in general, the trend is from rural to urban to a bigger urban, kind of an upward move towards urban. And maybe going abroad after that if, you know, possible. Upward doesn't necessarily mean America, it means many other countries. But it's a process going on in many families."

Beyond rural-to-urban-to-international migration, a reason why these statements might contradict one another is that India is a complicated place; like anywhere, two people are likely to view their own country or even their own city through different perspectives. In slightly different terms, two people could view the same *person* differently; similarly, multifaceted identities could be used in describing a *place*. These and other perceptions toward India can be relevant considerations behind people's attitudes about the retention of IMGs in Delano County. In addition, there are individuals, organizations, and state and federal laws that complicate the issue of retention even further.

To show another side to retention, consider the following statement from a U.S. medical graduate regarding the race of IMGs:

White people leave. [laughs] They do. I'll give you one good example. There are two IMGs, FMGs really. I guess you call them, or foreign medical graduates, one is white from like some Russian based country, girlfriend is white, purely white, and the other one is Indian, and his wife is Filipino. So you have the Asians and whites, and both are FMGs. They both came here at the same time, brought here by the hospital, had thriving practices, and they both really kind of liked the area. And when their contract was up, the Indian guy stayed, the white guy left. And why did the white guy leave? His girlfriend thought this place was not cosmopolitan enough for her, and because he was white. And you know where he went? Maine. Good God! You know—But she—I had talked to her,

> and she just couldn't make it in this town. You know, not enough theater, not enough whatever. So white people can leave.

Actually, the IMG did not move to Maine but to another state in New England, and he was one of the waiver physicians discussed earlier. Nonetheless, the physician quoted above perceived that nonwhite IMGs from Asia might be more likely to stay than are white IMGs from Europe.

This next example will contradict the previous statement that IMGs who are from Asian countries are sedentary in their practice locations. An IMG from South Asia told me about the importance of family toward his retention in the area:

> What happens, Lenny, is that when people are trying to look for that job, they're looking at a long term goal of possibly—for different people it's different, I might not stay in the U.S. for more than ten years. I might decide to go back to [country in South Asia]. And there would be family reasons, children growing up, I want them to grow up like [people from the South Asian country] rather than Americans, or whatnot, my parents are aging in [country in South Asia], things could change for them. If the situation is good enough and I can find a job, sure, I will go back.

Again, as shown twice now about physicians from South Asia, examples can have counter-examples. Therefore, it becomes difficult to make a generalization even about people from the same world region; there is cultural complexity, regional diversity, and individuality that further complicate the issue of retention. Nonetheless, people also form perceptions toward heterogeneous groups such as IMGs, and make statements that serve to categorize people easily.

Favorable Perceptions on Retention

Certainly, the issue of retention is considerably more complicated than in Quincy, where it was rare for any IMGs to leave. Many of the concerns in Delano County focused on retaining IMGs over the long-term. At the same time, IMGs in Delano County have also earned a reputation among some members of the medical community for having staying power. In the words of a U.S. medical graduate:

> We tend to have a higher retention value with the foreign medical graduates than we do with U.S. graduates. Now it may be because their opportunities are more limited and they're not gonna be wooed away by better offers or more competitive towns. But the FMGs do tend to stick it out. They tend to stay once they get here and get their practice established, and they're very busy. I mean, in this town they have full practices, to my knowledge.

Another U.S. medical graduate expressed a similar sentiment about IMGs:

> From the ones that I've seen, they try very hard to fit in, and I think probably do a pretty good job of doing that. A lot of them who come, I find, sometimes have been from diverse backgrounds themselves, and not all of them have necessarily been on the higher socioeconomic status, so I guess they realize the difficulty in getting some jobs and opportunities, so they work very, very, very hard to find them, you know, to fit in. Whereas a lot of the American grads, they know they're marketable other places, so they say, the hell with it, I'm out of here, I'm going somewhere else. They don't realize this has to be the only stop, I mean, this is the only stop. Whereas see, with the foreign grads they try hard to blend and to make where they land home. They try real hard. Sometimes they're successful and sometimes they aren't.

IMGs appeared to be cosmopolitan in the sense of coming from so many different places and having variability in terms of their interests, ideas, and thoughts about the future. The future often looked very bright for long-term practice in the area, especially when I was talking with an IMG from Southeast Asia working at a large group practice. He used to be on a J-1 visa waiver, and told me that he was fortunate to have such a good practice opportunity:

> Hamilton is close, reasonably close to bigger metropolitan areas, like, you know, [names of places in the state]. And very few—That's, you know, for the geographic part. For the professional part, very few underserved areas are going to have practices like this in which you take call once a week, you have midlevel working with you at night, taking first call, and having several days off. You know, working only four days a week and doing all these other things, other perks. Most of my colleagues in underserved areas are either on every day call, every other day call. They're lucky if they go on every third night call. I think it's going to be very hard to attract National Health Scholars or loan repayment people to these sites. This place in particular is able to attract people from Johns Hopkins, from the powerhouse programs, because it's a very livable practice. You know, you're not carrying the beeper twenty-four hours a day, seven days a week. You actually pass on your pager and you don't have to worry about holding on to the pager until a week later. So professionally speaking, this is a very good place to be, even for a non-IMG, even for a non—Yeah, even for a non-IMG.

In a nearby small town, I interviewed an IMG who told me that she was tired of moving. She went to medical school in her home country, practiced medicine briefly, and moved to Texas where she worked in a health care related job, took her medical exams, and applied for residency programs. Then she moved to Chicago where she did her residency, and then moved to

Hamilton. Meanwhile, she and her husband did not live in all of the same places; now they are together living in Hamilton and, after a year, still working on unpacking boxes. As the IMG explained:

> Actually right now I don't think I'm moving because I—moving, it was very stressful and I have not even finished unpacking, [laughs] so . . . it has to be a very big enticement, you know, somebody has to really entice me with a big benefit and all that, you know, to have to make me move my whole family again. Well, it's hard to approach yourself, your family, like if you have made friends, you have known the people around, you know, it's just like starting all over again, you know. I mean, there has to be something very compelling to want to make you to do that. So like, I'm really getting—like I say, I've just been here one year. I'm getting comfortable here, so, knowing the people, and knowing my way around. So it's going to be difficult for me to move, even though I've just stayed here for a little over a year, I don't foresee that, but for me to be able to move it's going to take a lot of [laughs]—a lot to move me, that's right.

The fact that there are so many opposing and complementary perspectives on retention is revealing about acceptability. There simply are no easy clues to categorize who feels a greater sense of belonging. On one extreme, some physicians are less open to hiring IMGs because of perceived problems with retention; on another extreme, IMGs have earned a reputation for staying put.

COMPETITION

A concern expressed in policy circles is that IMGs are taking away jobs that otherwise might go to U.S. medical graduates. Perhaps because Delano County is medically needy, concerns about IMGs trespassing onto the turf of U.S. medical graduates surfaced on only a few occasions. A community member talked about the influx of IMGs to the area:

> The only thing I can relate it to is what's happened to like our textile industries here. We had a very fine textile industry in this country til it all went offshore, and now it's benefiting Mexico, but our people have been hurt. This is not true everywhere, but it is true in here. It has hurt us here, our jobs were given to foreign countries. If bringing more—increasing the number and bringing more foreign doctors in here eliminates jobs for our own, you know, I don't know how to make those kinds of decisions. But I don't know the numbers. Maybe by increasing—Maybe we still have such a need for physicians, maybe by having more foreign doctors maybe it doesn't eliminate American jobs, I don't know, you know.

Another community member who recalled a *60 Minutes* report on IMGs took a different standpoint on the issue of competition:

> From my understanding, they're not interfering with their space, they are here way out here in the boondocks somewhere where people—All out in Texas and all over. So what do you do, just leave these people? They have to go—Anything can happen and then you have to get somebody a hundred miles away before you can get to the first doctor? Only thing, I'm like the state—Okay, and even if you made it more appealing, American doctors still might not want to go into these rural areas.

A U.S. medical graduate who is active in recruitment raised similar points about IMGs going to areas that have physician shortages:

> A foreign graduate is probably more likely to come to an unappealing area because they just want a job. Our American graduates are much pickier about where they're going to go, and they want to go to a place that has a good standard of living, that's a pretty place, that there's a lot of things to do, that has good schools, that has—a community that has a great deal to offer. And not all communities meet those standards, so consequently, the ones who don't, have trouble recruiting. And when you have trouble recruiting, you're going to probably get a less desirable group of people. We've tried to react to that by making this a much more desirable place to work and give them great call schedules and good benefits. We can't pay them any more than they'd get anywhere else, but they have a life if they work here. And that's how we attempt our recruiting, but for a lot of them—There's a surgical practice in town that's been recruiting forever and they can't get anybody to join them, and they don't understand why. And the reason they can't is because you're not coming to a great place, you've got to have something to offset it. Those guys go to work at five o'clock in the morning and work til ten or eleven every night. You know, somebody can go anywhere and work like that."

A premise for the argument that IMGs are taking away jobs from U.S. medical graduates is that there are not enough jobs for physicians who otherwise would come here. The issue of whether to hire new physicians can be controversial, even without considering IMGs in particular. The hospital recruiter told me that it can be difficult to persuade physicians that there is a need for hiring more people from a particular specialty; some physicians worry about new competition. He explained that, with input from the medical staff, an outside consultant makes recommendations about which specialties need to be hired. With a written report supporting the need to hire particular specialties, it is more difficult for physicians to say that recruitment is not needed.

Many of the medical practices are so busy that they are not taking new patients. For example, an IMG of Asian Indian origin told me, "We have one of the few practices, well, actually the only practice at the moment accepting new patients, so we have a wide variety of patients coming through." She works in a two-person practice with her husband, another IMG. The two physicians appear to be filling a need for services that otherwise might not be filled. At the same time, it is easy to sense that a practice can grow and become popular through word of mouth and patient satisfaction. She continued:

> We came at a time where other practices were closing the door. And our biggest—you know, we advertise three times a week faithfully, we advertise in the yellow pages, but you know our biggest source of referrals is our own patient load. Not even other doctors. We have generations of families coming here. You know, like I have a great-grandmother all the way down to the great-grandchild. And it's not just one family. It's many families that do that. [laughs] You know. So I'm rewarded that way. I like that. I'd rather they came that way. You know, I really found a good doctor, I like what she does, go see her. Versus, oh yeah, I saw your ad in the yellow pages and I picked out, you know, just because your ad hit my eye better than the others did, you know. To me it's more rewarding.

In attracting new patients based on word of mouth and advertisements, it could be argued that these two IMGs are actually competing with other physicians for patients. A physician assistant at a clinic in a nearby small town told me that he was concerned that competition with IMGs could eventually cost him his job. I asked him if he thought he would still be practicing in the area in ten or fifteen years. Here is how he replied:

> I hope so. But I worry about the hospital bringing a new grad or an FMG in here who's willing to work for less money than an established physician, but a little more money than I do. He can establish himself and then move on because he or his family don't find living in this small community appealing. He might even live somewhere else and commute. That would not make him a part of this community like I've tried to do. You know, it's interesting that you contacted me about this. Every day I worry about someone taking my place, so I try to do a better job. It's always an ongoing thing. It's a matter of economics for the hospital, a matter of economics for everybody.

I asked, "Do you worry about that specifically with regard to the international medical graduates or —"

> Well, it seems that an FMG would be willing to get started anywhere and then move on. I chose to take on the role of a family practitioner and to me that means being a part of the community you live in. At least to me it does. So I'm concerned

that whoever takes my place is not going to do as well as I do, he's not going to do it with the feeling I do about these people. But nobody cares about that but me.

There appears to be a fine line between competition for jobs and providing care that reduces underservice. The wife of a U.S. medical graduate explained to me that it was an asset to have an IMG in the same subspecialty as her husband:

I think it would be very lonely to be the only GI doctor in the community, or the only pulmonologist in a community cause you don't have anybody else to consult, or to even run something by. And how litigious our society is, lots of times it's a lot easier for them to pick up the phone and say, this is what I've got, and this is what I'm going to do, what do you think?

Some health providers might instinctively protect their own turf. This attitude of protectionism surfaced in an interview with an IMG of Asian Indian origin. He claimed that the hospital favors hiring U.S. medical graduates over IMGs, and said that he would do the same thing in India. I asked him why he would give physicians from other countries a hard time. "Because you think they're going to take your opportunity," he said.

I found no indication that the hospital favors hiring U.S. medical graduates over IMGs, although his assertion indicates that such issues may still surface in hospital politics. His rationale for giving others a hard time in India seems consistent with the original exclusion of IMGs from the hospital. It is as though there is an aftertaste from the original exclusion of IMGs that still lingered, even if the IMG did not experience such exclusion in Hamilton firsthand.

A few participants expressed a concern that, with more and more IMGs coming into the area, there might be less room for U.S. medical graduates. A lawyer who works closely with the hospital told me that he was concerned about the influx of IMGs:

The more international physicians we have may create a physician community that would militate against attracting white physicians here, because of the makeup of the medical community, because they may not want to socialize with international physicians. And it may be, you know, if that medical community that's been here forever, I guess, dwindles and decreases in size, my guess is they're going to have more trouble attracting those physicians to come to Hamilton.

A U.S. medical graduate, who had been practicing in Hamilton before the arrival of the first IMGs, expressed far greater concern about the influx of IMGs. The physician explained to me:

It was good at one time because they filled a gap when we needed physicians. Now, they're building up their own little clique of foreign medical graduates so

> the American medical doctors are not coming in. So when they fill up the town and get their group, their nephews and cousins and uncles to come over here and practice with them, that closes the town out for the American doctors to come in and practice. So in that regime, I feel that it is not good."

"When did it stop being an asset to have the international medical graduates here?" I asked.

"Oh, I would think in just the last two or three years when they got so many of them to come in."

The last two or three years was the same time period that saw the hiring of the first waiver physicians; i.e., IMGs hired specifically to help reduce underservice.

We talked further, and I said, "So ideally if an area is to have international medical graduates, it would be best to have only a small percentage, is that right?" He responded: "But you can't control things like that. You'll never be able to control that. You might say it, you might think it, but you can't control it in any way possible. And that's what happened to the foreign medical graduates, just one or two came, but they brought one or two more, and then one or two more, and then one or two more. And now we've got what, fifteen or twenty or twenty-five of them here?"

I asked if a town should resist hiring IMGs in order to prevent a future influx.

"Well, that's hard to do too. It's hard to control that part of it. As long as they have a state license in [the state] they can practice anywhere they want to in the state. You can't tell them they can't practice, see. And you can't keep them out of the hospital, particularly if they have their boards, and most of them do." He went on to say, "We don't need them anymore, we've trained enough. And those doctors really ought to go back to their own countries and help their own people. You know, we have plenty over here, they need to go back where they're needed, but they don't do that. But they should. And it'd be better for their people and their country if they did. They could go back to India or South Africa or Guatemala and be the best trained physician in the country in whatever they're doing, cause they're American trained."

APPRECIATION FOR INTERNATIONAL MEDICAL GRADUATES

Appreciation is an event that is deeply interwoven with acceptability, and it can be difficult to discuss one without discussing the other. The same mechanisms behind acceptability also influence appreciation (e.g., retention, the role of pioneer IMGs, the role of the hospital). However, for the sake of this discussion, acceptability can be viewed on a broader sociological level; that is, acceptability of a group, whereas appreciation often takes place on a more individual basis.

Some of the appreciation for individual, pioneer IMGs has already been discussed, but additional comments from patients, physicians, and medical staff can show even further the extent of appreciation. For example, while looking at a bulletin board in the hospital, I saw the IMG pulmonologist's name with the word "winner" next to it. It was a "TLC" award from the hospital reflecting his treatment of patients. I talked about that with him. In our conversation, he added that he had been the first IMG to win an award from the local newspaper, which conducts an annual survey to determine the best doctors. "That was about three, four years ago," he said. "I was second on the list of the best three doctors. Best liked by the patients, not best doctor, but the most liked by patients."

A patient in Berry told me about her "love" for the IMG pulmonologist and his partner. Referring to the IMG pulmonologist, she said:

> When I go there, which I have to do blood work real often because of I'm on a blood thinner, and it's unreal to see—And of all races, all races too. And seemly there—I can hear him down the hall, and he's just as kind to one race as they are another one. In fact, we sort of have a hugging relationship. [laughs] Dr. [name] said, '[Name], you are old enough to be my mother.' I said, 'Well, good, son, I'll take care of you.' You know, it's that sort of relationship. Then if I stay out a long time and not go back. 'I was wondering if you were coming back to be my patient.' I haven't needed you, Dr. [name]. [laughs]

In a similar vein, an IMG from sub-Saharan Africa who practices in a nearby small town told me about the appreciativeness of her patients for her work:

> Actually they were very appreciative and they would ask me, I hope you're gonna stay, or how long do you plan to stay, you know. Are you liking it here? they keep asking me. . . . When I go to the post office in [the small town] I'm bound to run into one or more of my patients. This afternoon I ran into one of them, said, are you not my doctor? I said, yes, I'm your doctor. She came and gave me a hug, you know. [laughs]

The appreciation for individual IMGs came across as deep and heartfelt. A few weeks before quitting his practice in another nearby small town, a waiver physician said: "Now that I'm leaving, everybody comes and said, I'm sorry you are leaving. Some are crying, some are not crying, but saying that hopefully it doesn't work out for you up there so you can return back."

Later, the nurse practitioner who had worked alongside him told me about patients' reactions to his departure:

> There were patients when he left that were crying, sending him roses, cooking him cakes, pie. I mean, honestly. They loved him. Because as he sort of got used to what it was that it was going to take to communicate in there, he just fit perfect. He would sit down and talk to the patients and be very calm, take much time with elderly patients, which is what a lot of his patients were, and take the time to talk to them and try to understand them, which is not always available, and they loved that. They loved that man. I'm not lying, they just like—People were just like crying out in the halls. It was pitiful actually. And it's all very sad.

A senior citizen who had never been to an IMG before told me about accompanying her husband to see a general internist at a large medical clinic in Hamilton. The physician who took care of her husband was from Pakistan and has only been practicing in the area for a few years. She told me:

> And I thought that he was just god-sent. And I'm sure his god was not my god. [laughs] But I just was just so pleased with him. In fact, if it wasn't a hassle, I would like for him to be my own physician, but of course, when you're in a clinic, you stay with whom you're with unless you've got very extenuating circumstances for changing. So I'm happy with the one I'm with, who is Dr. [name of a U.S. medical graduate]. But I would really recommend him to anybody who is looking for a new doctor because I just thought he was just one of the most compassionate people, I just can't say enough nice things about him.

Some of the most glowing praise was reserved for an IMG pediatrician from the Philippines who has been practicing at another major medical clinic in the area. A community member in Hamilton said: "There's eight or ten or 12 pediatricians in one group, he's probably as loved or the most loved pediatrician there. He has a wonderful following. He is just very kind. And I talked with a new mother yesterday, as a matter of fact, with a week old baby, and she was real thrilled that she was allowed to—she was going to be able to see this gentleman, cause he has that kind of a following."

A U.S. medical graduate who leads the group practice at the pediatric clinic also spoke in glowing terms about the IMG of Filipino origin: "Everybody in this office immediately fell in love with him, patients, staff, everybody. They think he is absolutely—One of the girls told me the other day, I don't see why you don't quit recruiting, and just throw Dr. [name] in the copy machine. Said, if we could just get some more like him, wouldn't it be wonderful?"

The above comments are testimony to the extent of appreciation that has been achieved by individual IMGs in Delano County. An obvious implication of such praise is the role of the individual in furthering the collective acceptability of

IMGs. A handful of IMGs emerged as some of the most frequently praised physicians in the area. Exactly what causes such appreciation is another issue and can be explored more deeply by examining another related issue, trust.

TRUST IN INTERNATIONAL MEDICAL GRADUATES

A few participants talked of their trust in some providers who were born and raised in the local area. This was especially evident in Berry, which is predominantly Native American. Participants there talked of a special bond or connection with people who have a family history in the local area. A Native American physician explained:

"You know, my parents have good standing in this community, so there's a certain trust I came in with just because my mom and dad—I mean, I may be a terrible person, but because my mom and dad have a good standing there's a certain amount of trust I will have automatically. Unless I break the trust. Right? So that's that difference between maybe somebody who's coming in as an outsider or foreign graduate."

"And if you were to practice in Hamilton, would you have some of these advantages?" I asked.

"I'd have some," he replied. "I wouldn't have as many. [laughs] Hamilton's a different place."

A university student who was born and raised in Berry added her own thoughts about trust in local providers:

> Just say a doctor does, like you said, come from [a local neighborhood] and go through—become a doctor, and people have known him through school, they know him personally. And if he practices here they already know if—They've known him for ten years. They're going to be more open to go to him than somebody they've never seen in their whole life. . . . And somebody that they've never seen or doesn't know their background or where they come from, they don't know what to think about that person. Cause my mom told me yesterday that a European physician, they—I don't know if it's true or not, but they said that there was a European physician that had killed like over a hundred women by giving them heroin, overdoses of heroin. And somebody like that could come into our community and set up a practice and do that and nobody ever know. I mean, until it starts happening, nobody ever know that that's his main objective or, you know, what he's here for. So that would scare me to just to be that open and say, here, my life is in your hands, if I don't know you, than to somebody I've known twenty years.

Such statements need to be balanced against the fact that newcomers can establish trust as physicians. It is unknown how easy it would be for an IMG to base a livelihood on practice in Berry. No IMGs practiced in Berry except for one on a rotating basis who worked for a multi-site community health center. In Hamilton and other parts of Delano County, I learned that IMGs often need to establish trust as physicians upon arrival in the local area. In the words of a pioneer IMG:

"You know, people just want to be sure they'll treat me like everybody, somebody from locally. I think there are more kind of immediate trust on the local guy. He's our guy. He'll take good care of us. But as time goes on they'll realize that it doesn't matter. But once you get over those feelings for each other, then trust is automatically building."

Similarly, a nurse practitioner who has worked closely with IMGs emphasized the importance of the individual in establishing trust:

> I think that the trust comes from the one-to-one hookup, wherever the person comes from, and I think that that's exactly where it happens from the beginning, and doesn't have anything to do with anything else I don't think. I know the initial appearance, you know, may turn some people off for whatever reason, but if—You know, if you get that one-to-one communication right the first time or the second time, it's like a done deal. You earn that trust, you don't like get it just by who you are or what you look like.

An IMG of Asian Indian origin also underscored the role of the individual physician in establishing trust. At the same time, being perceived to be an outsider might actually be an asset. In his words: "To some extent some patients have actually come and told me that they trust me more than the previous doctor or the other doctor or whatever. So sometimes I think it's again person to person depending on what the doctor does."

In thinking about the above comment, I wondered whether it might be easier for some patients to confide in IMGs. The IMG responded:

> See, in a small town like Hamilton, a lot of things can be—You know, you can learn a lot from the gossip line, which may not necessarily be true. And certain things some people know that we're not going to meet with certain people and talk with them and tell them about this. So yes, it is easier for them to confide in me maybe sometimes even more than they would to their pastor. For the mere fact that I'm not trying to control their lives, but I'm just a vent, and may just, you know, give an objective answer to them what to do.

Building on the IMG's comments, a possibility is that patients may have greater confidence in someone who is an outsider. A few participants even told me that they prefer to have a physician who does not know their family. The issue of confiding information to an outsider was rarely mentioned by participants despite ample opportunity in discussing the issue of trust. Then again, except for the above example, I did not probe to find out whether patients might confide more sensitive, personal information to IMGs than to U.S. medical graduates.

Organizational Trust

At the same time that the individual influences trust, trust in a physician can also be achieved on an organizational level. For example, patients may have trust in the organization that hired an IMG. As a result, some patients who otherwise might not want to see an IMG would trust that the organization makes good hiring decisions; by extension, a newly hired IMG would be accepted more quickly as part of an established clinic or center. It may or may not be a coincidence that organizational trust surfaced only in interviews with older community members in the white community. A senior citizen shared with me her thoughts about trust in any IMGs who join an established practice:

"If they were a member of an established firm, I would expect that firm to have done all of the credential checking and I would feel very confident with anyone they brought into an established firm. I might have a problem with a doctor who is in independent practice, without knowing something about him. I would really want to know something about him before I went to him as a patient. But I would feel different with an established firm." A little later in conversation, she added, "I know anyone who comes without the sanction of the established medical society will not do very well, and so my advice is either to join a firm or make sure you have established yourself within the medical community. Because it does seem—I won't say it's a closed society, but it's certainly one that looks after its own, and protects its own, and you need to be a part of the circle."

She then tempered her remarks by saying that she may be speaking for how things used to be ten or fifteen years ago when she worked for a health insurance company. Nonetheless, the point that she was making about organizational trust foreshadowed other comments by participants about trust in a clinic that hired an IMG from Pakistan. For example, another senior citizen told me about an experience in which her regular doctor at the clinic was not available, and she ended up seeing the Pakistani IMG. She explained that she had "faith in that clinic."

A U.S. medical graduate also mentioned the same IMG:

> The young man that I mentioned to you who everybody is so fond of, the internist, is [in] a group, an established group that's been here forever. And it really surprised me because they're mostly older, white men. It really surprised me when they took this guy in, but he has been a big hit. And they've recently hired now a second one.

The clinic, which has seven full-time physicians and one part-time physician on staff, has built a sense of loyalty from a number of patients. In the words of a community member who is in his fifties:

> In case if I went let's say to the [clinic name] is where I go, and if I went in there and my doctor is not there and they say, you know, he was just called over to the hospital, but [the IMG of Pakistani origin] can see you right now, okay, no problems. And the reason being is that the people in that clinic are pretty competent, the ones that I know, and I trust their judgment. I don't think they would bring an incompetent in there with them. That they've done—They've asked the questions that I'm not smart enough to ask. I don't have enough medical background to figure out whether this guy's got the right training or not. But if they've brought him in there into their clinic and he's stuck with them three or four years, and they've accepted him, then that's okay with me.

A senior citizen talked about trust in the same IMG in relation to trust in the clinic:

> I don't know the man, but I know one of his patients who thinks very highly of him, and he's Pakistani, but he's part of the [clinic]. Well, that gives him a little bit of an in right there, I would think. For example, when my son, who hasn't had a doctor since he was a child, you know, and he went to look for a doctor, and of course, my wife and I both have doctors at this clinic. She suggested, well, call them and they'll get you in. Well, there was nobody there but this Pakistani doctor, and he accepted it without any problem.

The above participant also had a separate rationale for wanting to see a doctor who is part of a clinic:

> To me, one of the important things is for a guy not to be alone in a practice because if he's incapacitated or out of town and you need emergency help, it's nice to know that there is someone on call to cover his patients. So that would be a major consideration for me, if I were looking for another clinic or doctor or what have you.

The Role of Referrals

Beyond patients' trust in an organization or the trust earned by an individual IMG, there also can be substantial trust in the referring provider. This finding mirrors what participants told me in Quincy; e.g., that trust in subspecialists is often not as important to patients as trust in primary care providers. However, the majority of IMGs in Delano County are primary care providers; since they are not subspecialists, they do not get many referrals. Thus, referrals might not be as important an issue in establishing trust as in Quincy, where most of the IMGs were subspecialists. A related issue is that word of mouth or trust in others' advice can also factor heavily into a patient's trust in an IMG.

A family physician in Berry told me about a patient he had seen that morning:

> This lady came in, she didn't come to be seen as a patient. She said, I just want to ask the doctor a question. She's been a patient of mine for a long time, she's on Medicaid. She been being seen by one of the clinics down at the health department. They had referred her to [a hospital in a neighboring county] for a cataract. And they had told her she needs to have the cataract removed and had set her up a date to go in and have it removed. And she come—I had not sent her up there and I hadn't seen her for this cataract. In fact, I haven't seen her in a good little while. But she says, I weren't going to let them touch me til you told me it was all right. So the loyalty is tremendous.

An allied health professional who works closely with physicians at the hospital in Hamilton said that there can be some initial hesitance to see a new physician. She told me, "If their doctor tell them that, oh, he is good, you know, then they'll be fine. You know, that's the way, whatever they tell them. You know, they say, okay, I'm going to refer you to this doctor, he's a really good, the impression is completely changed, you know."

Comments from patients throughout the area confirm further the trust placed in primary care providers. The following comments came from interviews with whites, blacks, and Native Americans, and focused on patients extending trust from their primary care providers to IMG subspecialists.

According to a small business owner and farmer, "Well, you know, our family doctor, I would trust his recommendation. . . . He's in that business and I'm not."

A participant who identified herself as a homemaker said, "Say [name of a U.S. medical graduate] is my medical doctor, if he said, you know, so-and-so's a good surgeon, I think you could go to him and do it as well as with anybody, I'd take his advice for it."

A retired schoolteacher in Berry who is a patient of a pioneer IMG said, "I feel like if he referred me to them, that he thought he would do the job. I would trust his judgment."

In south Hamilton, another retired schoolteacher commented, "I trust my physician enough to know that when he refer me to someone, he knows me, and I think he would do the best thing for me. If he suggest that I go to him, I trust him, that he know what he's doing and this must be the right guy for me to go to, or the right woman."

A resident of a homeless shelter said, "If [name of a U.S. medical graduate] sent me to him, I know he got to be right."

A participant who works in public relations for the public school system talked about having been referred to an IMG. "No, I had no problem with it, I assumed, since I was referred in both cases, I assumed that the person referring me to them knew that they were capable."

From the above comments, it is notable that all but one participant spoke about referrals to IMGs as a hypothetical situation rather than as a prior experience. Of course, some of the IMG subspecialists do primary care, as do most of the IMGs in the area. Unlike most patients in Quincy, people in Delano County have not necessarily come into contact with IMGs while seeking health care. Sixteen of twenty-seven community members interviewed in Delano County said that they had been patients of an IMG. However, the extent of interaction between doctor and patient varied substantially. For example, a few participants had been the patients of pioneer IMGs for decades; numerous participants had only seen an IMG one or two times, or had difficulty recollecting whether they ever had seen an IMG.

Another consideration is that all but one of the above quotations from patients were from senior citizens. The fact that trust in the referring provider surfaced primarily as an issue for seniors could simply be a reflection of the sample. Of twenty-seven community members interviewed for the study, ten were sixty-five or older.[2] Senior citizens are more likely to be health care consumers. Consequently, they might be more familiar with what it is like to be making an important health care decision, or simply to be referred to a subspecialist.

Without much managed care penetration, primary care providers do not act often as gatekeepers who can allow or disallow patients to see IMG subspecialists. Also mirroring findings from Quincy, it did not appear to be as important for a subspecialist to establish trust as it was for primary care providers. For example, an IMG subspecialist of Asian Indian origin told me that he does not have to be as concerned as primary care providers in developing patients' trust.

"They're already referred to me," he said.

"Referred patients," I said.

"Yeah, referred by other physicians. So they already tell them that, you know, Dr. [Name of self] is good and this and that, and go and see him. But for a primary care provider it could be different. Because if an American graduate is referring the patient to me, so he definitely have trust in me to send his patient over to me. So my situation is a little different."

A community member in a nearby small town made a similar point:

> As a general practitioner, a level of confidence is probably very important. Seeing a specialist, may not be so important to me. I have always been fairly healthy, so I don't know what type—My impression of seeing a specialist would

probably be a very limited amount of contact, maybe see them a few times, half a dozen times at most, and then that would end contact. So in that sense it would sort of be like visiting the Coke machine, you're just going there for a service and then you leave, it doesn't matter whether it's a red Coke machine or a green Coke machine.

Trust in All Doctors

At the same time that individuals and organizations play valuable roles in trust, some participants talked about a more general trust in doctors. In the words of a community member in south Hamilton:

> It takes a lot to get a degree in medicine. I think you work hard for that. And I don't think the board would accept you if you are not prepared to do that job. And that's the way I feel about anything, any profession. I figure this man or woman is out here, they passed the test, and that job is just as important as mine is as being a teacher. And I respect that, and I'd be delighted to go to him as a new doctor, as a regular doctor.

Meanwhile, many of the less educated patients in Delano County might be especially trusting of doctors, according to an IMG of Asian Indian origin:

> The more literate a patient, the more you can explain and the more they can comprehend about the complexity of the disease they have, the easier it is for them to accept it. Of course you need to reinforce it from time to time, like for everybody, we do it to everybody, but the initial acceptance of any kind of regimen. On the other hand, you do find sometimes that there's this blind acceptance of what a doctor says in this particular population too. The lower the literacy rate, there is a section of patients who accept you blindly and who will follow you to a tee. And then there's this other group of patients who simply are noncompliant, will not follow up on visits, will not follow up on medications. And it goes either way. And there is this one group of patients, either at a lower literacy rate, for whom whatever you say is the gospel, you know. They'll do exactly what you tell them to do. It gets difficult treating both kinds of patients, because the patients who accept your work as 100 percent expect the same kind of results back. And it's difficult to explain to them that, you know, that's not always the case in medicine. You never get 100 percent results. It can vary depending upon the disease. Try a medication, you know, in a hypertensive, you try one medication, it doesn't work, you shift to another. It's kind of difficult to explain to them that that may be the case. Or why an allergic reaction takes place. So their belief is if a doctor's given it to me, I should be well, nothing else should go wrong. So those kind of complexities, it sometimes gets difficult to deal with. Even in patients who are very, very accepting of what you tell them to do.

Thus, among many other factors mentioned above (e.g., role of the individual, role of the clinic, word of mouth), trust can be influenced by individual or collective belief systems about the medical profession. Such trust was demonstrated further in an interview with a Hispanic participant who works as an interpreter for Spanish-speaking patients. She told me about the initial trust that patients have in their doctor:

> If you have a sign there that say it's a doctor, we trust in you. [laughs] Okay? As long as you—we go there the first time, and if we want to come back, we have to be treated with respect, you had to be listening to our needs and take care of our needs, and the medicine that you prescribe the first time, it works for us, that meant that you're going to be our doctor for life.

The reverse can also occur; that is, some patients can be afraid of doctors. In the Hispanic community, there are many people who come from very poor, rural areas in Mexico that lacked easy access to a medical doctor. Going to a doctor's office can be a new and unfamiliar experience. There are some Hispanics who feel more comfortable seeking care from "hueseros" who heal broken bones, or to other alternative providers, according to another participant in the Hispanic community. In addition, most of the Hispanics in Delano County are on the lower end of the socioeconomic scale; many work as unskilled laborers in a poultry processing plant. For patients who do not speak English, referrals via interpreters can also have a substantial influence on trust in IMGs in Delano County.

The Role of the Interpreter

Two Hispanic participants told me that they act as interpreters for non-English-speaking patients. I interviewed them in a Catholic church in Pierce, a small town of approximately 4,000 people. Mass had been conducted entirely in Spanish to over 300 people. According to one participant, there can be as many as 450 people attending services at the church. Both participants told me that most of the Hispanic immigrants only speak Spanish; my own efforts to communicate with others at the church confirm that many Hispanic immigrants in Delano County do not speak any English. The town has seen an influx of Mexicans in the last few years, and now has several stores and restaurants catering to Hispanic residents. Having said that, the Hispanic participants also told me that the recent influx of Hispanics is not concentrated primarily in just one town but, rather, is dispersed throughout the area.

I said to one participant in the Hispanic community, "Well, one of the things I was wondering about is whether it might just be difficult for people to go to a doctor." She replied:

> It is, they don't trust them. Here we function with trust. If I tell them, they know me. Okay. I tell them, okay, this is a good doctor. If you want, I'll go with you. Okay? I take them the first two or three times and then they get to know the doctor, they feel comfortable, then they'll take the whole family there. See, it all works by word of mouth. Now they know me enough to know that if I tell them that somebody's good, they can trust me. But they won't go on their own to a regular doctor unless—I don't know, not on their own.

Still, the interpreter needs to earn the trust of the patient. She explained further:

> Many times these people understand everything that the doctor says, yet they're waiting for you to translate what the doctor says to see how much they can really trust you. Okay? Cause I used to go out with this woman, and—her baby was really sick and I went out with her and one day I couldn't go, and she asked somebody else to go with her, a so-called friend, and she said that she would never trust her again because she wasn't telling her—translating actually what the doctor said, she was telling her something totally different. Sometimes they can't speak the language, but they understand it. So even if—They bring you to communicate, not to hear what the doctor has to say, but what they want you to tell that doctor, that's what's important.

Thus, the need for an interpreter adds yet another component to trust in an IMG; that is, trust needs to be established by the interpreter in order for the patient to feel comfortable following the interpreter's recommendations.

Competence

In Quincy, virtually no one wanted to say anything negative about the competence of IMGs. In Delano County, participants were much more forthcoming in discussing competence with regard to the qualifications of IMGs to practice medicine. Such contrasts in the openness of participants could have many possible explanations, including different political sensitivities between Quincy and Delano County, differences in my degree of entry into or acceptance by communities, and the fact that people generally seemed more straightforward in Delano County in saying what was on their minds.

I often came across one of three general mindsets about the issue of competence, not necessarily exclusive from one another. Participants commonly said that IMGs are just as competent as U.S. medical graduates to practice medicine in the area, some participants said that IMGs are actually more competent, and some expressed concerns about the competence of IMGs.

A rationale for viewing IMGs as equally competent physicians is the trust in U.S. standards for health care. For example, licensure as a physician can lead to trust, regardless of where the physician was trained. Similarly, being hired by a clinic that is held in high regard, or being referred by a respected physician, can increase the perceived competence of a physician. Furthermore, participants in the medical profession are often familiar with the preparation necessary for IMGs to practice medicine in the United States. According to the hospital recruiter: "I'm always amazed because so many of them not only did a residency or a fellowship in their native country, come here and then maybe repeat that. How better trained can a person be, by national or international standards?"

A person who works with the credentialing of physicians expressed similar thoughts about the competence of IMGs: "And then I think that what you have to understand is, is that they get their pre-med and their medical school in another country, but they come and train in their residency programs here in the United States. So they become acclimated to the standards of medical care that we expect here."

A lawyer in Hamilton also viewed the competence of IMGs in the same way:

> I think if he's accredited by, you know, the Certifying Board of Surgeons or Internal Medicine, here in the United States, they've done that job and I wouldn't be worried about whether he could diagnose me better than some American doctor, I don't believe I would go into that. If I felt like that I'd been referred properly and the fellow had a good reputation, I wouldn't—The fact that he'd gone to school in India as opposed to Canada or the United States, I don't think would weigh heavily with me, if he's, you know, accredited, has the credentials.

An IMG originally from South Asia told me that in other places, he has sensed that IMGs are often expected to practice substandard care. He has not sensed that in this area: "And it really doesn't matter to patients where you trained. I have yet to find a person—or, you can feel it sometimes, and I've yet to feel anything like that, that somebody might think that I might not be well-trained enough or whatever, just because I didn't train here in the U.S."

A community member in a nearby small town said that his concern in seeing a doctor is about feeling better, and not about where the physician was trained:

> You know, a sick person don't care. You know, they're not going to be asking you for your credentials, they're going to come in, can you make me well? Can you save my little kid? You know? What is wrong with my baby? What do I have to do to stop my baby from crying? If you have those answers, that qualifies you. That's really the only important issue, you know, with that.

Some of the participants viewed IMGs as more competent than U.S. medical graduates, and often based their opinions on the hard work that must have been necessary to practice medicine in the United States. For example, I asked a community member who is an immigrant from Latin America if IMGs were as competent as U.S. medical graduates in Delano County. She replied:

> Of course. Of course. And sometimes they're even more competent. Because here, we Americans are very accustomed to taking the easy way out. When you go out of the United States—Somebody who becomes a doctor in India is a real doctor. Okay? There's no BS in this because these people go there and it costs them a lot of money and they have to work for it. I've seen people who become doctors like in the Dominican Republic, they have to study their heads off. They are real doctors and they are as competent, or maybe more than the doctors here. Because to them it cost them more, so it's more important. You know, whatever costs you in money or in effort, it's more important, you value it more.

A pharmacist also saw differences in schooling as a reason why IMGs might be more competent. Some of his comments also reflected some of the racial divisions in the area. Referring to IMGs, he said:

> I'm not familiar with all of them. But them I am familiar with, they're generally just one step better than our homegrown. I don't know what the reason is. I think maybe it is because their chance to become a doctor was much less than our natives, Native American and all the others here, and I think they took more pride in it. And I think they only ship us the best ones. I don't know whether that's true or not, but that's been my opinion. Of course that's the way opinions are, not always correct, but they're my opinions. But generally I've found that most of them are just a notch above the general MD. And I understand part of it, from what I have learned, is that they take school more seriously.

A community member in Hamilton also raised the idea that it might be better to seek care from someone who is not from the local area. I asked her about the competence of IMGs, and she told me:

> I'm sure they would be as competent. In some cases I feel like they may have had to work harder and may actually be more willing to listen. I know some local doctors, they feel like they already—It's like so rote. And then they already know who my whole family is. And they don't necessarily communicate with me, they just sort of treat and they're gone. And other doctors who don't do all that just see me as a patient and tend to communicate a little better. I have sort of a bias against some of the local doctors.

At the same time, some of the major concerns about the competence of IMGs focused on the quality of medical education in developing countries.

This relates to an idea from a few participants that physicians who come from a medical school that is well-known, or at least well-known locally, might be viewed more readily as competent physicians.

I asked a U.S. medical graduate for advice on how to handle myself if I were a new IMG in the area. Her response dealt with the issue of improving others' perceptions of my competence:

> Well, I would say that the first thing that you should do is to try to build an alliance with the other members of the medical staff. You certainly should become friends with them, go to County Medical Society, go to every meeting that the hospital has, start to get on committees as soon as possible, talk to people in the hallways, be very available for consults. Treat your initial patients just as well as you possibly can because it takes about two years to build a reputation, a good reputation. It takes about two minutes to get a bad reputation. And so I guess the first thing I would say is for about the first two years, you have to be just as perfect as you could possibly be. Treat your patients well, try not to make any glaring errors, don't suddenly become absent from the call schedule when it's your turn to be on call and dump something on your colleagues. That would be the main piece of advice I would give them.

I asked, "Do you think that the international medical graduates might need to hear that advice more than the U.S. medical graduates, or is it something that just should be heard all around, that no group is better at heeding the advice than others?"

> Well, someone who's a foreign medical graduate may have to even be more careful about being perceived as someone who's a very high quality physician. If I had a fellow who came to town who had done his residency at [a prestigious U.S. university], and was from the United States, I would probably perceive him as being well-trained, even though he may be the worst doctor on the face of the earth. If somebody came in who had gone to medical school in Pakistan I wouldn't automatically assume that he was a terrible doctor, but I wouldn't assume that he was a great one either. It's sort of like, well, I'll wait and see how he does. There's going to be that period where you have to see them prove themselves.

An IMG pediatrician who is held in high regard in both the medical and nonmedical communities told me that he can sense sometimes that there might be doubts about his competence:

> This doesn't happen very often, but sometimes you talk to a parent and they kind of give you this look like, do you know what you're talking about? So that's—To me, that means, you know, you're not—you're probably not as

qualified to be an M.D. as somebody else. Now I don't know if that was because my professional judgment really was in error at that time, or it was the way it was delivered, you know, an Asian person saying those words.

Such concerns were based on subtleties rather than anything explicit, and there could be many possible explanations why the parent did not want his advice, such as chance or individual personalities. In addition to concerns about language barriers, racism, or xenophobia, another possible explanation for not wanting an IMG's advice might be that most people are not aware of the standards that are necessary for IMGs to practice medicine in the United States. Even in the medical community, there can be a misperception that IMGs do not have to undergo residency training in the United States.

A U.S. medical graduate told me about his preference for physicians who received at least some of their medical training in the United States:

> I would be much more attracted to somebody who's well-trained, who perhaps had been to medical school in another country but had a residency or specialty training in America. I would much prefer that because that's something we know about. Whereas if they're trained all outside of the United States, I won't have any experience or point of reference to know how reliable a training that is.

A community member in a nearby small town had a similar comment about the competence of IMGs: "The only drawback that I see, and my perception is, that foreign physicians may have come through a training where technology or whatever was not as advanced as here in America."

Most people did not express a concern that IMGs were any less competent than U.S. medical graduates. Sometimes though, participants assessed the competence of IMGs based on the perceived economic development of other countries. I had the following exchange with a senior citizen.

I said, "So if a physician says to you that he's from India, would that make any difference to you?"

"My main concern would be the quality of his education," she replied. "I think sometimes we think of India as a third world country, and you would wonder if his medical knowledge was the same as it would be in the Western civilization, particularly the U.S."

"And if the person said, just to choose another name of a country, England?"

"Well, of course, that's more similar, so you wouldn't have quite as much misgiving, or you wouldn't question the qualifications as much, I think."

Complicating matters, there may be some differences in exposure to some aspects of health care that are more common in one country than in another. For example, nurse practitioners and physician assistants are used heavily in Delano County, but nonexistent in much of the world.

Nurse Practitioners and Physician Assistants

The issue of the role of nurse practitioners and physician assistants in providing care in rural needy areas was controversial to several IMGs in Delano County. Some physician assistants worked without a physician onsite most of the time, and therefore had a relatively high degree of autonomy as health professionals.

The ability of midlevels or "nonphysicians" (e.g., nurse practitioners and physician assistants) to maintain quality of care was a major concern in some interviews. While no participant objected to using such health providers alongside physicians, five IMGs expressed a concern that nurse practitioners and physician assistants should not be replacing physicians. Concerns about whether nurse practitioners and physician assistants should be considered equivalent to physicians are not limited to Delano County (Cawley, 1996; Fowkes, 1993; Spitzer et al., 1974). Furthermore, there was no reason to think that Delano County IMGs were particularly notable in expressing concerns about nurse practitioners and physician assistants. Indeed, a nurse practitioner also agreed that she would work best alongside a physician, rather than as a stand-alone health provider. A U.S. medical graduate also volunteered similar concerns about nonphysicians, but I did not check to see how everybody felt about them.

Some IMGs noted that other parts of the country were not as dependent as Delano County on nurse practitioners and physician assistants. For example, in some residency programs, physicians have had only minimal exposure to them. Consequently, concerns about nonphysicians may have more to do with a physician's background in the United States than with a lack of exposure to them in another country.

An IMG of Southeast Asian origin told me that there were not any nurse practitioners or physician assistants in his country of origin. He explained:

> It was a novel concept, it took a little bit of getting used to. I guess the reason I say that is, coming from a residency program, we considered, or I considered myself as sort of a midlevel. You're doing the doctor's work and you're getting paid much, much less than the doctor. But at first I thought of them as, well you know, I treated them with a little bit of suspect because I didn't know how they could cram four years of medical school and three years of residency into two years. But the PAs [physician assistants] that I work with today, you know, I have utmost faith in them. I talk with them about problems that my kids have. So you know—And I talk with them about, you know, certain things. Like if I have a patient that I, you know, needed a second opinion, I would actually talk to them. So they have my respect. I would not be working here if I had a big issue with PAs, because these PAs take call with me, and so they actually see the patients first at night, and if they felt that they needed to communicate with us, then they

> would talk to us. So I liken the relationship to when I was a resident. There's a difference between a senior resident and an intern. An intern is the person that gets pushed into the battles, first line. So they do all that, but the only difference is our PAs' judgment is so much better than a first year intern's judgment, cause they've been doing this for years and years and years.

This idea of adapting over time also emerged in an interview with a nurse practitioner who had worked alongside an IMG. She told me:

> It was so funny, we laugh about it now cause we're very good friends. But in the beginning when he was new to the United States only a few years and then he was really new to here. And he had never dealt with working with midlevel providers and he did not like it. In fact, the first conversation we ever had—When I met him I was in my residency actually, and he made it plain that he did not like having to work with midlevel providers. And we had—But he felt like he didn't have a choice, was what he said. So I was somewhat stressed by that. But we agreed that we were going to get to know each other very well, and then by the time we worked together—When he was getting ready to leave and setting up a practice, he wanted me to go with him. So it was like we made a very good working situation and a good relationship. I learned a lot from him. I learned a lot of medical stuff from him, and he learned a lot of American politics [laughs] and how to survive around here from me. And it was a very good relationship and a good time, I'm going to miss him a lot.

Earlier, the IMG who was working with her told me:

> She works in the same office, and every problem she has she calls me so I can see the patient. That's a different story. Most of the other PAs, nurse practitioners I have been asked to supervise, or the other physician was asked, were working solo in the other clinics. They can call you on the phone for problems that they think exist. But the other thing, working in the same building, if you care to learn, it makes a lot of difference, cause you can pull over the nurse practitioner and say, this is what I'm going to do now with this whatever problem, so she knows how to do certain things that she probably wouldn't be able to learn if she was on her own, how to manage certain problems, how to deal with certain situations, skills. So I have pretty good relationship with this particular nurse practitioner. She also has fifteen years of nursing practice, which makes a substantial difference when you're talking about taking care of people. She's been through the mill, she's been taking care of ER, ICU, as a nurse, and she's seen a lot of problems. True, from a nursing perspective, but as far as patient handling is concerned, it's very important to have worked with sick patient so you can have some idea what's going on.

This brief focus on IMG-nonphysician relations has shown some of the difficulty in making static generalizations about IMGs in relation to other health professionals. Professional and social attitudes vary from individual to individual, and change over time, too. The adaptability of individuals transcends the ability of two people to work alongside one another, and points to a much greater issue of adjustment to life in a new area.

NOTES

1. Consistent with the previous Quincy chapters, I will not be labeling items as mechanisms or nonmechanisms. At the same time, it is still important for the reader to keep in mind that mechanisms are central to this chapter (see Chapter 2).

2. Among Native Americans, it seemed more likely for me to be referred to respected elders than to young people. Also, I usually did not know that a participant was a senior citizen until age was disclosed during the interview.

Chapter Eight

Contexts and Hamilton, Part I: Issues and Nonissues

So much depth underpins ideas about contexts in Delano County that two chapters are needed just to discuss them; the divisions between this and the following chapter are only for organizational purposes.[1]

THE AMERICANNESS AND FOREIGNNESS OF PHYSICIANS

The terms "Americanness" and "foreignness" refer to people who are perceived to be American or not American, respectively. Quincy had many different conceptualizations of Americanness and foreignness, bearing on considerations of race, language, familiarity, and the status of doctors. Similar conceptualizations were also found in Delano County, albeit with different nuances because the locale, individual participants, and my community entry were different.

Participants shared different ideas in thinking about who is an American or foreign physician in Delano County. Citizenship surfaced in several instances as a criterion for Americanness, although I saw no indication that people were aware of everyone else's citizenship status. It was common for participants to say that country of birth or education determined a physician's Americanness or foreignness. Yet there was also room for a gray area in which people from some countries might be considered more foreign than those from other countries.

Race and Nationality

In a few interviews, the idea of race made it difficult to determine who was an American. Consider the ideas of a nurse:

"When I'm meaning foreign, I'm meaning foreign people that come from other countries to come to United States. That's what I mean by foreign. So basically, the rest of the doctors of different races are from this area. When I think of foreign doctors, I think of others that's come from other parts of the country besides United States."

I asked her, "What if a physician comes from Canada, would that be a foreign physician?"

> Well, it would be foreign in the sense [laughs] of outside of the United States. But as far as [laughs] race, I guess it wouldn't be foreign, because people—I mean, a lot of people, you know, such as Canadian, England, countries like that, you know, their language, the way they speak, gives them away. I mean, if they never said anything you wouldn't even know that, you know, they did come from another country. But to be from India, I mean, you know, you can't help but notice. I mean, we just don't have too many people—I guess you just don't see too many people from India in the United States. I mean, of course, more and more are coming in. But that's what I mean, something that you see with your—see visually, you know. If they're from Canada, you don't really see it until they speak to you, you know. But I don't know. [laughs] Oh Lord.

At least two issues emerged from the above quote about Americanness: one was visual image, and the other was sound. Both seemed intertwined to muddy the issues of race, language, and nationality. On the one hand, a person who has a particular skin color might be seen as more likely to have some difficulty communicating in English. On the other hand, anyone who speaks English with an accent not perceived to be common in any part of the United States can also be seen as a foreigner, regardless of visual appearance. As the nurse explained further about perceptions toward international medical graduates (IMGs):

"The visual difference is what seems to make more difference to me, I mean, to the patients, than any other quality. Because usually when they say things, it's concerning—it's not concerning them being foreigners, it's concerning the way they talk, you know, if they can't understand them."

A community member in south Hamilton also raised the idea of a dual approach to considering foreignness, including both visual image and sound. I asked him, "And do you always know that the doctor is foreign or—"

"No," he said. "You don't know, but accent will give them away. You can see—You can tell—You can look at a person and tell if they're foreign, most of the time, you know. Sometimes you can't. But it doesn't really matter, but sometimes you can tell by the accent, sometimes you can tell by the look."

A senior citizen linked the idea of skin color more directly with Americanness. She had defined "foreign doctors" as physicians who come from countries besides the United States and Canada, consistent with the academic literature. Then she added that some physicians originally from Europe can be American doctors, too.

"Well, even London, say," she said.

"London?"

"You see, if I—I would—I know they would be foreigners, but you wouldn't think of them as a foreigner. So . . . I think—bad as I hate to say, it has a whole lot to do with the color of the skin."

A similar idea of connecting race with nationality came up in an interview with a man who had just eaten a free lunch at a soup kitchen. He said, "In all nationalities, you got a lot of prejudiced people."

"Right," I said. "In all nationalities? What do you mean by nationalities?"

"Nationality's race," he replied, and then rambled off topic.

A pharmacist raised similar points about nationality, telling me, "I'm sure that there are many people that consider anything except white Eurasians to be a foreigner. See? That's the way the South is."

Whether a local or regional conceptualization of Americanness, it appeared as though a few participants regarded whiteness as an American trait. A black participant in a nearby small town compared being black to being foreign:

> Twenty-five years ago, a foreign doctor would only been able to wait on black people. No white person would have trusted their life to a foreign doctor. Okay? By the same token, they wouldn't have trusted it to a black doctor. See, we were foreign to them also, if you see what I'm saying. That has changed, but then that's just a change of our attitudes in the country, you know. I don't think that's just Delano—You know, it's not just Delano County.

In short, there can be variation in the linkage between race and nationality over time. Social changes occurring beyond just Delano County can influence who is or is not a foreigner within Delano County. Changing attitudes in the South and the United States toward foreigners and blacks could have added further to considerations of Americanness.

The Foreignness of Non-Native Americans

Prior to coming to Delano County, I had become accustomed to calling IMGs "foreign physicians," for ease of explanation. One of my contacts who was Native American and a professor at the university in Berry suggested that I use the term, "foreign physicians" because it would be understandable to participants.

Near the end of my fieldwork, I spoke briefly to a group of Native American students in Berry and told them that I would be interested in interviewing people to get their perspectives on "foreign physicians."

A student asked me what the term means, and I answered by explaining that I like to ask participants that question to get their insight. I explained also that, for purposes of this study, my focus is on international medical graduates, and I defined the term. At the time, I was unaware that I may have offended some sensibilities regarding the issue of who is or is not a foreigner.

Later, a Native American student who volunteered to be interviewed told me her thoughts about foreignness:

> I think foreign means anybody that didn't originate from this country. So even if they've been living here, their parents lived here, their great-grandparents, even—I mean, anybody that's now—to me, I mean, I'm Native American, so anybody that's not native to me is a foreigner, even if—Not like I'm racist or anything, but that's the way I see a foreigner. Like if I go to China, I'm foreign, or if I go to England, I'm foreign because I did not originate from there, nor did my parents, nor did any of their parents. So that's the way I see English, or African, or Chinese or anyone. If their parents did not originate from here, from this country, then they're foreign.

As we talked further, I asked, "And the whites, they would be considered foreign physicians too?"

"Yeah," she replied.

"I would be considered a foreigner too?"

"Basically. [laughs] Not—It doesn't—It's not a racial thing. I mean, it's not anything like I don't want to be in contact with anybody that's not from my country originally. That's not even how it is. It's—That's just my definition of a foreigner, not—It doesn't have anything to do with the way I feel about somebody."

I asked her to explain about some of the consequences that I might face as a foreigner relocating to Berry.

She replied, "I think people just might be a little hesitant to switch doctors. Like if they have a native doctor, they might be hesitant to say, well, I'm going to go over here and see how he practices. Well, if they hear a lot of good things about that person, that might alter their decision. I mean, they could have a Native American doctor and they not treat them the way they want to be treated, so maybe this physician could offer more things."

An important consideration is the role of family lineage in determining Americanness. Based on the above conceptualization, people are not simply American on an individual basis but on a family basis.

A white community member considered the idea of foreignness more succinctly in saying, "You know, we're all foreigners, when you get back to it." Consequently, except for Native Americans, the United States can be considered a convergence of foreigners; to be foreign might even be considered an American trait.

On a few occasions, it seemed that participants considered Native Americans to be foreigners, or to have some foreignness about them. For example, a senior citizen in the general community remarked that Native Americans are not "western":

"I think Native Americans in Delano County are more eastern in their thinking than western, so it isn't necessarily totally geographic and foreign. Because, if you deal with Native Americans, pretty soon you come to realize that their approach is eastern rather than western."

During fieldwork, I thought that there had been several instances in which participants referred to Native Americans as foreigners. In reviewing the transcripts later, it was more difficult to detect any overlap between people's thoughts toward who is a Native American and who is a foreigner. For example, a lawyer talked about attracting physicians to the local area:

"But I do know that we have attracted a number of attractive foreign physicians here. There are two or three here I think who have a reputation of being top-notch physicians."

"I probably know which two or three you are referring to, but who are you referring to?" I asked, expecting him to name the two pioneer IMGs.

"I'm referring to [the two pioneer IMGs]. I think that they're looked upon in the community, along with [a Native American physician] with [another clinic]. You know, I think the people in [the clinic] would not have brought in a fellow like—And of course, he's a Native American. He's not a foreign doctor, he's a Native American doctor, so he's really not in the same category as [the two pioneer IMGs]."

There might be nothing to the idea that Native Americans and foreigners are somehow grouped together, since the lawyer did make a distinction at the end of his comment. Possibly, the blurred line between IMGs and some Native Americans could simply be a result of my own misunderstanding of people's perceptions at the time of fieldwork. If, in fact, some participants confused both populations, one explanation could be that people might simply group "others" together.

A Hispanic Perspective

This point can be illustrated further through a Hispanic perspective toward IMGs, in which all physicians (not just all IMGs) are grouped as Other. A participant in the Hispanic community told me when we first met that everyone is a foreigner to Hispanics in the area. She continued to make the point when we sat down for an interview in the front pew of a church after mass:

> And as I said before, for the Hispanics, everybody here in the United States is a foreigner, even another Hispanic. Because if you're Mexican and the doctor is Cuban or Dominican, I mean, they're a foreigner, because it's the same language, but a slightly different culture. I mean, we all speak Spanish, but we're not—we don't all act the same.

She raised the idea again and again that everyone in the United States is a foreigner. For example, when I asked her about trust toward "international physicians," she replied, "As I told you, they're foreigners to us anyway. So it doesn't matter if it's a foreigner from the United States or from Mars, it's still a foreigner, so the mistrust will be there. Now, it's up to the physician to gain the people's trust."

Later in the interview, she raised the idea that everyone is a foreigner yet again when I asked, "Is the issue of communication with foreign physicians something that should be a special concern?"

"No. No, I don't think so. Cause as I said, they're all foreign to us."

A participant in the same small town in Delano County offered a similar idea about Hispanic perspectives, albeit without reference to the many Hispanic cultures: "To them, everyone is going to be foreign, unless it's a Hispanic doctor."

The majority of Hispanic immigrants in Delano County came from Mexico, but none of the IMGs in the area received their medical degrees in Mexico. Only three physicians received their degrees from medical schools in Spanish-speaking countries, including Argentina, Guatemala, and the Dominican Republic. The "foreignness" of a physician might be an inconsequential consideration to many Hispanics in this context of not having any doctor available from their same country of origin.

U.S. Citizens as Foreigners

As in Quincy, the distinction between a foreigner and an American did not cut precisely along geopolitical boundaries. Most of the time, people did not confuse U.S. territories with other countries. However, without being prompted, a couple of participants volunteered that physicians from Puerto Rico are foreign. For example, a physician in a small town told me about his residency training around foreign doctors:

> And so recruitment of physicians for house staff at this large medical center, [name of medical center and location], a thousand-bed hospital, a large percent-

> age of internal medicine staff were foreign. They're from Puerto Rico, they're from Guam, we had some from Nigeria. And me being an American grad, that was rather foreign to me, because I had not seen such a major portion of the medical staffing, house staffing that is, being foreign.

Some participants referred to Yankees as foreigners. For example, a pharmacist in Hamilton said, "There was a time when if you didn't speak our language, you were a foreigner. Well, worse than that, you were a damn Yankee."

An allied health provider expressed a similar viewpoint: "Here, anybody who's not from 'Delano' County can be considered foreign. You know, northern, anything north is foreign to a lot of the patients here. But I know that you're speaking particularly about foreign trained."

Similarly, a community member laughed and told me, You could be from up north and be foreign to some folks down here, but I'm talking—I'm assuming you're talking about they're not Americans, they're from out of the country."

A couple of participants raised the idea that people who are from the United States can have a foreign attitude. Foreignness can represent negative traits in a person, regardless of country of origin, citizenship, language, race, or any other issue. According to a participant in a nearby small town:

> Your attitude towards me makes you foreign. Okay? If you—If we were talking geography, then that's another thing. But if you have a, you know, a nasty disposition, I don't care if you're black, you're foreign to me, because I don't see the reason for that. If we're talking geography, then you know, anyone that's not an American is my definition of a foreign physician. I mean, born in America, is more or less what I'm trying to say.

Uncertainty about the Distinction between Americans and Foreigners

Unlike Quincy, not everyone seemed to notice that there had been an influx of physicians from other countries to the area. This became apparent to me in several interviews, particularly when participants tried to consider how many IMGs were in the area. For example, the following excerpt is from an interview with a senior citizen who volunteers at the hospital. She told me that she had just received the hospital physician directory.

"What were some of your reactions in looking through it?" I asked, referring to the hospital directory.

"Well, I haven't really had time to complete it, but what I decided I would do, since I was coming in for this interview with you was to go through and just mark the foreign doctors that we have, and I was just halfway through and I'm completely surprised at how many. See. Just marking those few, look a'there."

"You missed some though," I said.

"I know."

"You missed her."

"Well, yeah, surely did. Nigeria. But see, I did this hurriedly because I had to give a speech today. [laughs]"

As we talked further, I said, "Well, you say you were surprised that there are so many foreign physicians here."

"Yes. Yes. I surely was. I really was. I knew, you know, we've had them for quite some time, a spattering of them, you know. I can remember an orthopedic man was one of the first, [name of IMG orthopedist]. I don't believe [he] is here now. But we have had them and I knew they were available, but I just did not realize that we have as many as we do in Delano County. And connected with the hospital."

The social status of physicians further blurs the line between IMGs and U.S. medical graduates. According to an IMG's wife, "And I would definitely say that doctors, just the profession itself, you know, gives respect. You know, that profession is so respectful that I think doctors would be more accepted than any other profession being a foreigner. I think that's definitely true. You are respected more, definitely, if you're a doctor than any other profession."

The status of doctors obviously varies from one country to another, and could even vary from one part of the United States to another. A hospital recruiter told me that he thinks the status of doctors is a motivating factor for people to practice medicine in the area:

> Whether they come from Germany or Romania or India or Africa or wherever, again, they want to know that they'll be accepted, and I think they sense that when they come, that this is a friendly area, that there is a great amount of need. And to a large degree they'll be put up on a pedestal as a physician, because we don't have nearly enough of them, and that usually rings clearer to them than it does some of the American medical graduates who have maybe a greater realm of selection.

A nurse who is also the patient of an IMG reflected that the social status of doctors can be much more important than perceptions of foreignness. Talking about her physician, she told me, "Well, my experience has been a positive one because to me I don't see him as foreign. I mean, he's just my doctor, you know."

The distinction between foreigners and Americans appears to be uncertain or, in many cases, irrelevant. As in Quincy, Americanness is a composite of many different influences that have local meaning. In Delano

County, the meanings of Americanness and foreignness transcended race, language, family heritage, familiarity, professional status, attitude, and changes in perceptions over time, among other issues. Thus, as was also the case in Quincy, the lines that are drawn on a map to distinguish between countries can be irrelevant in considering who is or is not a foreign physician.

SOCIAL CONSTRUCTION OF RACE

As a researcher who had never lived in the area, I always felt like I had something more to learn about racial divisions, social networks that cut across race, and complexity in people's perceptions on race. Even now, after sifting through transcripts and field notes and reflecting on my personal experiences in Delano County, I am not authoritative in any way about the intricacies of race in Delano County. At the same time, it is difficult, if not impossible, to disentangle the issue of race from virtually anything else in Delano County.

Tri-racial Advantage

As discussed earlier, Delano County was reported in the 2000 Census to be 38 percent Native American, 33 percent white, and 25 percent black. Participants often referred to the area as being one-third Native American, one-third white, and one-third black. In my first interview in the area, a U.S. medical graduate talked about the lack of a clear racial majority as a positive characteristic for Delano County.

"So from what you're describing it sounds to me like a very tolerant, open town," I said.

"I think—well, I think—It is to me," the U.S. medical graduate said. "There are people who are not, there are pockets. But compared to what I see and hear in comparable towns I think this is a more open—If nothing else, just because of the mix that's already here. The absence of a majority makes a big difference. Nobody is in control. It's not like I'm big daddy and I control this community and I can get you. That's not right. That does not—I really don't think that exists here."

One consequence of "the absence of a majority" is that people are accustomed to seeing others who look different. As a result, IMGs from India might not be considered outsiders, at least not based on physical appearance. According to the hospital recruiter: "The fact that we're a tri-racial community I think allows for people to be more understanding to some differences that may exist. Our medical staff, over the years, have come from all parts of the

United States, as well as from other parts of the world. And I think, without exception, they've all been embraced and felt to be welcome, to a large degree."

This point about the advantage to IMGs of working in a tri-racial community was reiterated in an interview with a social worker. I asked her if she thought that the town was open to outsiders. She replied, "I really think so, and one reason I think so is because we are a tri-racial anyway. So therefore, you know, we—That's just a everyday occurrence to us, we don't think about, he's from India."

Whether or not it is an advantage to have a "tri-racial" county is an open question that is far beyond my comprehension. Several participants suggested that it is advantageous for IMGs to be moving into an area where, theoretically, no one is othered based on color of skin. Yet race still has strong meanings, and people make classifications or judgments of Others based on perceptions of race. Race still is constructed but it is often not tied directly to color of skin. Based on physical appearance, there is no clear way to know who self-identifies as white, black, or Native American. Thus, it becomes even more difficult to determine the race of IMGs with different skin color.

Problems with Racial Distinctions

Throughout my fieldwork, I realized again and again that race has different meanings to different people. Although many whites and blacks consider color of skin as a major component of race, many Native Americans view race much differently. The difficulty distinguishing race based on physical appearance was made especially clear in an interview with a nurse practitioner. The following excerpt from our interview begins with the nurse practitioner discussing the importance of kinship:

> You know, like my last name is a very common name here, and so people see that and say, oh, we're probably related somewhere, you know. And you know, so there's not an opportunity for somebody who's internationally trained or who is from abroad to come in and do that, so there has to be another way for them to connect with people here. But the concept of relationships and family, even very distantly removed family is something that's important to people, and I find that when the dynamic with somebody who is originally from this area, you see that take place again and again and again, and it's something that people really connect with here.

"Is it just coincidence that you have a last name that is very common among the [name of Indian tribe]?" I asked.

"Well, I am [name of tribe]."
"You are [name of tribe]?"
"Yes," he said.
"Okay, I didn't know that," I said.

> Right. And you see, and that's another thing like for internationally trained, whether it would be a doctor, physician, nurse practitioner, whoever, is understanding that the [tribe], there's not necessarily a characteristic phenotype you can look at somebody and say, oh, there's a [name of tribe], because, you know, the [tribe] can be very fair complected or they can be quite dark in their complexion and that's just the nature of [name of tribe], and the way things are. And people sometimes are pretty sensitive about that, so I'm very careful to find out what their ethnicity is before I start making any kind of statements about this is a forty-five-year-old black female or Indian female, or whatever the case may be.

I felt as though I had just made a tragic mistake in not realizing that the participant, who had white skin, could be Native American. Shortly after the above exchange, the participant looked frequently at his watch, and I felt that his answers to my questions became clipped. The next day, the participant e-mailed me to apologize for scheduling difficulties that had caused us to cut the interview short. Later, in reviewing the transcript, I wondered whether there had been no tragic mistake in my interviewing but, rather, simple concerns about scheduling that had nothing to do with race.

Immediately after the interview, I had an appointment with a professor at the university in Berry. In giving me advice, the professor told me that a major mistake that newcomers make is assuming that people are white or black based on skin color. I felt as though I had inadvertently stepped into a sensitive issue in the conversation quoted above.

Later, I interviewed a leader in the Native American community in Berry who told me that race is an issue that cannot be avoided: "But for race, you can't really make any decisions here without taking race into account, cause it's real and it's not even subtle. I mean, it's palpable. You can touch it and feel it if you hang around long enough. Sometimes you have to hang around a few weeks or months, sometimes even years, to really sort out how people live and feel and do, and so that has a lot to do with it."

Although, for many people, race is often too sensitive to be discussed openly in Delano County, it is an extraordinarily important consideration affecting people's self-identification, choice of residence, and social interactions. Within this context of different cultures and social networks, a U.S. medical graduate told me about the importance of meeting the needs of people in a racially diverse area: "Well, you have to be adaptable, that's true, you have to be a chameleon. You know, a chameleon, he gets on the wall and he can be a brown brick or a white brick, but yet deep inside he's a lizard or whatever. Deep down inside, you know that you are a provider, but you have to be able to adapt."

If race is so much a part of culture, history, and identities, it stands to reason that some knowledge about the different races in the area can help a provider to be a chameleon. However, it is often unknown whether a person is white or black or Native American. I certainly did not always know the race of participants prior to interviews, and learned quickly not to make any assumptions about the race of anyone based on physical appearance.

An IMG of Asian Indian origin explained, "In this county, in particular, my experience has been that people maybe a white person will look like an American Indian person, or a Afro-American person will look like a—You know there's kind of a little bit of give and take on each side. So those things, skin tones and all, eventually take a backseat when health care is concerned, I think. My treatment is same to all of them."

Most participants did not group IMGs into a general, racial classification. However, on a few occasions, participants said that IMGs belonged to a separate race, or that IMGs were not white, or not black. In one interview, a pharmacist told me about the different racial categories in the area.

"I found out quickly there were not just one, two, three races, there was half a dozen, and all of them were different and all of them equal."

Later in the conversation, I said, "You mentioned earlier that this town has something like six different races."

He laughed and replied, "It's hard to tell."

"Were people from India included in that?" I asked.

> I would say foreign-born probably is one set, the Native Americans is another, the blacks are another, the whites are another, and then there's the mixture of blacks and Indian, and Indian and white, and all grades in between. And I never knew—I used to—When I went back home—When I first came over here I said, I saw a lady going down the street today and she had four children, and none of them were the same color as she was, and that's just sort of true. I'm not opposed to that, but it's just strange cause I never was used to that, you know. It was either black or white and that was it. But now, it's—We're all becoming so integrated until I think the whole thing will be more or less melded together, sort of like.

In an interview in a nearby small town, I asked a community member if he thought that a physician from India would be of a different race. The participant replied, "Not necessarily a different race, just a different cultural background. You know, I guess skin—I guess appearance factors in to some degree, but not so much race."

Later in the interview, I asked him to explain what he meant by the term "appearance," and he told me:

> I guess I'm trying to use that as a phrase as opposed to "race." I wouldn't necessarily, and maybe I'm being a little ignorant in my use of that, but I wouldn't necessarily consider an Asian as a separate race like I would a black. But I guess, you know, that would be my label for someone that was different from me in appearance, whether it be in skin color or whatever. And I go on the basic assumption that appearance would be neat and well-groomed. I mean, I would be just as uncomfortable if I had an American physician that looked like he'd come in off a seven day drunk, as I would [laughs] someone else. So I guess that's just my label for trying to distinguish race.

Again, it appears that there is no precise racial categorization that applies to the entire IMG community, or even to one fraction of it.

In the same small town, a participant talked about the difficulty in classifying immigrants as white or black.

"All right, Italians will come here, they will be Italians, but they would be considered white. And as you know, Italians aren't white."

"They aren't white?" I said.

"No, they're not. Okay? And, someone from France who come here, they would be considered white. An Indian comes here, and his skin is the same as mine, he's not considered black."

"You mean an American Indian or an Eastern Indian?"

"Eastern Indian. He comes here, he's not considered black. If you're not white, then you are allowed to be whatever you are. If you are white, or you know, what they consider white, then you are grouped into that category. I don't know why, you know. And it would probably be insulting to a East Indian if you called him black, and I find that to be a little off the wall."

A member of the hospital staff speculated that some people might consider some IMGs to be black. "If their skin, if it's very dark, they may be considered of the, you know, the black race." The participant also noted that she did not share such views.

At the same time that some whites might classify Asian Indians as black, an IMG with black skin might not necessarily be considered black to some members of the black community. According to a "black" IMG, "As a matter of fact, it was very interesting, a person came to me, African American, came to me and asked me if I'm black? [laughs] I thought—It happened—I mean, the first time I thought, well—But it happened twice, they said, you know, are you black?"

The physician explained that, before asking about his race, patients would tell him not to be offended. He would brace himself for the worst.

"So I braced myself, why did you say that? Are you black? I was like, why are you asking that question? Well, you speak different."

As he recounted the story, it seemed amusing in conversation, as though he had been expecting patients to ask a serious medical question but instead he only received a question on racial identity. Without any clear pattern in the racial classification of IMGs, a complicated issue is that community members often told me that they prefer to see a doctor of the same race.

Preferences for Racial Congruence between Doctor and Patient

Many participants explained to me that the race of the physician is not an important concern. However, it was also common for me to hear that it is better to have racial congruence between doctor and patient.

Comments from an IMG serve as a good introduction to the importance of race in choosing a doctor:

> If you look at the population, people want to go to people of their own sort. African American would like to go to a black doctor. I would like to go to an Indian doctor if I had—or a Pakistani doctor, if I was a patient. Whites would probably like to go to a white doctor. I don't know how that is, that's human nature probably. Native Americans would like to go to a Native American doctor. It's probably easier for them to relate, whatever we're talking about, things that we don't—at least I don't know, like cultural beliefs and stuff like that. Or just knowing the person as he was growing up in the community and stuff like that.

The rationales for preferring a doctor of a particular race varied from individual to individual, and also from people preferring one race to another. In the words of a Native American physician in Berry: "Like for Indian people, Native American people best relate to Native American people, especially in the area of health care—especially in health care. That ability to relate is what makes a medical encounter a great one. It's a difference between a poor one or a good one, or even a good one and a great one, the ability to relate."

He explained further that racial preferences can vary from one place to another: "Some of it depends on how strong your identity is of who they are, and Berry being the seat, the heart, of our tribal government and what is looked at as the center of [name of tribe] culture, you know, people identify very strongly as Indian. But as you go outside of this area, it's maybe a little bit less so. You know what I'm saying?"

"Uh huh," I said.

"So somebody in the far eastern part of the county who knows they're Indian, but yet doesn't do anything as it relates to their Indianness, it may not matter as much. But now in Berry, that's a different matter."

Thus, a geographic concentration of people from a particular culture might foster a greater cultural identification than in an area in which people of the same culture are more geographically dispersed.

The Native American physician explained further: "Some people come just because they know I'm Indian, and some people say, you know, I wouldn't take my child to a person who's not an Indian. I remember one time being in the hospital and a dad said, my wife's about to have a C-section, but I don't want that white doctor, I want an Indian doctor, when my child is born I want an Indian doctor to be the first person my child sees. So I was there."

"Is there a native OB/GYN?" I asked.

"No, not yet, working on it," he said, and he laughed.

Preference for racial congruence also surfaced in an interview with a participant who works in health care administration. She talked about the benefit of being the patient of a doctor of the same race and gender.

> I like the fact—First of all I like the fact that she's female. I just think females understand females better, number one. I think there's things that females go through that males just don't go through, and I think another female understands the psychological impact of that much better than a physician can, regardless of how much education and training they've had. But I just like the fact that she's Native American, she's had my experiences, she knows where I'm coming from and she understands me when I talk to her and what I have to say. She understand immediately what I'm talking about. And those are some of the communication things that can be missed out if you're even not from this—Even not necessarily a foreign medical graduate, but not from this area, and not knowing what the background of the people are and where they're coming from culturally and, you know, in terms of the way they were raised and your belief system and all that kind of stuff. You know, I can say something to her like, you know, I've been having problems or whatever and I went to the church last night and had the elders to pray for me, da, da, da. And she'll say, well, that's great, keep it up. You know, whatever. Whereas, you know, somebody else might like, do you really believe in that stuff? Yeah, I believe in that stuff, I believe in it.

Preference for seeing a doctor of the same race cannot necessarily be disentangled from other important issues, such as preferences for seeing a doctor of the same gender, or concerns about religion. Race is just one nebulous issue that cuts into a composite of many other contexts for health care in Delano County. At the same time, race can be of extraordinary importance in choosing a doctor.

In interviews, I usually sought to learn whether people had racial preferences when choosing a physician. One participant who identified herself as Native American responded: "Well, say there's an Indian and a black and a white in the same area of medicine, if I thought the Indian was just as good, I would choose the Indian, the [name of tribe]."

"All things being equal?" I said.

"All things being equal, right. So does that answer your question?" Later, she added, "You see, it's why I said if they were equal, I would choose [name of tribe]. It hasn't always been where we could get Indians into medical school, and it wasn't because they didn't have the brains, it's just because they didn't let them in. And I guess that makes you have a stronger feeling for the [name of tribe] who have gotten in and come back and done well."

As indicated by the above response, people might consider, in at least some way, past geographic and social exclusions when choosing a doctor. After a community has been excluded from an important opportunity like medical education, there can be a grassroots reaction in support of the accomplishments of people from the group that was excluded. In slightly different terms, Jim Crow has a lasting legacy for some patients who do not want to be excluded anymore. Pride in the accomplishments of Native Americans has added further to preferences for racial congruence between doctor and patient.

In the black community, I learned more commonly about a sense of disempowerment, as evidenced by the lack of a health clinic until recently in south Hamilton. Beyond south Hamilton, blacks are relatively dispersed throughout Delano County, without comprising a majority in any town. Such dispersion may contribute to disempowerment since there is not a core geographic concentration of blacks in Delano County. Meanwhile, there are geometries of power between whites and Native Americans, with whites more centralized in the eastern parts of the county, and Native Americans in the west.

A black U.S. medical graduate explained to me:

> We've had to go where Caucasians have gone all our lives and accept whatever we've been given. We had no other choices historically. So we've not had that empowerment that we could go somewhere else. We just took what was given to us and then dealt with it. It's only that a large percentage of the Native American population in the Berry area are a lot more powerful. And obviously there's more power in their numbers, okay.

Meanwhile, a black community member referred to disenfranchisement as a reason for wanting more black doctors:

> Well, that's one of the things that the black community do not do enough of, which is patronize their own race, and that's the reason why we're poor and we are getting poorer, [laughs] as a race. But individually, there's some of us that are overcoming financial problems, but as a race, we're poor. And I think one of the biggest things is because we do not patronize one another. When we have

> businesses, we do not patronize one another. We can't get the pastors to respect our businesses. And of course if another person has been in business for fifty years and you've been in business for five years, of course they're going to have more revenue to have nicer things. But we can't—So back to foreigners, I think that it's important that we patronize one another, and allowing foreigners in does not encourage blacks or people of—American people to go into—to become a doctor. If we're going to accept foreigners in, we're less likely to see the need to encourage our children to go to college and become doctors.

In the black community, some people might even prefer to see white doctors, although no black participants told me of any such preference. As in Quincy, the issue of black community members preferring white doctors surfaced only in one or two secondhand accounts. A nurse practitioner who works in a small town in Delano County told me about having a patient base that was predominantly black:

> Even having done the rotations in the clinics and worked in the Hamilton area I was not used to seeing patients, so many black people. And it took some getting used to for me cause things are a little different in the communication, and that sort of stuff. So I've adjusted to it very well. I mean, I feel very much at home doing that, and I think [name of IMG] did too. But the patients who were predominantly black—Well, our office manager, who is from the area, she said, you know, when [name of another IMG] comes, it's going to take a while for the people to get used to him. And I said, what do you mean by that? He's new, yeah. She said, well, you know, he's black, and the black people don't want to see the black doctors. I said, I didn't realize that, I would think it'd be the other way around. Why is that? And she said, I don't know, they seem to think they're not as smart. Now I have no knowledge of that but it seems so unusual. I would have thought that they would have been better received by their own race.

Preferences for white physicians surfaced in some interviews with white community members. For example, a senior citizen told me:

> Probably your first choice would be your own kind, I think that's natural. Just as a Native American would choose a Native American physician as opposed to a white physician. And I think the white person would choose the white physician. But limited choices dictates that we reconsider that. And I would not have chosen any of these. If I had been looking for a doctor I would have gone with who I was accustomed to and who I knew. But my experience has been very positive when I have fallen into one of these other situations, and it's been accidental, not by design, but very good results.

I asked, "So if you had your choice, all things being equal, would you choose a white physician?"

"Simply because you seek your own kind. Like, I don't know, likes are supposed to repel and opposites attract, but I don't think that is true when you're looking for a doctor. I think just human nature would dictate that you would seek someone as similar to yourself as you could find."

Once again, it is difficult to disentangle preferences for racial congruence from other concerns, such as the ability to make a physician choice. Without much choice (e.g., seeing the only available physician at a clinic), a patient who otherwise might not seek care from an IMG now has that exposure, and views it positively.

The issue of racial preferences is not always a matter of preferences *for* a particular race but, also, *against* particular races. According to a health care administrator in a nearby small town:

> Even though there is mistrust amongst the other groups, but in terms of levels of mistrust, I think the white population would probably—They still have problems around here dealing with African American and Native American physicians, so when you bring a foreign medical graduate in with brown skin and speaking a heavy accent, you know, they really have—You know, why can't you get us some—I mean, they'll tell you, why can't you get us some white physicians in here?

"Have they said that?" I asked.

"Oh yeah! Oh yeah! Why can't you get us some white physicians in here? Uh huh."

In another interview, a nurse practitioner recounted working around the hospital emergency room:

> We had doctors of all races there, more than anywhere else in the hospital. And there would be patients who would want to see the white doctor, who might be the worst doctor in there that night. But they would say, I don't want to see that person at the desk. And I don't know where that comes from, but I have seen it."

Similarly, in the words of a lawyer:

> I think it would be difficult for some people in this community to go to an international physician or a black physician, or maybe even an Indian physician. There's a lot of—In this county I'm sure there are a lot of what is generally termed redneck territory, and they're just not going to go to physicians that are not American born, white physicians.

Although such concerns were often expressed in the third person, several participants still talked about preferences for seeing doctors of "your own kind." Based only on my own reflections, I think that participants had some recognition of the limits of what might sound more acceptable. Some participants may have found it acceptable to say that it is only natural to prefer someone of similar background, but still unacceptable to claim a preference for one race over another. The line separating what is an acceptable and an unacceptable perception on race (i.e., what should be disclosed to a researcher) varied not only on an individual basis, but, I would suspect, between Quincy and Delano County.

At the same time, differences in perceptions toward race do not appear to exist on a straight line or continuum. In other words, the ideas that people expressed about race were not simple or one-dimensional but, rather, complex and multifaceted, especially in Delano County.

Consider obstetrics and gynecology (OB/GYN) as an example of the varying, multifaceted nature of the findings from one part of the study area to another. Delano County has nine obstetricians or gynecologists, none of whom is an IMG, and only two of whom are black. The issue of the OB/GYN's race did not even come up in Delano County, even though this issue was mentioned frequently in Quincy. In Quincy, in which all but one OB/GYN was black, preferences for white OB/GYNs led to outmigration of patients for health care. In Hamilton, I asked a white gynecologist if patients express a preference for doctors who are white or black. The physician replied, "No, I've never had anybody that requested a physician solely on the basis of race."

Yet people make health care choices that are subtly or indirectly linked to race, as when people prefer to see a physician in a white neighborhood for any number of reasons (e.g., close to home or work, loyalty to a clinic, past experience). There might also be differences in patients' racial composition from one clinic to another. Such differences can be minor and incidental, as when one office has a slightly higher percentage of white patients than another. According to an IMG of Asian Indian origin, differences in the racial composition of physicians' patient bases can be significant. We had just been talking about racial separateness in churches, and he told me:

> And, if I can add, there are practices of physicians which are predominantly catering to whites, there are practices of physicians which are predominately catering to Indian Americans, American Indians, and I guess there are a group of doctors who also cater predominantly to Afro-Americans. Indian doctor community actually ends up getting all three into their clinics.

From my limited perspective, IMGs appeared to be part of the broader landscape of multiracial inclusion in patient care, rather than a special case of being more inclusive than anyone else. Then again, the track record of pioneer IMGs suggests that inclusiveness of patients of different economic, racial, and cultural backgrounds has been particularly noteworthy, based on comments from participants.

Fitting International Medical Graduates into Race

In Delano County, contradictory statements about "race" (or what many perceive to be race) appear to be true. Differences in physical appearance do not matter, and differences in physical appearance do matter. Despite the fact that people's appearances do not fit easily into racial classifications, IMGs might still face some concerns through people's perceptions that there are differences or similarities in physical appearances. An IMG of Asian Indian origin explained, "In New York, as a physician or as an Indian guy, I could walk on a street and no one cares. Here, if I walk, they would think, hey, what is this guy doing here? So that kind of difference of perception, yes, exists. And that doesn't apply to just physicians, to any foreigner who would come in."

I asked, "There's a perception if you were walking down the street somewhere in Hamilton, that people would say, what is this guy doing here?"

"Maybe I am already known. But say if I was a new guy, and if I went into, say, a residential area of white guys or, say, of black guys, or any community for that matter, obviously they would be amused to see a—Just like if you were in India, went into a community, you'd be, you know, kind of—People will curiously. Not necessarily want to hurt you or anything, but they'd be curious, what are you doing here? What are you here for?"

Meanwhile, with social circles divided largely along racial lines, it becomes complex to consider the place of IMGs socially in Delano County. According to an IMG of Asian Indian origin:

> I may have only few blacks as my close, good friends. Few American Indians, local Indians as good friends. But most of them are white somehow. I don't know why. It's not that you do it purposefully but I think they try—I think they try—don't come close to you. I don't know why. I get a feeling they don't really initiate that. They kind of, you know, stay aside in these relations. I don't think it is any race, I think it's just people try to mix within themselves. . . . I feel like Indians stay in their own community, whites stay in their own community, blacks in their own community. There is some interaction but not to the extent of between themselves. There is some kind of, I think, groups that make their own barriers themselves.

The "barriers" between races do not simply fall because a physician has a different color skin, or does not fit neatly into a particular racial classification. Simply by having a social life, an IMG can have friendships in a racially divided area that fall more on one side of such barriers than another. Yet, an indefinite number of variables besides race can influence social circles, too, such as individual personality, age, or the social circles of friends. In another interview, an IMG told me that his friends were mixed among different races, more so than when he was living in New York. Again, there is no easy classification that IMGs fall more onto one race than another.

Racial divisions in Delano County may in fact have some similarities to the caste system in India, according to one IMG, "I think India is similar, based on the caste. Here we are races, we were caste systems. Everybody tried to be more comfortable in their own caste. They marry in their own caste. So same thing here. The races here are the castes there."

There can also be first impressions that people from India or other countries belong to a particular race in the local area. Three IMGs of Asian Indian origin told me that they have been mistaken by patients to be Native American. Similarly, a Native American physician in Berry told me that he had just hired a physician assistant who was born in India: "The PA who's coming to work with me, if you didn't know he was from India you would assume he was a [name of tribe] Indian, if you saw him. He's got black hair, he's about my skin color, you've seen him."

I told a member of the general community in Berry about the possibility that some IMGs of Asian Indian origin might be mistaken for Native Americans. The participant, who was Cherokee, replied, "I don't know about that. No, I don't know about that. I think—I don't think any of them that I've ever seen, I don't think you could get them mixed up with [name of tribe]. [laughs]"

"I was surprised—" I said.

"[Name of tribe] was—You know, there's blue eyes here and blonde there, and there's something else over here and here. So you can't just say, hey, what you are, when you look at [name of tribe]."

The issue of similarities in physical features still surfaced in other interviews, despite the fact that Native Americans in the area are diverse in skin and hair color. An IMG of Asian Indian origin told me about her experiences being mistaken for a Native American:

> Well, I've been mistaken for [name of tribe], a lot of times. And they want to know if I'm related to the [common family name] and, you know, [laughs] I've been stopped in the hallway when I'm doing rounds, said, honey, are you so and so [another common family name]'s child, or you know, [laughs] you favor her. I say, no, why? And they say, you favor her. You know. I've had a lot of patients that say well, you look like the [common family name] side of my family. [laughs] So it's happened. And I think it's cute, I mean, I don't take offense to it. I just laugh it off, you know.

Another IMG of Asian Indian origin told me, "I know a lot of the local Indians think I'm a local Indian, Native American."

"They think you're a Native American?" I said.

> Yes, some people, because I have some of the coloring which belongs to them. I very often have the question posed to me, you know, they want to know which family I belong to and so on and so forth. And then I kind of explain. You know, we're called Hindu Indians, regardless of whether we are

> Hindu or not, we are called Hindu Indians just to distinguish the Indian from the Native American population. That's what the Indian, [name of tribe] Indian community usually refers to us as, and that's the way I tell them, you know, when some of my patients ask me, they're Indian, whose kin are you? So I'd say, no, you know, I'm a Hindu Indian, I'm not a [name of tribe] Indian. But that's kind of interesting.

Such mistakes about Asian Indians being Native American might be merely incidental, with no bearing on the actual doctor-patient interaction. Then again, if similarities in physical appearance help in forming bonds between people, it is possible that IMGs and their patients may actually benefit from such mistakes.

Having said all of that, and having discussed so many details of racial perceptions, other issues besides race can be of primary importance in health care. According to a Native American physician in Berry:

> Now when a person is drowning, they're not going to be too particular about what color the straw is that they grab onto to save their life. So, so far as the acceptance of more or less other races among the people here, or foreign graduates, if that's all they've got, they're going to accept that, you know. So I think the people in underserved America don't have much choice, they have to take what comes, you know.

In discussing the issue of race in Delano County, an IMG of South Asian origin told me that patients are simply more concerned about getting well. In his words:

> You have sheriff elections, there's an Indian sheriff and a white sheriff, and people will be talking about whether we need an Indian sheriff or a white sheriff. You go to [university] chancellor, they want an Indian chancellor or a white chancellor or a black chancellor. [laughs] So obviously there is race issues. Those are for politicians. Those are not for doctors. I don't think people—I don't think they think about that when they're going to see the doctor, to tell you the truth. They have other things on their mind. People think about these things when they're well fed and not in pain. [laughs]

An IMG who is originally from Eastern Europe expressed a similar viewpoint:

> If, let's say, I'm going to refer a patient to somebody, and there is like two or three options and they tell me one of the physicians, I wouldn't ask them, well, why are you choosing this one, because he's of your race? It just doesn't come up, you know. You don't like the other ones, fine. Believe me, when you have twenty-something patients a day, and you have nurse practitioner pulling on the

> sleeve and saying, come see this one, you don't really care about these issues. You only care to plug in the patient in the right path and get them fixed or get them as close as fixed as you could.

Thus, this discussion on race has now come full circle. Race is both central and peripheral in health care, important and unimportant in the doctor-patient interaction. Race can be a barrier to health care, or unrelated to health care. Race can be based on physical appearance, or not based on physical appearance. All the while, IMGs enter into the racial equation knowingly or unknowingly a part of internal divisions, and yet separate from the racial divides of the area.

THE ROLE OF WOMEN

A thorough study on the acceptability of women as physicians in rural America should include many complex issues, such as economic changes impacting opportunities for women, equal rights, perceptions on interpersonal relationships, the social construction of gender and gender roles, changes in medical education, and feminist theory. Obviously, I cannot discuss all of those issues here while maintaining a focus on IMGs. However, the social construction of gender roles—in particular, the role of women as physicians and as spouses of physicians—is far too important to be ignored.

The area's twenty-five female physicians included five IMGs. My sample in Delano County had six female physicians, including three IMGs and three U.S. medical graduates. I also interviewed two wives of physicians, one the wife of an IMG, the other the wife of a U.S. medical graduate, and a husband-wife couple who were both IMGs. In addition, participants included two people—a nurse and a community member—who had once been the wives of U.S. medical graduates. These and many other interviews yielded a fuller picture about gender roles than was available in the Quincy findings.

The Context of Being a Female Physician

An interview with a U.S. medical graduate who is a gynecologist was particularly helpful to me in learning about the context of being a female physician. In her words:

> I probably have a skewed population, because the people I talk to are the ones that choose to come to me, so that's a pre-selected group. It's not just an unbiased population. These are women who automatically have selected a female physician, so they show a bias towards us. But I think that in general, women

> physicians are perceived as more willing to listen. Today is a good example, that's the reason why you had to sit out there and wait for so long is instead of just a lady who comes in for a routine yearly physical examination, oh, her world is falling apart and she's miserable and you have to sit and listen to them and try to sort through the problems. Otherwise, you know, it would be very easy to cut people short, very easy. You can do it in a heartbeat, and they know when you're cutting them short, they know when you don't want to listen. And I think women are perceived as more willing to listen. And also, for better or for worse, people perceive you're not as busy. When I was in a practice with two other male OB/GYNs, and we would see pregnant patients, and we would rotate, oftentimes, the women would come in to see me on their rotation, and they'd say, well, I've got this problem. You know, it would be a non-acute problem, just an ongoing little minor thing. But they'd say, I didn't want to talk to doctor so and so about that last week, because he's so busy. Well, I'm just as busy, but you don't mind taking my time. Women are perceived as more willing to listen regardless of race. And I think that, at least among your female patients, we're perceived as maybe a little bit more understanding and we don't view their complaints as not serious, therefore, I'm not going to really waste my time delving into it sort of thing. It's serious to the person, but we know it's not anything that's going to kill them. That's something that's a benefit to the foreign medical graduate if she's a woman, she's going to have people who say, well, I want to talk to you about my husband, or something like that. Nurses don't like female physicians as well as they like male physicians, they just don't. Women don't like taking orders from other women. I don't know what to say about that, but it's true. You really have to treat the nurses very nicely.

As the conversation continued, I asked her about the acceptance of female physicians by other physicians.

> You have to prove yourself. I was the first female surgeon who came here. I'm not a general surgeon, but I operate. I'm the first female who came here to operate. And I'm an excellent surgeon, I will just tell you that off the bat, I'm an excellent surgeon. But I can promise you if I'd have had any kind of problem in my first year, I would have not been given the benefit of the doubt, and fortunately I didn't. I'm trusted. But it's like I told you, if somebody had gone to a prestigious medical school I would have the assumption that they were a good doctor until they proved otherwise. A male who comes down here and is a surgeon, I think there's an assumption that he's a good surgeon until proven otherwise. A female has to prove herself. I don't know why, but it's true.

"And a female international medical graduate then would really have to prove herself?" I asked.

"Yeah. Depending on what specialty she is in. If she was in a soft specialty—If she was a pediatrician, yeah, nobody's going to hold her hand to the fire and say, oh my God, you've got to correctly diagnose the first 500 kids that walk into the office. But if she's chosen a surgical specialty, probably she would be scrutinized a little bit more closely."

Based on the above comments, there are overlaps between the experiences of IMGs and female U.S. medical graduates. For example, both groups of individuals may have to prove themselves to varying extents, depending on specialty. Comments about soft versus hard specialties are particularly instructive in considering a social hierarchy among physicians. The fact that no IMGs are surgeons at this time may or may not be reflective of the social status of IMGs in Delano County. Another insight gained from the above comments is the idea that female U.S. medical graduates may have some problems in their working relations with nurses. As demonstrated by these few examples, understanding more about the experiences of female physicians can be insightful in thinking about the possible experiences of IMGs.

In another interview, I learned from an IMG of Asian Indian origin about being a female physician in Delano County. She explained to me:

> The problem I have found is rather than do with nationality, it's to do with sex, with the fact that you're a female. That certainly was somewhat difficult to overcome initially, especially with patients, not so much with the physicians, but with patients, because the concept around here was a female was a nurse until otherwise, you know, no way could you be a doctor. So getting them to accept what you said with authority was somewhat difficult. But now as we go along, most patients know you well enough, and after you've kind of built up your experience, you know, they've kind of trusted you, it's much easier.
>
> I mean, it's just that some of the old-timers, and I don't necessarily get upset, it's just some—it's just a common—it's just an observation you make. And most of the time I kind of work around the problem. I either—I don't know that—as patients, you go along having more experience with patients, they build up trust in you. And most of the time that's the case. There are still some die-hards who will not see a woman. . . . But by and large, now it's okay. But when I first came in here, it was like, where's the real doctor? You know. So, in a smaller town—this never happened in New York. I mean, that was one thing which I never had to face there, whereas in a smaller town, yes, when I first came in here that always was the case. And I'm not the only female physician who's had that kind of experience.

A U.S. medical graduate shared her perspective on being a female physician in Delano County:

> Well, some perhaps would not perceive being confused with being a nurse as a negative thing. . . . But there are also positives to being a female. Certainly, you

> know, you have the issue of being a role model, I get to talk to Girl Scouts and things of that nature because I'm a woman and a physician. Certainly some patients prefer to see a female, so it's not all negative that I'm a female and a physician. And I have not felt as if I were not accepted because I'm a female, but certainly other physicians have not felt that way.

I commonly met female participants who expressed a preference for female doctors. Furthermore, as indicated by the female gynecologist, many patients may have a perception that female physicians are more caring. Such issues obviously influence the acceptability of female physicians. Nonetheless, the impact of such issues becomes more complicated by considering cultural variation from one country to another. The roles of women in different countries enter into people's expectations of female IMGs and the spouses of IMGs in Delano County.

Geographic Variation in the Roles of Women

As different cultures from different parts of the world converge in an area, the potential exists for conflicting views on the roles of women in society. For example, perceptions toward women in India vary from perceptions toward women in the United States (Cole-Kelly, 1994; Pulsipher, 2000). Further variation in the roles of women takes place over time and within individual countries.

A nurse practitioner explained to me:

> We have several international graduates who are females, and most of the patients—female patients particularly have liked them. And I think that tends to be more of a gender understanding. . . I've seen just as many sexists from New York as I have from India, so. [laughs] Or from Delano County. [laughs]

In another interview, I talked with an allied health provider of Asian Indian origin who works at the hospital. She told me that she has given advice to physicians from India about how to treat women:

> Some people when they come they feel like, why is it the women are so, you know. Because, you know, especially—In most of the other countries, even in African countries, or in India or in other countries, women are not—do not have that much importance like men. So the men have always the feeling in their mind that, oh, okay, I am the supreme. Okay? Ladies comes second. But in this country, it is different, so I feel like when I talk with them, okay, don't think like that, think everybody's equal here. So don't think that you go first, or she goes first, you know, or I had to go—No, no, no, don't think like that. Okay? It is the same. And respect ladies more than—[laughs] So I had to—Sometimes I had to tell them like that.

> Sometime they feel like, you know, these overpowering, you know, that kind of feeling, oh my God, why the, you know, the nurses are doing this or that, you know. Sometime they feel like that. Then I tell them, no, no, no, you don't have to think like that, you know. Here everybody, you know, act in the same way, and your culture may be different. But once you come to this country, or you know, once you are in another country, you need to change it. If you cannot change it, you should not come here then.

At the same time, it would be a mistake to consider every place in India as identical in terms of the treatment of women. A male IMG of Asian Indian origin explained that there is variation by place and people in the social status of women:

> I come from a middle income or middle class, upper middle or middle class Indian family where ethics are important. Women are treated equally. Many women are equal breadwinners for the family, and they are treated—And they have the opportunity to work—The social conditions, like, there are certain things, there are certain taboos or certain ways that, you know, you don't want to get out of your marriage if you can, only as a last resort you seek divorce, that kind of thing. That's different from here, where, you know, even if they get along on a few points but sit down together and say, we can't, you know, work this out, let's just separate. There's a difference there. And my perception—If I'm not aware of the culture initially, when I come in as a resident, it may be different from that after a few years.

As we talked further, he continued, "If you go into Indian scriptures, into Indian mythology, women have a very unique place. They have reverence towards women in certain—It might have, you know, some black spots somewhere because someone's misperception or—There was a time when the ruling class had a custom of sati. I don't know if you're familiar with that."

"How do you spell that?" I asked.

"S-a-t-i," he said.

> And that was something which made the outside world think that the women were persecuted in India because the system was that if a king died, his wife would immolate herself in his funeral pyre. And that was something which was actually considered like she's wedded to him for lives, for subsequent lives. We believe in rebirth and all that which is—But that, plus, I don't know, certain organizations in India which might be, you know, trying to bring women together and—I think it differs. In rural India, maybe women are kind of oppressed, but I come from a urban place, and I haven't really seen any woman—I've seen women actually ahead of men in places.

The wife of an IMG of Asian Indian origin shared a similar perspective about women being ahead of men:

> In fact, women are more educated in our culture than men these days, you know. So the opportunities to the women are just as open to men, because they are more educated. But—And I'm sure there's always going to be few men who want to suppress the women, and that happens in any culture, you know. So there's no such thing that women are not respected as much as—In fact, they are more respected than probably men, because they take care of the family.

A complicated, related issue is that this discussion on gender roles has the potential for misunderstandings stemming from the imposition of one culture's norms and values on another. What makes sense in one culture often raises questions in another. Perceptions on respect for women serve as one example, and the "puja" or Hindu prayer meeting in Quincy warrants further exploration. At the puja, which was discussed in Chapter 5, men and women occupied different spaces in the same room. To my initial thinking, the unseen partition between men and women must have had some grand explanation, but none was offered to me other than socialization. In Hamilton, I revisited the issue of gendered spaces by asking a few Asian Indians for their thoughts on why the men and women sat separately at the puja.

Here was the explanation from the male IMG of Asian Indian origin who was quoted above:

> Why is that? That is a tradition in India. It's a—If you go to any function anywhere in India, the majority of the time, you will find—It may be that—When you see any function going on, most of the time you'll see people talking more than paying attention to what's going on. And the talking, they're more comfortable if a man is sitting and he's talking to another man and maybe he's catching up on social things and other things. Women are trying to catch up on some other things. And somehow, this is how it is. Even if you, you know, sit them together, eventually at some point they would probably like to mingle in that way, because there are certain common things the men would have to talk with each other and women would. So, but it's no hard and fast, it's just—it just happens, I can't explain it.

The same statement could conceivably be made about the separateness between men and women at many social gatherings in the United States.

I also talked about the puja with the wife of an IMG of Asian Indian origin. I told her that I had asked a man at the puja why the men and women sat separately, and that he had explained it was just a matter of different interests. She agreed, and told me:

> It just happens. It just happens. That happens to all our social gatherings, the women get separated and the men get separated. It's nothing—no prejudice or

no—nothing. I mean, just somebody coming from outside probably noticed because here, all the functions, everything is together, you know, everybody's together. But even in weddings, men would sit on one side, women would sit—Like the women would be around the ceremony that's going on. The men would be out talking and, you know, just socializing. It's nothing—You know, they're just different—You're right, exactly, whoever said that. You have different interests, you have different—And when you get a chance to go to this social gatherings that when you have a friend that you might want to sit next to that you don't talk on a normal basis, you know, you haven't seen somebody in a long time. So they get—They do get segregated, you know. Women go together, children go separately, they're playing in their own little world, the men talk about probably whatever stocks and sports and all that, and the women talk about probably clothes, [laughs] and cooking and, you know, it's different interests, you know, exactly. So it's nothing—There is no rule or anything. You could go sit next to a man, you know. But it's just like in our culture it's—Other than your spouse, you don't just sit next to anybody, you know. So they just get separated, you know.

Cultural norms in South Asia have been transplanted to rural U.S. settings, influencing different interpretations of how IMGs treat women. As in Quincy, some participants expressed a concern that women are not treated well in Asian Indian cultures. According to a senior citizen:

Well, maybe it's just my perception because I think of them as coming from a country where women aren't as independent, or they accept what their—It's a male dominated society, and they are—I view them as being accustomed to accepting whatever the males of society dictate. And you know, Pakistan had a prime minister who was a woman and so has India, but I still think it is a male dominated society as a whole, and women do not—they are not as independent. Maybe that's just a misconception on my part.

A retired U.S. medical graduate also perceived differences in the treatment of women: "I don't think a lot of foreign trained people respected women as women, you know, as American people do."

I asked, "Is that something that you've had experience with in terms of interacting with physicians who while—"

"Yeah, in a—Yes. Yeah, really, yeah. Particular I remember an orthopedic surgeon that was foreign trained, he had total disdain for women. I mean, really."

"Could you explain a little about that?" I asked.

"Well, he just—as far as in my experience with him treating some people, he treated them as if—no different than if it was some animal or something. I mean, he just gave them no status. He would talk with their husband or talk with a male but, you know, wouldn't talk with them. And that was my experience. Now this is not true with some of the later people that have come along. They seem to be very cognizant of what's going on with—But that was an early-on impression."

Similarly, in the words of a nurse: "Of course, the American culture is a little different than the culture from India. You know, the American women just do anything they please. [laughs] You know, it's like the India woman is always trying to please her husband. You know, she stays at home and more or less takes care of the family and the extended family and—I've seen that."

I asked the hospital recruiter whether there was a perception that IMGs might treat women differently than do U.S. medical graduates. His response: "I think there was at least initially, and I think as people have grown to know that population, they realize that is not the case at all. That difference may have existed in their previous life, living in that other country, but that it was a perception that was ill-perceived."

Thus, the issue of the treatment of women is highly variable, not just between or within countries, but over time as well. Complicating matters, differences in the treatment of women are not necessarily understood through fact but through perception of unfamiliar cultures.

The Spouses of International Medical Graduates

One of my own perceptions in Delano County, as in Quincy, was that many of the wives of IMGs were putting their own careers on hold for the sake of their husbands' careers. I commonly learned that IMGs' wives worked in their husbands' offices or as housewives. Less frequently, I learned about U.S. medical graduates whose wives put their careers on hold, although this appeared to be more common among older physicians. For example, a U.S. medical graduate told me:

> Thirty years ago no doctor's wife would work, that would be totally unheard of, and now that's not the case. There are a lot of couples who some of them—We've got a lot of these couples where there are two physicians who are married and they both—they all—People don't have the time that they used to have. But it's—I don't think that they're excluded, it's just that nobody's breaking their neck to include them.

IMGs enter into this changing dynamic of spousal employment with values and ideas that can be indicative of cultural differences. In one interview, an IMG's wife told me that she has a bachelor's degree in engineering, and she manages her husband's office.

"And have you had the opportunity to work as an engineer?" I asked.

"Right out of school, we moved to New York where he was doing his residency, and I haven't had a chance—While I was at university I was doing sort of an internship, but I haven't had a chance to work in my field. And then when we came here after his residency and we set up the office and everything, I started helping him and I enjoyed it, so I sort of didn't go looking for anything in my field. So it's worked out good, it's worked out."

"Did you plan to return to engineering?"

"No, probably not, probably not. And there's not many opportunities in small towns anyway. So. My career wasn't sort of that important anyway, so. [laughs]"

"It wasn't?" I asked.

"It wasn't. I mean, I just—I enjoyed, you know, engineering, and I studied it, but then I really wasn't that keen on working, you know, in the field, so sort of that got put on the backburner, and I'm enjoying what I'm doing right now, so the discipline and everything that helped me become an engineer helped me, you know, figure out a lot of what I needed to do here too, so it's worked out good. I don't regret anything."

As we talked further, I raised the idea of putting family first.

> Family first. Oh, that's definitely true, especially, you know, in the cultural background that we have. You know, we're from India and family comes first. No, we don't have any children as yet, but his parents and they all stay with us, and it's really like a big family, so we have—All the time we have family visiting and, you know, coming and going. It's like an open house. So it's a big family. And that definitely comes first. Especially—You know, I'm not like into all this feminist, you know, move, that they're saying, you know, that you have to be fulfilled if you [have] a career, and you know. I'm—I enjoy the fact that, you know, his priorities come first. And his priorities are my priorities. So, I mean, I don't feel that I'm not able to do what I want, you know. It's—I guess I get that from our cultural background maybe, you know.

In another interview, I spoke with an IMG of South Asian origin. His wife has a medical degree and is working as a housewife. In his words:

> I don't know how to say it . . . but you just have to have the right place for both the spouses to keep them in a certain place, and unfortunately Hamilton just doesn't provide—most of the rural communities don't provide that. But spouses who decide, whether it's the male or otherwise, who decide, like my wife, if she decides to work I'll be in trouble. [laughs] Because she would want to go—she's decided on herself that first we need to raise the kids, for at least the early formative years, and then pursue her goals. That's her goal for now. So it is easier. I don't know what it will be like five years down the road.

"Why would you be in trouble?" I asked.

"Because where would I find a residency for her here in Hamilton?" he said, and explained that it would be more difficult for him then to stay in Hamilton.

In another interview, I mentioned the importance of the happiness of the spouse to an IMG of Asian Indian origin. The IMG responded:

> Yeah, I think as I said, we have very good support in Indian communities in this area. So that was not a problem. Fortunately my wife was very busy. We had kids keeping our time. Then we had friends and a lot of Indian friends. So really that wasn't a problem. She was very happy here. She was very hesitant to come here actually in the beginning, but now, she is very happy that she came here. She actually, she did law in India. Then she decided not to do anything here. She wanted to do housework. Take care of children, family. When there are two professionals in the family, she thought it would not be good for the children. So she decided to sacrifice herself.

I talked with the wife of a U.S. medical graduate about similar issues. In her comments to me, she offered additional insight about the role of women:

> I can think of several foreign graduates' wives who themselves are physicians who are not practicing, by choice. They want to stay home with their families and raise their children. And the two that I can think of readily both participate in how they want to participate in the community. I also know some who are highly trained who stay at home and have no interaction, or limited interaction in the community. But I'm assuming that's because if they're doing that and are happily doing that, that's because that was the role in which they felt they were structured prior to coming to this country. They can fulfill that role wherever they are. I think a lot of what happens though sometimes that causes some difficulty is that the women come and realize that that's not how things are in America. So there's some role differences, and they may come with one idea and one cultural background, and the further they get from the time they spend in their native land, then they start having some real confusion.

As cultures converge, the roles of women in different societies are transposed against one another, but not as opposites or inconsistent ideals. Rather, since cultures undergo change, so, too, does the role of women. The line between treatment of women in India and the United States can thus become blurred, since people adapt to new expectations and societies. Still, not everyone adapts identically with regard to gender roles, and there were some instances in which an IMG would have his wife walk behind him.

"I have heard about that," an IMG's wife told me. "That's totally wrong concept about our culture. So, I mean, he was—No disrespect to him but he was really orthodox, really orthodox."

We talked further, and I said, "You've never heard of anybody doing that in India?"

"Oh no! Absolutely not. Nn nnh. He had like, I don't know, archaic [laughs] ideas about . . . I never heard anything."

According to a U.S. medical graduate:

> I recall an Indian orthopedic doctor who was here, he's not here now, but his view of women was a definite impediment to his getting along very well with the nursing staff, for example. He was—When his wife was here with him, she would walk right behind him, and that was the way he expected other women—That was his attitude toward all women. And that got on the nerves of some of our nurses on the floor who didn't like being spoken down to. That was a cultural difference.

A social worker also referred to the same IMG:

> But this [name of IMG], there's certain things he couldn't do. Like for instance, he couldn't walk behind a nurse, he would have to be first and she'd have to walk behind him, things like that. And his wife was becoming too Americanized, and I think they sent her back—he sent her back to her country, [laughs] things like that. So his culture was too—The doctors that learn to flow in with our culture I think do better probably.

A community member who used to serve on the board of directors at the hospital also referred to the same IMG:

> And another thing I could say, of all the doctors that came in, international doctors, we at the hospital had to tell one doctor that he couldn't practice at our hospital because he was cruel to nurses. He would have them crying, he would speak to them very sharp and all. And that's the only doctor that I think has been a black mark by his name. But he was a good doctor, if you could just stand his—the way he did things. And I think he finally just moved away.

Thus, concerns about the treatment of women were often personally directed toward an individual physician, the IMG orthopedist. Furthermore, the concern that his wife might walk behind him was sometimes interspersed with concerns about his treatment of female nurses. Whether concerns about his treatment of women could have influenced perceptions toward IMGs in general is uncertain.

Obviously, there is not simply one Asian Indian culture but many. Yet, some people may have a perception of an entire culture, or group of cultures, that leads to stereotyping or generalizations about how Asian Indians treat women. Some perceptions could be based on limited experiences, even as cultures undergo change.

Across all cultures, it appears that the happiness of the spouse is a basic issue for the recruitment and retention of physicians in Delano County. The hospital recruiter said to me, "Three things that are very important in physician recruitment, number one, you please the wife, number two, you please the wife, and number three, you guessed it, please the wife. The spouse, whatever, because now there's a greater number of, certainly female physicians than in the past, but still."

It might be complicated for a recruiter to help ensure the happiness of physicians' wives if people have so many different backgrounds, cultures, and life experiences. However, no one suggested that the spouses of IMGs are more likely to be discontent in Delano County than the spouses of U.S. medical graduates. On the contrary, one idea that was raised in Delano County, as in Quincy, was that IMGs' wives might be more willing to move to rural areas that lack the social and professional amenities that can be found in a larger city.

Most of the IMGs interviewed for this study are married, and the importance of the happiness of the spouse cannot be underplayed. I often heard about physicians who left the area because of problems experienced by their wives in adjusting to life in a small town. I met two IMGs whose spouses (in one case, a significant other) had left the area because they did not like living in Hamilton. In one case, the IMG was about to leave the area himself, and be together with his significant other in a different part of the country. In the other case, the IMG's wife was an IMG herself who had moved along with their children to another part of the state, and he traveled frequently to visit them. I also met an IMG couple who were husband and wife, and they had conflicting views on how long they wanted to stay in the area. Meanwhile, an IMG's husband had moved to the area and could not find work; the issue of spousal employment is by no means limited to IMGs' wives, but to husbands, too.

As always, this discussion shows that the issues involved are far from straightforward. Even while contrasts in gender roles can appear to be strongly pronounced, they can also appear to be indistinct and changing. Social adaptation, cultural changes, individuality, and social and geographic variation in India and other countries contribute to the complexity of gender roles in Delano County.

THE ROLE OF RELIGION

During my fieldwork, I attended Diwali (the Hindu New Year's festival) in nearby Filmore, and also several churches in Delano County—a Hispanic church, a Native American church, and a black church. In every church that I attended, people went out of their way to make me feel welcome, primarily by being attentive and caring hosts.

Non-Christians in Delano County

The IMGs interviewed for this study came from different religious backgrounds, including at least five Hindus, four Catholics, and two Muslims. Another IMG was Christian although the precise denomination was not clear, and two other IMGs did not disclose their religion. The physician community appeared to be more varied in terms of religious background than was the case in Quincy. I sensed that the religious diversity of the physician community may have contributed to a greater sense of openness in Delano County, including public displays of religious beliefs. Two Hindu IMGs had a picture of their spiritual leader in their offices, including one IMG who had printed out speeches from the Internet by his spiritual leader to give me in our second meeting. After one meeting, I expressed an interest in learning more about an IMG's religion, and he seemed so delighted to tell me about his beliefs, his spiritual leader, and about meetings with others to hear the words of his leader. I was impressed by the IMGs' religious devotion, and I think he was pleased to find someone so interested in learning about his beliefs.

A social worker told me that she teased a Hindu IMG in a friendly way about his religion:

> Well, for one thing, you know, we have your traditional, Baptist, Presbyterian, Methodist churches around here. We don't have any of your Hindu, Buddha, or any of those other, I call, way-out religions. And we don't turn toward Mecca five times a day or anything like that. And I—You can kid [name of Hindu IMG] and them about that. I said, I know, you turned towards Mecca five times today, and they laugh.

A senior citizen told me that there are some concerns that stem from having a different religion. "I think it is one area of discrimination that hasn't completely disappeared. I don't think that we're intolerant, and I say we, I don't think it's that the people are intolerant of someone else in their religion, I just think you don't meld into the mainstream as readily."

"And are there particular religions that you're thinking of?" I asked.

"Yeah, I'm probably thinking of the Asian religions because it's something so new to us, we just did not have these religious influences until, well, certainly since World War II and particularly probably since the 60s and early 70s. It's a relatively new thing here, even though there are right many now. And maybe I'm out of step more so than a younger person might be."

An underlying current in the above passage is that exposure to people of diverse backgrounds can lead to greater openness. Consequently, increasing global connections through migration or even war can make the unfamiliar seem familiar, and therefore more (or less) acceptable. Meanwhile, openness to people of different religious backgrounds can still vary in social settings from one part of the county to another. According to a health care administrator:

> My experience, because I'm thinking right now of a couple of Muslims that I know who have moved out into the county, the unincorporated areas, is if they—Once they've been in a community long enough to show the folks that they don't have two horns sticking out of their head, and they're willing to stand around, joke and talk, and da, da, da, and then people begin, well, he's okay, you know, he's not so bad, you know, he doesn't believe the way we do, but he's okay. But it takes—It's tough at first, but there's eventually—And again, that's like I was saying earlier, you know, if you're coming from outside the county moving in, you know, there's this barrier you have to break in order to be accepted into the community, and I think it's the same thing with people who are non-Protestants. Once they get to know you, they will accept you, but it takes a while, and it's not easy. It's not easy.

Again, exposure to religious differences can break down social barriers, which could conceivably alter the range of places where a person with a different background might feel accepted more easily. Most of the IMGs interviewed for this study lived in Hamilton and therefore did not face concerns about living in unincorporated parts of the county.

In Berry, a U.S. medical graduate considered that religious differences could pose a problem in some doctor-patient interactions:

> Now, the people in this area, and in a lot of areas, particularly in southeastern United States and southern United States, are highly religious, and they're real concerned about their doctors being concerned about their dying and their going to heaven. And of course, as you know, some of the other religions aren't that concerned, so they're not going to cotton too much to a person that says, well, when you're dead, it's all over, just burn them up and get rid of you. And if they know that that doctor has that kind of feeling, they're not going to trust that doctor, cause that doctor, he doesn't care much for my life, cause human life doesn't mean much to him. So from that standpoint, I can see where cultural beliefs might have some influence.

The patient's belief system needs to be considered in doctor-patient interactions, and it can be a problem if the physician is not familiar with some beliefs. For example, an IMG referred to Jehovah's Witnesses in discussing health care:

> It's important to understand the beliefs of a person because if somebody believes that they're going to suffer eternity, that's much longer and much more important than a lifetime. So the question becomes how important are you as a physi-

> cian to save their lives, quote unquote, or are you doing some other damage to their eternal soul or whatever they believe. You have to know a little bit of all those things.

A nurse practitioner also saw problems if a physician is not familiar with a patient's belief system. The provider told me that some patients discuss experiences at church while seeing physicians:

> A prime example of that that I remember very vividly was a physician who was talking to a client and then was later sharing this experience with me, who thought that this person was actually psychotic, when in fact what they were sharing with this person was a spiritual experience and what is commonly referred to as speaking in tongues around here. And for anybody who is from this area and knows the culture would know exactly what that means. But to somebody who is not necessarily familiar with it, it can seem quite strange and bizarre, and can lead you to a very different conclusion than was the reality.

The nurse practitioner explained further that the physician who was unfamiliar with the idea of speaking in tongues was an IMG.

To non-Christians in a social setting, questions that most Christians might take for granted can be unsettling in some situations. According to a community member:

> But if you're not involved with a church, then one of the first questions they will often ask you is, what church do you attend? And that will put some people—make some people uncomfortable maybe, if they don't. In my case, I happen to be Jewish and so, you know, when they say church, they're not thinking synagogue, they're thinking church. And if I say, I don't attend church, without any further explanation, then they might consider me as—do I really want to know this person too well?

The area's Jewish population is so small that there no longer is a synagogue. At the time of fieldwork, there was at least one Jewish physician in the area, according to an article in the local newspaper, and he was a U.S. medical graduate.

The Questionable Importance of Religious Distinctions

Distinctions between religions are not necessarily important for some IMGs. It simply might not matter if a physician comes from a different religion, according to a Hindu IMG:

"Personally it makes no difference to me being of a different faith from most people. I may not get to go to the church, it doesn't matter to me as long as I have an intensely strong faith myself in God or whatever. Our Hinduism is basically a—it's a—what do we call it? It's not religion per se, it is a way of thought, a way of life, and it's called Sanatan Dharma, I don't know if you're—"

"No," I said.

"Sanatan Dharma," he said, and he spelled the first word for me.

> And our philosophy by itself—You find thousands of sects and there are thousands of different, you know, deities being followed by different people, and this and that. But the entire one philosophy which comes from the vedic philosophy and that, to some extent, is common. Recently, I was at one religious discourse, and I was listening to a story which is exactly the same as Noah's Ark story. Exact same from our scriptures. Now, you can go on debating which came first, this one or that one. Who learned it first, who came—It's immaterial. What it boils down to is that, you know, it's just which group you identify with, which group you feel comfortable with. Frankly, I feel I have no need to be identified with any group, as long as my faith in my god is intact.

Religious differences might be part of social barriers only to the extent that religion helps form social circles. The IMG explained further about being a Hindu in Delano County: "It's same as a American guy who's vegetarian has a difficulty when he has to mingle, say, with a group of persons who, you know, eat meat. Or the same thing that an Afro-American person would have if he goes into a crowd full of white guys, and he may have certain difficulties initially, like relating to them. I think it's no different."

Another IMG also told me that differences in belief systems between religions are not a concern for him. We were talking in his office, and he showed me a picture of his spiritual leader:

> I hear people tell, yeah, I go in this church, I wish you can come too. But I'm busy with my religious activity, he is my guru, and these three pictures are my god pictures. And he teaches different—he doesn't name any religion, like we are Hindu, but he's—these religion is world religion is going to be accepted by the whole world in next 500 years. You don't have any name for it. He doesn't want to give any name to that religion, that we are Hindu or we are Baptist or anything. If you believe in his philosophy, you spread his philosophy. If you don't like his philosophy, don't do anything. But what his philosophy, that if you are Christian, you become a true Christian. If you are Hindu, you become true Hindu. If you are Baptist, you become true Baptist by his philosophy. That is what—So that's why, you know, I stay busy with my activity with him. He is in India.

We talked further, and the IMG described himself as Hindu by birth, "but after listening to him, I'm human being."

Again, distinctions become blurred, and it no longer can be so easy to differentiate one religion from another. According to another IMG of Asian Indian origin:

> Well, I think we create our own church. We have church. We go every Sunday to Filmore.We have created our own church. And you know, people will do that, they have their own activities, church activities. We have classes for kids about the religion or education, all that. But in general, Indians don't go to church on a regular basis like Christians. They have their temple in the house, they do their rituals at home. And then they go to temples which are maybe a hundred miles away sometimes. So it's different.

Explaining further about the temple in the house, he said, "That time we're there, that room becomes our temple. It's a feeling rather than structure."

The actual, physical structure of the temple appears to have little to do with the meaning of a place. Instead, a place is created as a "feeling" by people who gather in a particular room. Moreover, being a non-Christian in Delano County could be a non-issue, since people can create their own sense of belonging by achieving a critical mass of people who share similar social or religious backgrounds.

Creating a sense of belonging within a community can be important beyond the social group that participates in the religious activity. A minister's wife in Berry told me, "It was good to hear that one of the physicians from India, I think, on Tuesday night I think it is, he said that his house is where they meet to have their services. And this was a local person that was talking, so that was good to know."

"They meet and have Hindu services?" I said.

"Yes. Uh huh. Something like a Bible Study, which we have at our churches on Wednesday night."

As in Quincy, it can be an asset to have strong faith, which can further a sense of belonging both within and across communities. In addition, based on my own limited experience as a non-Christian in Delano County, I did not get the sense that a newcomer needed to be a Christian in order to feel comfortable in the area.

Religious Differences as a Possible Non-Issue

In Quincy, I had often felt uncomfortable as a non-Christian. I felt more comfortable in Delano County, where Christianity was tightly woven into the area's identities, too. Perhaps my experience in Quincy had prepared me for other rural areas in which Christianity is of paramount importance in many people's social and professional lives. The diversity of Delano County, particularly with regard to educational backgrounds, also made me feel more comfortable. Some comments from participants added to my own impression that religious differences were not necessarily a barrier to being a newcomer in Delano County.

According to an IMG of South Asian origin:

> Just being a physician, you really don't need church to socialize, to tell you the truth. A physician just gets you whatever you want to, just because of the work you do, people come here, open their hearts, talk about everything. And then they're the elders of the communities, and they're every kind of person. So for physicians I don't think that—to get a stepping stone in the community, you really don't need that, because you have so much interaction with all classes and—well, hopefully there are no classes in the U.S., but still. [laughs]

Another IMG told me, "People that I see as my patient love me, and I never been to any church around here."

In some interviews, participants emphasized that there are other avenues besides church that can lead to being active in the community, such as schools, work, or social organizations like Kiwanis or the Rotary Club. The importance of church to community entry can vary, according to a nurse:

> It just depends on the individual, I think. Because as for me, I may have a conversation with someone, and church would never come up in that conversation. I mean, but I have met different people that, you know, discussed their religious views. If it's something I don't know about, you know, I will listen, but basically I think it depends on how strongly you feel about church that you'd even let that enter into your conversation. Cause a lot of people it doesn't even enter in the conversation. I would probably be one of those people that church would never be an issue.

Similarly, a community member saw religion as a topic that was often not discussed openly. "In the South, you know, there are certain things you talk about, and certain things you don't talk about, there are certain things that are taboo, and religion is a lot of time one of them. Unless they're really close friends and you got a pretty idea of where they're coming from to start with, you don't get into religion."

Arguably, the privacy of religion is not generalizable throughout the entire South. For example, I felt surprised repeatedly in Quincy when people publicly shared their strong Christian faith. Some people in Delano County also openly discussed religion in casual conversation, and, according to a participant in the medical community, would ask health providers to pray with them. Nonetheless, the attitude that it might be taboo to discuss religion openly in some situations may have contributed to my own sense of comfort as a non-Christian in Delano County.

A Hindu IMG told me:

> The only few questions I did have from some patients were about my religion, which was amazing, which was about my religion, about what church I went to and what kind of religion I practiced. And that seemed to be one thing which, I guess the church is such a predominant factor here, I understand that, you know, but apart from that, I've had no problems in being accepted by most of the people outside.

Variability in people's openness to discussing religion was consistent with the idea that church is simply more important for some people than for others. According to a U.S. medical graduate in a large group practice:

> This is a very church-oriented community. We find that many of the physicians who come here, foreign medical graduates and otherwise, have very little interest in church. Some are very interested in church. We've got such a broad spectrum right here within our own practice. We have some who would not go within a hundred miles of a church, and others who are there every time the doors open. And largely, I think the ones who are involved with church, I feel like they're much more likely to be here five years from now. And of course, I guess that could conceivably be a problem with some of the foreign graduates because their faiths are not represented.

The Perceived Role of Church

Religion plays an important social role in Delano County, as explained by a Hindu IMG:

> If I belonged to a church, I probably think it would be easier for me to get into the community, and the fact that I don't belong to a church does make it a tad difficult, even for people to approach you. I mean, I look at it even from the other way, for, you know, the community can't reach out to you til they have a forum for a connection to form, and that is definitely one of the areas where you start off, you know, a starting point, especially in small areas like—small towns like Hamilton.

A community member in a nearby small town also told me about the importance of church to the area. "Well, I think you hit the nail on the head when you're saying the church being a vital part of the community, because it's really probably the bloodline of most of these communities. And you know, you're in what they call the Bible Belt, you know, so yes, church is a very important part of everybody's life and daily living here for the most part."

A Catholic IMG told me that there are only a few other Catholic physicians in the area. I asked him if being a Christian was helpful socially, and he replied: "Well, yeah, if we're regularly going to church and all of that I think that would be helpful. Cause I know one of my cousins who actually became Baptist or Presbyterian, [laughs] after being Catholic for so many years, [laughs] because he want to get involved with the community, and this and that. But he may be a businessman. [laughs]" The IMG went on to say, "I think because most people are, you know, Baptist or Presbyterian around where he is, then that's what he did."

"So he changed his religion to be more accepted in the community?" I asked.

"That's what it looks like," the IMG replied. "I don't know whether he hates Catholics. I don't think he does. But maybe just wanted to go with the flow there."

The cousin was an IMG, too. The motive for the cousin's conversion seemed apparent, even if the exact denomination was in question.

One way for a newcomer to gain entry into a community is by attending church. As in Quincy, I found that people whom I met through church were especially open to talking with me. A senior citizen in south Hamilton explained to me about the importance of the black church for accepting newcomers:

> I think if you come to, say for instance from India or anywhere, and you want to feel welcome, that you would come to church and make yourself known. And then—You know, just like you now, you went to church Sunday, and if I hadn't known anything about you, but you just going to church, and nobody hadn't told me anything, and if it hadn't a-been [a mutual friend], I wouldn't have accepted you.

We talked further, and she told me about an IMG who came to her church.

"[Name of IMG] came to our church a couple of times, Dr. [name] did. She did. That's where I got acquainted with her, through [a mutual friend]."

I said, "Oh, okay. So [she] has helped open doors for foreign physicians."

"Well, she did that one, I know. She did that one, cause she told me about her and I went to her. Then she got other patients through me. You know. My sisters both went to her, and a friend, so I've helped her too."

A parishioner in the same church told me that he decided to see an IMG who is married to the one discussed in the above example. "Well, when he was at the church, he was standing at the door, so I told him, I'll be by to see you, doc. He said, oh, fine."

The IMG told me:

> They invite you to their church and so on. That is quite remarkable, cause you don't get that up north, you know. It's like—Obviously, I'm Catholic. I don't

> guess that's obvious, but I was born and raised Catholic. And it's a little different in the Catholic Church. You don't have other Catholic calling you and saying, hey, won't you go to church with us Sunday? [laughs] It doesn't happen, so I thought that was very interesting. More than just interesting, I thought that was excellent to have people from—I mean, inviting you—Why don't you come to my church, you know. And I thought that was—I mean, I end up going to different churches. You know, every so often I go to somebody else church cause they invite me. And I feel that if you find that, you know, take the time to invite me, I should take the time to go. I mean, I've never seen that happen before, so that was a novelty to me. And I thought that was very, very powerful. I thought that was very, very powerful statement on how people viewed their church, you know, so to speak.

The Catholic church can also be a useful entry point into some communities. I asked a Hispanic participant if it would be helpful for me as a new physician in the area to attend mass at her church, conducted entirely in Spanish.

"Yes," she said. "It does. Because that shows that you're interested in really serving the community, regardless if they're white, black, or Hispanic. You're here to serve. [laughs]" She did not think that any physicians had ever attended the church.

A Native American physician in Berry also told me that physicians are invited to church services:

> A lot of times it's been my experience that people in this area will use the church as a way to try to introduce people into the community. Because church, of course as you know, is a place where, you know, you don't just get fed spiritually, but there is a social part of that. And you know, certainly Berry, a Native American community, it's—Native American people are very spiritual people and the church here is a big part of people's lives. So I know that folks who have been in the community who are not from here, providers, they get invitations all the time to go to church from patients or from staff members, unless they're not from a religion that's from here. Then there's your obstacle, if you want to call it that.

I often asked people whether any IMGs had attended their churches before, and usually the answer was no. There were certainly exceptions, and ambiguity in people's minds about who is an IMG, but my sense was that attending black or Native American churches was uncommon for most IMGs. A Hindu IMG, who has been practicing for many years in the area, told me, "In fact, a few preachers, which were my patients, they asked why don't you come to our church and talk to them. Initially I didn't want to do that but I feel like I can do it now. Open up with them, you know, have so much different to share with them. So, but I don't have enough time for that. Wish I could do that."

I asked another IMG, who has also been practicing for many years in the area, "Do your patients invite you to church ever? Does that happen?"

"They spoke to me about that. And I explained to them that we go to temple. I'm a Hindu. And it's like a church. I believe in God. But I have gone to church or something sometimes, with some of the functions and other things. But not as a regular church, just to visit."

The de facto segregation of many churches along racial and class lines complicates the ability of people to use church as an entry point into the area. People have different impressions of different churches. The social circles that spring from one church do not necessarily overlap with another, even for people who perceive themselves to be of the same race. In short, there are unseen boundaries between communities, as reflected through attendance at different churches. Consequently, it becomes difficult for newcomers to use church as a tool to gain widespread entry into all or even most communities in Delano County.

As with most issues in Delano County, the role of religion for IMG acceptability is ambiguous. Churches can be a valuable entry point into communities, but so can physician's offices that have diverse patient bases. Hindus, Muslims, and Catholics might all face some difficulties simply by being different, but I found no evidence that such difficulties were insurmountable. The diversity of religions in the physician community, combined with the diversity of social networks in the general population, might add to the openness of the area to religious differences.

NOTES

1. As always, the items discussed will not be pointed out in the discussion as contexts or noncontexts. See Chapter 2 for further information on the role of contexts in this study.

Chapter Nine

Contexts and Hamilton, Part II: Peering into the Hologram

DOCTOR-PATIENT COMMUNICATION

In a place full of extraordinary complexity, the context of communication is surprisingly uncomplicated for the acceptability of international medical graduates (IMGs). Many of the same issues that surfaced around communication in Quincy surfaced again, but without as much nuance and complexity in Delano County. For example, participants in both areas said that IMGs are good doctors but "we can't understand a word that they say." Scratching beneath the surface in Quincy showed that difficulties with communication could often be a mask for bigotry. This seemed rarely, if ever, to be the case in Delano County. Instead, people in Delano County came across as more forthcoming in expressing their opinions.

Consider the idea that patients might have difficulties understanding IMGs. Certainly, physicians everywhere can face problems communicating with their patients. For example, physicians often use medical terminology that is not understood by patients, fail to pick up on nonverbal cues, seem too hurried to spend time with patients, or simply have difficulty teaching the patient what needs to be done (Gesler, 1999). Having a physician with a different accent or word choice can add to problems that already exist with communication.

The overwhelming consensus among participants in Delano County was that difficulties for IMGs with communication were merely a nuisance. In a few instances, participants considered such difficulties to be a serious issue that can affect health outcomes. Based on my fieldwork, there did not appear to have been any court cases or public accusations of health problems stemming from problems with communicating with IMGs. There have been times though when patients have not wanted to return to an IMG because of difficulty understanding a foreign accent. According to a nurse practitioner:

> Some of the issues that have been somewhat troublesome, I guess you would say, is for foreign trained physicians who may have had a fairly heavy accent, non-English accent. And in this area where there's a very strong dialect in and of itself of the English language, sometimes that was a barrier. Because I've had folks in my own practice, at my previous practice, who have seen some internationally trained physicians, who were very good physicians, but because of English being their second language, and there being some communication difficulties, clients would come to me and say, I don't want to see that person again, I have trouble understanding them. And that's not across the board, but that's a very frequent thing that would come up.

A nurse explained to me about some of the difficulties with communication:

> You know, a lot of people, if they talk real fast, you know, they have a problem with that, just like foreign physicians when they talk real fast. It's easier to understand them when they speak slowly because their words don't quite sound right. I mean—I don't know. Because of the way they pronounce the syllables, I guess, I don't know. The way that sometimes they'll run them together it's sometimes hard to understand—if you speak your words distinctly.

Difficulties understanding IMGs can also be a source of concern outside of doctor-patient interactions, for example, when health providers communicate with one another. An IMG of Asian Indian origin explained to me, "I mean, I know my other Indian colleagues, some of them here speak very fast and they have a thick accent and I can't understand them, you know, because India's so diverse too. They come from a different part of the country, their accent's different. I can't get them either. I'm, what did you say?"

A U.S. medical graduate told me, "We have some international medical graduates who are bright, who are nice wonderful people, you can't understand a word they say. That's a real problem in the medical community. They stand up at meetings and talk and I'm sure what they're saying is very relevant. I don't have any idea what they're saying, and most other people don't."

Similarly, a nurse practitioner told me about communicating with a pioneer IMG who is very highly regarded in the area: "If you're sitting down like we are, in close proximity, and concentrating, and he's speaking slow, it's easier. If you go to a meeting where he's speaking or conducting, or even talking to him on the phone about a patient, he's difficult to understand for me, and he is for other people that I know too."

For patients, problems understanding the physician can be intimidating. I frequently learned from health providers that patients were too shy or embarrassed to ask the doctor to repeat himself. Conversely, I also met many patients who told me that when they do not understand something, they ask the doctor to say it again.

An IMG of Asian Indian origin recounted some problems with communication: "You know, patients do this little go round the block deal, you know, with doctors. And they'll come and say, well, I'm glad I understand you, cause I sure didn't understand him, I never knew what he was saying. I said, well, did you stop and ask him? No, no. We were just too embarrassed or too shy, or you know, whatever the term is that they use."

Another IMG of Asian Indian origin told me that sometimes patients came into his office expecting problems with communication.

"Certainly there are some patients you don't know, they say, no, I don't understand you, before you open your mouth. [laughs]"

"Oh, yeah?" I said.

"Yeah, there are a few. I just tell them that wait for a few minutes, if you don't understand then you can tell me, I can tell you ten times. You still don't understand, I'll get someone. Like jokingly, you always try to make them feel that way."

In another interview, an IMG of Asian Indian origin said, "Well, some people are hard of hearing, and they find it hard to understand me, but people who are—Normal people should not have any problem. [laughs]"

Problems communicating with IMGs often came across as minor, at least within the context of our interviews. For example, in one interview, a senior citizen who has been seeing IMGs for decades recounted an experience she had many years ago. She told me that, during a medical exam, she had mistakenly thought that an IMG wanted her to raise her leg, but a nurse cleared up the misunderstanding. In another interview, a patient told me about going to the emergency room with an asthma attack and being cared for by an IMG. The patient said that he had been given a printout with medical instructions and, based on the visit, clearly understood how to care for his asthma. He spoke highly of the IMG, and acknowledged that there were some minor problems with communication: "A couple of times I had to ask him to repeat hisself. A couple of times I just did not understand what he was saying. Sometimes it is difficult to understand a foreign doctor. . . . Maybe I didn't hear him, his words didn't come out clearly. Maybe because I was laying down my words didn't come out clearly."

As in Quincy, several IMGs told me that they have taken more time with patients to make sure that everything was clearly understood. Patients also told me that they have paid closer attention to IMGs to make sure that there were no misunderstandings. Thus, except for extreme misunderstandings, a problem with communication could have some benefits on a psychosocial level, e.g., doctors might spend more time with patients, and patients might be more attentive. Individual IMGs have also improved their ability to communicate with patients, and nurses have worked to make sure that patients understand medical advice from both IMGs and U.S. medical graduates.

I also learned that individual IMGs had faced initial difficulty with communication that was soon overcome. According to an IMG of Eastern European origin: "Usually what happens is—And I'll tell you, initially I came over here, started seeing patients, I had to call—For every third or fourth patient I had to call the nurse to translate. I couldn't catch their accents. And the nurse also wouldn't know sometimes what they're saying, and that would confuse me totally."

A nurse practitioner who worked closely with the above IMG offered a similar perspective about some early problems with communication:

> On many occasions, [laughs] either the nurse would be with him or sometimes when he was in the room with me to help me with a patient, he would tell them something, and they would look at me, and he would say, tell them what I said. And his English was perfect, it was just the phraseology of how he put his words together. Then sometimes with the patients, he would have to say, what did they say, you know, because it was different. That didn't take too long to overcome though. You know, a matter of months, I think, actually.

An IMG of Asian Indian origin also told me about difficulties with communication that had been resolved.

"Like when I was new, I had a patient or two walk out and talk to my staff or nurse and say, I didn't understand much of what he say. And then—But at least I have been able to tell them that if there was a problem, come back and ask me. So the nurse came to me and I explained what I said and solved the problem."

I said, "Do you think that was—Well, did that happen more at first than it does now?"

"I had only one or two episodes. It's kind of almost an aberration. I didn't have much of a problem."

I did not hear any complaints from nurses about their role in clarifying IMGs' instructions to patients. However, in one interview, a health care administrator explained that there can be some frustration stemming from the nurse's role as a translator. Referring to an IMG who no longer works in the area, the administrator said:

> His English was so broken and so poor the patients simply did not understand him. You know, they would come out of the room, the exam room with him, and go to the nurse and say, you know, I don't know a thing this man has said to me. And so, you know, the nurses get frustrated because then they have to

go back and try to talk with the physician and then be the translator between the patient and the physician, and it just didn't work out.

Obviously, nurses are not the only ones involved in clarifying instructions for patients. Other staff, pharmacists, and family members can serve a function in making sure that the patient of any physician (i.e., IMG or U.S. medical graduate) knows what to do. According to an IMG of Asian Indian origin: "If I have a problem, I tell the family to come, especially the older people have problems hearing and all that. Makes it more difficult. They cannot tell by lip reading, and if you don't move your lips the same way, they don't know what you're saying. So I think family helps in those situations. But it's not a major issue. Minor problem."

A social worker told me, "I was talking to this [name of IMG of Asian Indian origin], and a nurse jumped into the conversation and tried to explain to me what he wanted, and he pushed her away and he said, no, I want her to understand what I'm saying, she is going to have to work with me. And as a result, I was able to learn how to interact with some of the doctors."

A pharmacist told me that he makes sure that physicians' instructions are clear on prescriptions. Referring to an IMG who received his medical degree in Taiwan, the pharmacist told me:

> Well, this friend of mine who I have to call almost—Inevitably, if I get a script, I call him, cause I don't want to make a mistake, cause I know he's—You know, most physicians will not give you the time of day, and this guy's nice and he answers the phone. And if his wife answers, she'll put me on right then. He writes—And I'm sure in the Asian countries, I don't know where he's from, Korea I think, they must write to the left, from the right to the left, instead of from left to right. And he gets a lot of directions that way, you know, written from right to left. And all you got to do is just turn it around. But it'll say, pills number so and so. It'll have number sixty pills. Different from what we see here. And then I'm sure they're used to writing in—What do they write in? Not Sanskrit, it's —

"In Korea?" I asked.

"Yeah."

"It would be Korean," I said.

"Korean I guess it's good enough. And a lot of his writing looks like Korean figures. [laughs]"

These examples present a mixed picture of communication. Often, communication is merely a nuisance but there can be isolated instances in which the active involvement of another health professional is required to avoid more serious problems (e.g., a physician who reportedly writes prescriptions backwards, or a patient who walks out of a medical office not knowing what to do). Having said that, such active involvement should take place anyway; that is, nurses do clarify instructions to patients, and pharmacists do make sure that their prescriptions meet the doctor's specifications. At issue is not simply doctors communicating with patients, but multiple interactions involving patients and providers who each play a role in ensuring proper communication.

Complicating matters somewhat is the fact that patients vary individually in their ability to understand what a doctor is telling them. As in Quincy, the two groups of individuals who appeared to have the greatest difficulty with IMG communication were the uneducated and the elderly. However, a slightly different—or at least fuller—picture emerges in considering that many of the problems with communication in Delano County may have been related to some patients' lack of exposure to other places. For example, consider the following ideas from a U.S. medical graduate:

> From my experiences with patients who have seen the foreign medical graduates, they have by and large liked them. The only problem is the language and ability to understand. And especially in a rural community, when people have had very limited access to outside folks, are used to hearing just one accent all the time, even somebody from Detroit may be perceived as having a foreign accent and they would have difficulty understanding what they say. And someone who is from Bolivia, it might be even more difficult when they have a heavy accent. So when I have patients who are seeing a doctor who is from another country, they don't come in and say, oh, I just don't think he gave me the right medicine. It's like, well, I really liked him, but I just never understood what he said. [laughs] That's a big stumbling block.

The physician then added that more educated people have less of a problem with communication.

Based on the above quotation, it seems that people whose social networks are mostly limited to the local area have more difficulty communicating with IMGs than do people who have much more experience beyond Delano County. Other statements from participants support this idea that patients' limited exposure beyond Delano County can impede communication with some IMGs. For example, the wife of an IMG explained why she thought that, at first, some patients had trouble understanding her husband, "Cause they have just listened a certain way, you know, in the area, and then somebody with a different accent comes, it's hard to comprehend." Patients would then adjust over time to the physician's accent. A U.S. medical graduate told me, "I don't know if the ears of the listener change or the mouth of the speaker gets clearer, or both."

An IMG of Asian Indian origin explained:

> I wouldn't say that there's any one particular group which I'm able to communicate with better. It's more to do with the literacy rate. The lower the literacy, the more difficult it gets to communicate. Sometimes it takes really long to get there. And I think that runs across all three, or all four, however you may put it, communities. And it's more to do with the literacy level than with race, at least from what I find.

Participants frequently mentioned the elderly as potentially having more difficulty than most groups in understanding IMGs. According to one senior citizen, "I would think that for some of the senior citizens that might be a major issue. Getting accustomed to perhaps a new way of speaking than a person has been used to hearing for a lifetime."

Another senior citizen spoke positively of her experiences as the patient of an IMG. She also added:

> The only thing I think I could say that wasn't positive, some of the older people cannot pick up on the accent and understand what they're saying. And where I would say, hey, back up here and let's say this slowly and tell me what you mean, while some of the older people wouldn't. That's the only criticism I think I would have. And I think they're probably improving, once you get used to it, you know.

A few health providers also told me about personal experiences in which elderly patients had difficulty understanding IMGs. For example, in the words of a U.S. medical graduate:

> My grandmother, who's ninety-eight, was being taken care of by one of the new Indian physicians this past year, she went in as an unattached patient, she had congestive heart failure. And an example of the language barrier is—My grandmother was probably in there four or five weeks, and my mom still could not pronounce his name, so she couldn't tell me—You know, who is grandma's doctor? [laughs] She couldn't tell, you know. Or what does so and so say when he comes in? She said, well, I'm not sure. And my grandmother's ninety-eight and she was not really in a state of mind to be able to question him and say, well, I don't understand. Do you know what I'm saying?

For my part, I usually had no difficulty understanding IMGs, although now and then I needed to ask some IMGs with heavier accents to repeat a word or sentence. As in Quincy, my educational background may have made it easier for me to understand different accents.

Most concerns about communication focused on difficulties understanding the physician's accent, word choice, or speed in talking. Such difficulties understanding the physician can be compounded by difficulties faced by any new physician—or any newcomer, for that matter—in understanding local expressions and accents.

Difficulties Understanding Patients

Although difficulties understanding patients appeared to improve over time, even longstanding residents of the area said that some accents or colloquialisms are difficult to understand. I usually had no problem understanding people in the general community, but I also recognized that sometimes people's speech patterns or even medical problems can make communication more difficult.

A health care administrator who grew up in the county told me that some people are difficult for anyone to understand. "I've run into some folks that I could not understand what they were saying. Their dialect was so far removed from standard English that I did not understand what they were saying. And it's just—I think it's fascinating. I mean, I'm like, man. You know? And to hear them carrying on conversations with one another, it's just absolutely mind-boggling."

At the hospital in Hamilton, an IMG of Eastern European origin told me, "You should probably come upstairs with me now on the fourth floor and I'll try to use you as a translator for a patient that I just got this morning from a rural clinic."

"To see if I can understand?" I said.

"Yeah. Even the nurse couldn't figure out what she was saying, and the nurse is, you know, Delano County, local."

I saw no evidence that IMGs had special difficulty understanding their patients. Furthermore, I never had difficulty being understood by IMGs, although I obviously did not speak with a local accent. Professionally, all physicians face the task of needing to converse in everyday language that can be understood by people, but socially some minor misunderstandings can slip by without any concern. For example, several IMGs told me about difficulties understanding jokes. According to one IMG of Asian Indian origin:

> It may be, like if I make a joke, to me it may be because I have a completely different perception from someone who doesn't find it amusing. And I feel that he didn't even understand what I say. He understands the words I spoke, but the context or why I made that joke may be totally foreign or too alien to him. So it may be that I may feel that he didn't understand. But as far as medicine is concerned, telling them about what to do, what not to do, what is the problem and all that, it's straightforward, and as long as you speak in simple terms they understand.

Another IMG of Asian Indian origin told me about some of the difficulty understanding patients:

> Well, you know, I say the country folk, I don't care what color they are, they have an accent that to me is sometimes difficult to understand. I mean, yesterday, I remember a lady was joking with me, and she said something, thank goodness it wasn't medically—If it was medically related, I would have stopped her and asked her to repeat herself ten times. But she said something and I kind of just laughed with her, but I have no idea what she was talking about, you know. And days when I'm really busy and, you know, they're making small talk, I just kind of laugh with them. Sometimes I really have a hard time understanding them, I really do.

Another IMG of Asian Indian origin told me:

> The English we speak, I speak, is from the British system, and there are some words which are totally different in the British English as opposed to the American English, some expressions which I still am trying to catch up with. There are some jokes which I don't quite follow because some of the slang is totally unfamiliar. And similarly some expressions I use are, you know, throw people for a six, because they don't know what I'm talking about. So yes, just complexities of the language were there. But that's more in terms of with . . . not in my profession. In my profession by and large, because you interact with so many patients, you do get to pick up the right expressions. This was more in the social sense than in my professional sense. In the professional sense more or less we manage to, I think, communication-wise we haven't done too badly off. There still are some patients who find it difficult to follow my accent. And I find it difficult to follow theirs. Some of the local Americans, the Native Americans, I do find some of the elderly ladies or elderly people I have some difficulty following exactly what they're trying to say. I've now figured out that it's just a matter of taking more time with them. It just takes longer. And most of the time we can manage to do fine.

Indeed, differences in word choice can lead to some delay in understanding what is being said, even without necessarily being problematic. For example, in one interview, an IMG of Asian Indian origin used a term that was new to me. He was telling me about the size of the town where he grew up.

"At that time the population was about four lakhs."

"Four what?" I said.

"Four lakhs. Means 400,000 probably."

"Is that British English, four lakhs?"

"Four lakhs. L-a-k-h-s."

"Is that a British expression?"

"I think so, it is a British expression, right. It's a British expression. Less than half million probably. Put it that way."

Later, I looked up "lakh" in the dictionary, and learned that the word is commonly used in India, and has origins in Hindi and Sanskrit (Random House, 1993).

As in Quincy, many health providers laughed about some of the idiomatic expressions which have surfaced in working with patients. Health providers who grew up in Delano County, or who have lived in the area much of their lives, also told me that they have often come across new idiomatic expressions in working with patients, too. The slang can vary from one "race" to another. In fact, a Native American in Delano County recently compiled two booklets on idiomatic expressions used by people in his tribe. He told me that people can understand such expressions when used within the context of a conversation. Some of the expressions from his booklets also surfaced in interviews with IMGs. For example, an IMG of Asian Indian origin told me about a phrase that, although familiar to me, was unfamiliar to him when he moved to the area.

"Lot of phrases, lot of words. I'm fixing to go, fixing to do. Yeah, I didn't know I'm fixing to do. [laughs] Grammatically sometimes they don't talk very correct English. You have to guess what they are saying. But I didn't really have a problem. I think it was easy for me to understand all these people."

Another IMG told me, "There was a lot of them, like fixing to do this. [laughs] A lot of different term that I have no clue what they—But I finally learned some of them. But I don't think that it kind of interfered with the way I practice medicine or my ability to communicate with my patients. I think maybe just some time I have a tendency to talk real fast. So I've learned to kind of slow down, and I'm still learning that."

Unfortunately, I lack the background in linguistics to differentiate between expressions that might be used predominantly among one group of people than among another. I cannot draw clear lines and say that a particular expression is limited primarily to the Native American, white, or African American communities. Moreover, different individuals might interpret some words to have different meanings. For example, two IMGs learned different meanings of the word, "drink," perhaps related in at least some way to cultural or geographic variation in the use of words. According to an IMG of Southeast Asian origin, "I was asking a mom what she gave the child to drink? And the mom repeated the word drink. And so I thought she was asking whether or not I'd said drink. I thought it was something in my pronunciation, so I said, yes, drink. And she said yes. And so she saw this puzzled look on my face and she burst out laughing and she said, around here, drink means Mountain Dew."

"Well, I wouldn't have known that," I said.

"I didn't know that either."

An IMG of African origin also told me about a patient's understanding of the word "drink."

> Oh, the other thing is drink, that's the one that I—that was one communication barrier that could have led to some, you know, potential medical—like when I tell them, like somebody's dehydrated or has urinary tract infection, I'll tell them you have to drink more, you know. Well, if I don't add more water or something, they think it's alcohol. Yeah, a drink is alcohol. So if you say a drink, that means it alcohol, it's not just any drink. So I had that incident, I told my patient to drink, he thought I meant to drink alcohol.

The slang expression "risin'" was mentioned by two IMGs of Asian Indian origin, with the same meaning interpreted by both physicians. One IMG told me, "When you come in on day one, you know what an abscess is, but you don't know what a risin' is."

"A risin'?" I said. "Okay."

"Yeah. And when you see it twice and two patients come in with the same complaint, I have a risin' on my back, then you know that it is a—what he's talking to. First time, you may not, but it doesn't take a long time. But it doesn't create a major situations where you don't understand at all, so it's okay."

Another IMG told me:

> They call a blister or a boil, they call it a rising, and I hadn't a clue what they were talking about. So I said, look, I really got to stop you, I don't know what this rising business is. What is this rising you're talking about? They said, don't you know what a risin' is? They point—You know, they pointed to something that looked like a rising. I said, ah, the risin', okay, okay. Or, to have a bowel movement, they say, I'm going to have an operation. So when they said they were going to have an operation, I said, excuse me. What? Where? Who's doing it? And he said, what do you mean, who's doing it? I am. [laughs] So we've had a few, you know, similar things like that. It's funny, cause I laugh about it later, but then I learn because then the next time I'm talking to somebody else and I'm looking for a word, and you know, carbuncle, doesn't make any sense to them, I'll say rising and then they get it right away. So they teach me too. I've got a colloquial vocabulary.

Another IMG of Asian Indian origin explained, "Well, it's not their phrases, but it's their accent and the way they, you know, speak. It's hard to understand sometimes. For example, instead of saying vomiting, they vomicking. But these things you can easily pick up. It's not that different from the normal pronunciation."

Meanwhile, problems with grammar can make it more difficult to understand patients, according to an IMG of Southeast Asian origin.

"There's sometimes a difference in usage of grammar which took a little bit of getting used to, but now it's more like second nature. I hear it and I understand exactly what they're saying. Like the use of the word be."

"Be?" I said.

"Be. B-e. You know, you can—There are several forms to it, like I am, right? It would be, 'I be.' So it's just very much—Again, this is mostly with the Native American community that they do that. So at first it took a little bit of getting used to kind of when they say, 'I be in pain.' So you know something was hurting. It's a little bit of difference in the way they use the grammar around here."

In one case, an IMG of African origin told me that some patients were difficult to understand because they were chewing tobacco.

"And tobacco is a big issue here, they chew tobacco. Like if you ask them do you smoke. No. But you have to find out if they chew tobacco. Some of them will have two balls in their mouth and they are speaking slurred, their speech is slurred, you'll be wondering why, maybe they have some—are they having a growth there, but they have two balls of tobacco, you know."

"In the doctor's office?" I said.

"Yeah, they have their cup and they are spitting into the cup. [laughs] They carry the cup around. It's not pleasant. So one of them, I was examining her mouth and she had it. I told her, please can you take that out, you know. And during that time you also would tell them the effect of tobacco. Like if you ask them do you smoke, they don't smoke, but that's not the end of it. I've learned to find out, do you chew tobacco. They don't think—they also snuff a lot of tobacco too, so if you just ask do you smoke, that's not enough. You have to find out the other thing."

"Did you know to look for that when you first came?"

"No, I did not. That was my first [laughs] experience with that."

Communication can be further complicated by nonverbal expressions that may be apparent to one person but not another (e.g., reading pauses in conversations, interpreting facial expressions, considering why something was not mentioned, knowing about activities in church or social groups). Nonetheless, concerns about nonverbal communication rarely surfaced as a problem mentioned about IMGs in Delano County. Instead, participants discussed communication mainly by telling me about words, accents, or expressions. In a few interviews, concerns also included the idea that IMGs might feel uncomfortable making small talk with patients, and the possibility of occasional problems for IMGs in finding the proper tone of voice in telling patients what to do. Difficulties in patients' grammar, differences in social mores or medical conditions that interfere with speech can add further to difficulties faced by IMGs in understanding patients. However, such concerns seemed far from insurmountable.

Adherence and Communication

All physicians face a difficult task in trying to get patients to adhere to medical advice. For example, the physician's instructions need to be clearly conveyed to patients so that they will know what to do. There are many complicated issues affecting adherence, such as problems with transportation, affordability of medicine, social mores such as dietary habits that conflict with medical advice, improvements in health that lead some patients to think that the prescribed medicine is no longer necessary, and use of more than one health provider for similar conditions (e.g., a patient sees an emergency room physician and does not tell her regular doctor that a medication was stopped). Indeed, concerns about gender roles, race, and religion can also affect a patient's willingness to follow medical advice. Yet, based on interviews, there did not appear to be special problems for IMGs with adherence, although there were certainly some exceptions. If medical advice was not understood, other people helped clarify it. Nurses, office staff, family members, and pharmacists all played a role in preventing problems with communication that could lead to problems with adherence. Furthermore, patients often received written directions explaining what they were supposed to do.

An IMG of Asian Indian origin told me:

> You know, the good thing about this community, if I can call it a good thing, is that I believe that a lot of people here are so set in their ways, whether they understand you or not really doesn't—Maybe it makes like one iota of difference. I don't really think it's a vast amount of difference that it makes. I can sit there til the cows come home and tell them, please don't eat fatback, you've just had a stroke, you shouldn't be eating this, it's going to increase your cholesterol. They'll look at you and say, yes, yes, I'm going to try. And then they'll go right home and cook with it. You know, it's just one of those—And there's no problems understanding me, truly. I can get down to the same level as the person that I'm talking to, not use big fancy words, you know, and still they don't listen to it. So I really think that in this community they're going to do what they're going to do. And there's a subset of people that will listen to you and do what you tell them, and care about their health, but a lot of folks there is just—If you don't believe me come see me in my office one day and I'll let you shadow me. [laughs]

In order for patients to change their diets accordingly, the physician's advice obviously needs to be clearly understood. A dietitian told me that some patients do not understand what the doctor is telling them.

> When I would speak with a patient I would ask them, well, what did your doctor tell you? Or, you know, what do you understand about this particular situation? And sometimes they would say, well, he told me but I don't know what he

> said. And so I do think that sometimes having the patients understand a foreign doctor or provider is a problem. I just think that they're not used to hearing that kind of accent, and sometimes I just think that maybe—I don't know, if they talk really fast or something, the patients just don't understand what they're saying, but they don't stop and say, could you repeat that, or, I don't know what you're saying. They just let the doctor talk, and when he's done then they leave.

I talked with a U.S. medical graduate about this very issue of patients not understanding what they were told to do. The physician told me about a patient who was scheduled to see an IMG for a stress test.

> And she was telling me that she had left the office and hadn't scheduled it because she had not understood that she was suppose to schedule it. And then when she came back, they said, why haven't you gotten this test? And she said, I didn't understand that you wanted me to schedule it. And this is an intelligent woman. And I think it kind of embarrassed her because she felt like she had not followed the instructions appropriately and they had sort of gotten on to her. So, no, I think it's truly that they don't exactly understand what it is they're supposed to do.

Additional Consideration

Adherence with medical advice that was given in a clinical setting is one issue, but IMGs must also establish credibility as physicians beyond the office. A lawyer discussed the issue of accepting IMGs' medical advice in a courtroom. I asked, "Do you think there's any difference in the perceived credibility of a foreign physician giving a deposition than an American physician?" The lawyer replied:

> I think it depends on how that physician presents himself. Most any witness, whether he or she speaks good English or poor English, is judged, I guess, on their demeanor, and how they respond, and how they act to questions. There's a lot to credibility beyond the spoken word, and so I think it would vary. I think if a jury could not understand what the physician was saying or the point he was trying to make, there'd probably be less credibility than if it was an English physician saying the very same thing he said. It may be just the lack of understanding.

"So is that ever a consideration in thinking about which physicians you want to call?" I asked.

> It's a consideration in the deposition if it's a video deposition. We have two types of deposition, you know, the video and the non-video. In the video deposition when you're actually having that physician's words come off of a screen toward a jury, you certainly want him to be able to come across to the jury so

they can understand him. If it's a deposition that's only in writing, and you have someone else to read what he's saying, then that changes it because that person who's reading what he says makes it a lot clearer to the jury than as if he were on the stand himself. And you certainly—If he's going to be a live witness, you certainly want to try to either ask the questions or phrase the questions in a manner that the answers that he gives will be clearly understood. And lots of times that's the lawyer's job to make sure that the proper questions are asked.

DISCRIMINATION AND STEREOTYPES

Overt forms of discrimination do not appear to be common against IMGs in Delano County. The patients who see IMGs are often pre-selected, in the sense that many patients already know something about the physician in advance of the doctor visit. The people who would be most likely to discriminate might be those who choose to avoid seeing IMGs, but IMGs do not appear to be at a loss for patients. There is no evidence that other health professionals avoid working with IMGs. Still, IMGs may perceive subtle forms of discrimination; other health providers may overhear a few critical comments about IMGs from patients; and people may react differently to foreign-sounding names. In addition, discrimination has already been discussed through considerations of race relations, gender roles, religion, and, among other issues, the experiences of the first IMGs.

In four of my interviews with IMGs, I learned that discrimination can be practically indistinguishable from everyday interactions that do not involve discrimination. One IMG of Asian Indian origin even told me, "It's not wise to go and pick the subtle things when you don't want to know."

Another IMG of Asian Indian origin told me:

No one has refused per se, put their foot down that I will not work with this one. I guess they are, I think, decent enough to reduce their interaction to minimal if they don't like me. And I per se don't get disturbed. I do my work, I know what I'm here for. I'm not here to cater to individuals' requirements, I am trying to help people's health, and that's what I—So I don't focus on those things. But I had only a few perceptions like that. Not very, very overt. Very subtle. And you sense them, but you really—Because there is enough to compensate against that. Because if one person did that and ten others welcomed you, you don't care.

According to another IMG in a nearby small town:

I have noticed a little bit of—maybe, first because I'm a female, secondly, I'm foreign trained, you know, so there is some reservation. Like we have the medical

> society, the [name of medical society] meetings, we have that once a month. I wouldn't say they're not friendly, but, you know, it's very, very—almost too professional, you know, that kind of thing. I've noticed a little bit some reservations. But I don't let that bother me. [laughs] Like I said, that's the kind of person I am. I don't go looking at people's faces to see how—if they like me or not. So unless you actually come up and, you know, do something really obvious [laughs] before I notice it. But I think there is some . . . I wouldn't say they don't accept me, but it's like maybe they are just keeping to themselves.

Later in the interview, the IMG commented on doctor-patient interactions that can be perceived different ways:

> I see mostly poor patients. And I don't know if that is anything, but I had one occasion of attending to a wealthy patient, white patient. The patient was admitted to my service by an on-call physician. When I came to see her, the family requested the patient be transferred to another service and this other person is a male, he's older, and he is white. Okay. And she's white. So I don't know. He apologized profusely, it wasn't because of me or anything, but they knew this other physician better and they would prefer for their mother to be taken care of by this other physician. So I don't know if it was because she was white and wealthy and that's why they wanted, or just because of the fact that I'm new and they knew this person better, as he said, you know. So, [laughs] that's one experience I had, you know. So that's—so I cannot—I wouldn't be able to make that general—I cannot come to that conclusion, but that's just one experience.

Thus, uncertainty is part of concerns about discrimination. The distinction between activity that constitutes discrimination and everyday activity that could be misperceived as discrimination is blurred. There are times though when subtle forms of discrimination come to IMGs' attention. In one interview, an IMG of Southeast Asian origin explained:

> You can more or less tell, going into a place or a room, by how they acknowledge you, or if they acknowledge you at all. You know, a lot of people around here, they go out of their way to say hi. Sometimes you're somewhere and that's not done, and when you know that's customary for the people here. And you know, I might take that as, you know, you're ignoring me.

In less subtle terms, a U.S. medical graduate in Berry told me that a few patients have spoken critically to him about an IMG from the Philippines who is very highly regarded in the community:

> So every once in a while I'll hear people who in a derogatory way will say, I didn't like the Chinese man. What they mean is they didn't like [name of IMG].

> And I'm supposing—It sounds like to me when they say in that tone, in that manner, they're objecting partly to whatever the medical issue was at hand that they objected to, but also to who he is, you know, the Chinese man. So maybe not in a referral sense, but I do kind of run into that kind of objection to a foreign graduate. You hear it all the time. I might hear somebody say, I didn't like the young white man, or I didn't like the young black lady. Sometime in not those nice a terms. You know what I'm saying?

In one interview, a community member in south Hamilton told me that she felt that she had been accused of discriminating against an IMG. She said that such an accusation was not warranted, since all she wanted was more information about the physician.

"I went to an office and they said that I had to see a foreigner, and so I started asking questions about him, and the person got so offended that she didn't want to give me any information. She thought that I should accept whoever he was and not ask questions. So I felt uncomfortable and decided not to go to that office . . . I had asked for the regular doctor and they said that he's no longer at this office, and that there's another doctor that's taking his place. So I asked what was his name, and she told me. And I knew it was foreign name from listening to the name, so I asked where was he from, and she got offended. And I told her that I didn't think that she should have gotten offended by me asking where he's from."

"That's all you asked?" I said.

"Yeah, that's all I asked, was where is he from. And she was a white lady. And I asked where was he from, and I was going to, you know, just ask some general information. Don't you want to know about a doctor before you pay him a hundred dollars for one single visit? It didn't mean that I didn't want to see him, it just meant that I wanted information on him. And she got offended and I didn't like her attitude, so I just decided I wasn't going to go."

In another interview, a senior citizen told me that she preferred to see a physician with an Anglicized name because it is better to see a doctor of similar background.

"The name is important?" I said.

"Uh huh," she replied. "Well, that's an identity."

I said, "There are certain names, maybe, that have a Scottish ancestry or something like that, that might be better?"

"Anglo-Saxon would get it every time. [laughs] As opposed to an Italian or a—It would always be if I were just, you know, just choosing randomly. Didn't know my bias was showing this much. [laughs] And I used Italian, because they're so obvious, you know, when you see the names."

Typically, such concerns are not expressed in front of the physician. Instead, the choice of a physician is, to a large extent, a private matter. It is difficult to discern publicly why one person privately makes a decision to see or refer to one physician and not another. Despite so much ambiguity between discrimination and nondiscrimination, there are still stereotypes about IMGs.

Examples of Stereotypes

Delano County and Quincy had some of the same stereotypes about IMGs, such as concerns about greediness, formality, and social hierarchies. The stereotypes that surfaced are telling of the criticisms that exist across places about IMGs.

Concerns about greediness can color people's perceptions toward IMGs, even though greediness is a stereotype that is often aimed at physicians in general. A U.S. medical graduate who spoke critically of IMGs told me, "When they come over here we see it in these doctors, their values are not the same. Well, I just want to make money and have a big house, and they're not interested as much in the community or the town or the profession as the American doctors are, I don't think."

In the words of a social worker:

> The thing that I was talking to you about, the income tax, they don't have to pay income tax. I think that's one reason [names of two prominent IMGs]—See, every so often they go back home for a month and come back because they have to do that. Somehow—something for their taxes, they have to do that. That's what I heard now, I don't know. I just hear things, and I'm just thinking about it. So I'm thinking they go back home because they're not American citizens. And therefore, if you're not an American citizen, you don't have to pay taxes.

As we talked further, I asked, "Where do these rumors get started?"

"I don't know, there's all kind of rumors around, you know, that you hear. And you know, you just listen, and say, oh, is that right? Somebody made the statement that they were mad because—or they just seemed to be a little angry because they said, well, get this, [the two IMGs] don't have to pay taxes like we do. So all the money they make goes in their pocket."

The two IMGs are actually naturalized U.S. citizens, and the allegation about avoiding taxes is clearly false. Later in the same day, I was talking with a senior citizen in south Hamilton. She told me, "I think that if I had my say, I think we got enough of people in this country, to run this country with doctors, and they should go to their country and work. And then I don't know whether this is a true saying or not, but they say they don't have to pay any taxes. They come here and work and get that kind of money and don't have to pay any tax, and I can't understand that."

"Hmm," I said. "That's the second time today I've heard that."

"And they don't have to—They earn the money, but they don't have to pay tax. And they're taking our money and I can't understand why they can't pay tax as well as we can pay tax if they're going to work and get the money."

"Where did you hear this from?" I asked.

"I heard it from the hospital," she replied.

"From the hospital?" I said. "From somebody working in the hospital?"

"Yes sir. She was working there, but she's retired."

Rumors about IMGs not having to pay taxes can serve to perpetuate a more harmful stereotype of IMGs as greedy or not interested in investing in the local community. Meanwhile, two U.S. medical graduates explained to me that many IMGs left socialized medicine in their home countries in order to make more money in the United States. Within the context of a lively, engaging conversation, I was not completely sure if a physician was exaggerating:

> Now the people I would limit would not be from India, I'd limit those Canadians. I'd take all of them back and send them back to Canada. Cause they're racist, they're only here for the money, and they're terrible doctors. You know, cause they ran away from a system, not because they didn't want to take care of the people, but purely for the money.

Another common stereotype focuses on the issue of formality. Based on my own personal observation, I sensed less formality in most interviews with IMGs from India in Delano County than in Quincy. Such a perceived difference may be attributable to my own improvements as a researcher, but also to differences in individual personalities and in IMGs' exposure to western culture while growing up. Perhaps more importantly, many of the IMGs in Delano County were younger than their Quincy counterparts. Whereas most of the IMGs that I interviewed in Quincy were in their forties and fifties, most of the IMGs that I interviewed in Delano County were in their thirties. Differences in formality by age group, combined with similarities in age between me and many IMGs, may have made interviews seem less formal and more relaxed. In addition, Delano County had a climate in which people seemed more relaxed and willing to say what was on their minds.

Concerns about formality still surfaced occasionally in Delano County. A community member in a small town told me that some people from India have difficulty acclimating to the area.

> They become a little standoffish and isolated. And maybe because that's just a defense mechanism, first of all, until they can get comfortable with their

> surroundings and their environment. But I would think that they need to be more, you know, maybe just a little bit more outgoing, you know, and take advantage a little bit more of maybe the cultural things and learning about other people's cultures as well, you know. One thing that I do know about foreigners, a lot of them, is that, you know, their upbringing tends to send them in a tunnel vision direction, and they don't—they're not very creative, and they don't sway one side to another. They pretty much, this is the tradition and this is how it's going to be and, you know, let's—you know, they teach their children the same way. And they're kind of like robots, you know. I'd like to see them kind of loosen up a little more. [laughs]

Also, as has already been noted, a few participants mentioned concerns about making small talk with IMGs who might be more accustomed to a more formal doctor-patient interaction. Some perceptions of formality can also be linked to social hierarchies, since formality can be characteristic of some interactions between people who are not at the same social level with one another.

Social hierarchies can be found throughout the United States and the world, with divisions in race, class, labor, and even medicine. For example, different medical specialties have varying degrees of prestige in relation to other medical specialties. Social hierarchies in medicine can also vary from one country or culture to another. For example, in Quincy, some critics of IMGs claimed that professional hierarchies in India contradicted a teamwork approach to decision making in the United States. In Delano County, similar concerns seemed to have a softer edge and could have been overlooked if I had not already thought to listen for them.

An IMG of Asian Indian origin said to me, "I think it would be harder for foreign graduates to accept criticism from people who are much below their level, or just the culture. But you have to realize that when you're in Rome, you have to behave like a Roman, you know. Otherwise, you're not going to be successful."

A nurse practitioner relayed some patients' concerns:

> You know, all I can speak from is my experience in what clients tell me. The internationally trained physicians that I have personally worked with in these rural areas, there were a few of them who seemed to come from more wealthy backgrounds, and I don't know a way to say this other than to say that clients said that they felt like they were looking down their noses at them. Which, you know, you can read a whole lot into that. I personally have not seen that to be true myself, but those are the things where a lot of the folks who had seen some of the international physicians and then would see me for different times would say those kinds of things. And let me be real clear, that was more the exception than the rule, you know, but it was a frequent enough thing for a few of them.

In separate interviews, two IMGs of Asian Indian origin told me that, in general, U.S. employers may be fairer than Asian Indian employers toward their employees. Such concerns were not focused on Delano County but, rather, touched on instances of unfair treatment (e.g., taking advantage of waiver physicians) in other towns. An IMG of Asian Indian origin told me:

> Actually, when we were looking for jobs after my residency, one of the things we would look for is not to work for people of our same—of the same country. Not necessarily needing to sound disloyal, but it just seemed like—Or at least not Indians. I wouldn't say not international medical graduates, but not Indians. Because there was this detrimental kind of, this negative perception of Indian employers versus the American employers. We all wanted to find jobs, you know. In the hierarchy of jobs the best job was finding an employer was American, who understood the system here and who was based here. And almost everybody wanted—that was the most desirable position. And the Indian—working for an Indian employer came at the bottom of the totem pole. So, it certainly is not the case. Probably what does happen is definitely you have a sense of community with the other Indian physicians and people tend to try and help people out. Not always because for positive reasons, but sometimes for negative reasons too, but most of the time they're trying to help one another out.

We talked further, and I said, "I don't know if this makes any sense, but when I was in Quincy some Indian physicians were telling me that culturally there's more of a hierarchy in how people work with one another. Does that relate to—"

> Yes, the U.S. perception of relationships is much more democratic. You know, a lot of the time, when we came—when I came into residency, for example, you know, in India we have the British system of residency, so you have a major, a big hierarchy between the resident and the attending. There's at least three or four steps before you become an attending. So the attendings are generally people who have been there in practice for like fifteen and twenty years. So, you know, the distance between a resident and an attending is tremendous. In some parts of South India people stand every time their attending is there. He will not sit in the presence of an attending. And so on and so forth. But that's the way the British system worked. As opposed to the American system where my director of medicine would encourage me to call him by his first name, which was absolutely unthinkable, I mean, it was just not part of me. It took me a long time to start calling him by his first name. The only thing which turned the tide was when he actually pulled me aside and told me that, you know, if you start practice and you insist on calling everybody by their last name, they'll think you're being very standoffish. And that's not the way we were taught. For us it was a sign of respect. It's just minor things like that. Now, this is from my perspective. On the other

hand, Indians who come here, when they take on an employee, have the same perception, you know, that that distance has to be maintained, because you are an employee and they're employers and that distance should be maintained. So yes, certainly that's part of—one of the reasons why you would not look for an Indian employer as desirably as you would look for an American employer.

Negative perceptions and stereotypes can also form based on one or more bad experiences, which then lead to false generalizations about all or most IMGs. Individual IMGs are sometimes de facto representatives of all IMGs, or at least of all IMGs from particular countries. A misstep by an individual IMG can have consequences for perceptions toward the entire IMG community, at least in the minds of some people who do not have much experience working with or seeing IMGs. A U.S. medical graduate told me, "I tell you quite honestly that my partners have said, when you recruit, you want American born, American trained, because we had two really awful experiences, we don't want any more of these people. And then we got [name of IMG], who's absolutely fabulous. So I don't know how we look at that."

In one interview, a senior citizen in south Hamilton was concerned about a misunderstanding with an IMG that seemed to influence her perceptions of IMGs in general:

I've had a doctor from India. I had one a while, but I left him. But it was all right, I reckon. But you know, you'd rather have home people. I know India's fine, with people from India, but I'd rather have people around that I know something about, that's going to work on my body and tell me something, that'll take time and explain to me what it is and what should be done instead of just wanting me to sign a paper and then go ahead and do what they want to do.

In a nearby town, a health care administrator for a community health center also discussed IMGs in general while referring to experiences on an individual level:

[The center] itself has not had very good experience with international medical graduates. I think they've come in with so many of their own cultural beliefs and they don't understand some of the things that our people do, and were unwilling to bend. And it's just made it very difficult for them to be accepted into the community, into the medical community, to the [name of center] community. Now I know there are graduates in Hamilton who have practices set up who have done very well. But we haven't—So far, we just haven't had good luck. And that may be because we serve such a high number of minorities, you know. Eighty-five to 90 percent of our population is Native American, African American, Hispanics.

When asked to elaborate about experiences with IMGs, the administrator explained that there can be problems in communication that can affect adherence. Such perceived problems included a lack of understanding of the need to "keep preaching" medical advice to patients, and limited familiarity with home remedies used by many patients. Again, problems with individual IMGs can lead to judgments about an entire community.

Nonetheless, problems with individual IMGs did not appear to be widespread concerns, and were often not linked to any generalizations about IMGs. Moreover, negative experiences with individual IMGs were reported only occasionally in interviews.

While there can be negative stereotypes, there can also obviously be positive stereotypes. For example, a good experience seeing an IMG can make a patient more open to accepting other IMGs. This certainly was the case when the pioneer IMGs paved the way for other IMGs to practice in the community. As was the case in Quincy, several participants said that IMGs are especially hard-working. In a couple of interviews, other positive generalizations in Delano County included the intelligence of IMGs, and their politeness in comparison with people from the United States. Still, subtlety was an underlying issue behind discrimination and stereotypes. According to the wife of an IMG of Asian Indian origin:

> Some things might be subtle, but I don't think we've ever faced anything like any out and out animosity towards us, you know. We have our different activities and we are still involved, you know, in certain community things as a group, you know, but mostly like we are—I guess we are separate, yeah, you could say. But I don't find that difficult or I don't take that as they don't include us. I think if we went seeking, you know, their community, then I think they would accept us. It's just we have all our cultural things going on so we really don't try that hard to, you know, meet them and build up a relationship. So I really can't say that if we went to do that how we would be perceived, because I don't think anybody has, you know, tried that hard to do that. And I think if we did, you know, go, I think it would be fine. I'm sure there's always going to be—You know, I don't take all this discrimination too seriously. I think there's always going to be difference between a white, a black, you know, the culture itself is so different. I don't make a big deal out of it, you know. If it's different, it's different. Just as long as each individual is treated like a human being and not superior or inferior to anybody, you know. Each of us are different, so I don't—It doesn't bother me that they don't include me, because my values, my stuff is different than theirs. I probably wouldn't enjoy what they do and they probably wouldn't enjoy what I do, you know. It's no big deal. I don't have all this discrimination stuff, I don't take that seriously.

Thus, the discrimination and stereotypes discussed in this section might have little impact on geographic or social exclusions of IMGs. Immigrant communities can help provide a sense of inclusiveness for new IMGs that might shield or protect them from feeling a sense of exclusion from the local area. Furthermore, stereotypes about IMGs can be subtle, and therefore might not even be considerations unless people actually look for them. In addition, there might be cultural or social explanations for the possibility of IMG separateness, unrelated to discrimination against IMGs.

THE QUESTION OF SEPARATENESS

Most of the preceding discussion focused on the assumption that IMGs can be considered separately from others in Delano County (e.g., in terms of race, religion, gender roles, language barriers, and discrimination). Despite my efforts to portray a full, rounded picture of IMGs, I risk accentuating minor social divisions or personal conflicts that would otherwise attract little attention. Even if policy makers and health services researchers must make decisions using precise definitions for IMGs and U.S. medical graduates, such distinctions become ambiguous in Delano County, as was also the case in Quincy. People cannot even agree on who is an American and who is a foreigner, and it is not clear that IMGs should be considered as a separate entity.

This same lack of clarity in considering the separateness of IMGs reflects broader concerns about immigration and assimilation, and underscores the complexity of being an American. At times, there is no clear line that separates IMGs from everybody else (e.g., when people simply want a good doctor) but at other times, the distinction becomes much clearer (e.g., when the medical staff systematically excluded IMGs). Such contradictions are part of the identities of Delano County. Just as every individual faces many internal conflicts, so too do places. Cultural and social differences add to internal conflicts, but also unite Delano County in the sense that difference is part of the landscape.

It is not so easy to take a legally constructed category of human beings and generalize about their behavior. Neither is it easy to take all immigrants—or people perceived to be immigrants—and assume some social or professional separateness from everyone else. A member of the hospital staff shared with me her thoughts on the issue of the possible separateness of IMGs:

> They don't set themselves aside or whatever. But I think they know that they're limited here, and they make their own socialization. I'm sure they probably have social gatherings that they do not invite some of the other physicians on staff. But they do not set themselves aside so much that it's a really noticeable drawing of the line, is my impression.

An IMG of Eastern European origin told me that he did not think that IMGs should set themselves apart from other physicians:

> The funny thing is when somebody sends you a letter that you are asked to attend such and such international medical graduate organization. That organization is going to, you know, provide for certain rights of international medical graduates. The way I look at it, you're segregating yourself from the group of physicians, because I have not felt, you know, any different than anybody else. People have treated me very fairly. You're competent, you're good, you do your things, they'll say, you know, okay, they'll appreciate your work. If you don't do well, they'll teach you, they'll help you, if you are in a teaching institution. Or, you know, if you don't do well, they will not tolerate that. I don't think I have felt like I'm an international medical graduate, except of course for the part that concerned the government. But with the people that I meet every day, I haven't felt—The most it will be they'll pick up the accent, they'll say, where you from and how did you come here? But that's it. So to me, participating in international medical graduate organization actually worsens the problem, if there is any problem. That's the way you put yourself aside.

Explaining further, he told me:

> I mean, I'm thinking about certain political movements, and I can't recall the name of the person who said, before we unite we first have to distinguish among each other, i.e., we have to understand our differences [before] we start acting together. There's no such thing in medicine. You can believe me that Bulgarian patients are exactly the same as [nearby small town] patients. [laughs] Exactly the same. They will tell you the same things, they'll be just as reserved in the beginning and then they'll be just as open when they get to know you. They'll be trusting you just as much so there is no difference.

In another interview, an IMG responded to my question about whether there was a separate community for IMGs:

> Oh, no, there is no separate community of international medical graduates. Where I am, right here in Hamilton, there are quite a number of international medical graduates and we try to, you know, interact with other people as well. We don't have a separate, you know. But we do have an organization of minority professionals that includes lawyers and health professionals, and that is in Filmore.

The IMG explained further that the organization of minority professionals includes blacks, Native Americans, Hispanics, and Asian Indians. In addition, she told me that she occasionally attended meetings, such as a "cultural display," in the city of Filmore with immigrants from her country of origin.

A community member seemed particularly surprised at the idea that IMGs might be considered a separate group from everybody else in Delano County. At the end of our interview, in which I had asked for her thoughts on IMGs, she told me, "But it's been interesting. And you've given me some food for—you know, things I hadn't really thought about before. Ah . . . international doctors have just been kind of part of the landscape . . . I just really hadn't much thought about them as a separate entity or an issue."

Despite the persuasiveness of the idea that IMGs are not separate from the rest of society in Delano County, there is a case to be made that IMGs—or at least some IMGs from South Asia—are separate to some extent. For example, there might be cultural differences, combined with a more sizeable community, that could have a greater impact on social relations for some IMGs from South Asia and other parts of the world. I asked an IMG of Asian Indian origin, "And do you think the Indian community, as in East Indian community, do you think it is separate from the general community, or do the lines blur?" He responded:

> No, it's unfortunate that there is a sharply demarcated line, and it's unfortunate that we don't kind of blend into it, you know. That's unfortunate part. We are now changing some, we are taking interest in other activities. But yes, no, it's kind of a sharply demarcated line which you can see that we don't involve with many local activity. There are several reasons for that, that you go in that activity and sometimes you get a warm welcome and sometimes you don't get good welcome and like those things do happen at times.

Another IMG of Asian Indian origin told me, "Some of us are from India. We have a couple of physicians who are not, but yes. Quite a few of us are from India."

I began to ask, "Does that lead to some special connection between—"

"Yes, unfortunately it does," the IMG replied. "I wish it wasn't so, but it does, you know. I mean, I probably don't like to admit this very often, but it does. You know. Being Indian does make things a little—you do look at—you probably find that you have more of a cultural similarity among the two. Though that's not always true, I mean, I do have a lot of Indian physicians who I have nothing in common with. But probably instinctively you'll kind of take the effort to find out whether you do have something in common, whereas probably the effort I'd take with a non-Indian international medical graduate would be somewhat less. It's just instinctive. I don't think it's something I've thought of, but it does happen."

"Why were you, well, almost reluctant to admit that there is a community—"

> I don't like to have it that way. I wish it wasn't, because I'd like to think that I'm able to connect to people regardless of which country they belong to. But it's just that sometimes you have cultural similarities, the way you look at things are somewhat similar, and that's how you manage to bond with some people better than others. And sometimes it's almost entirely because you belong to the same country. I'd like to feel that I could reach a point where the country doesn't really matter. It's just how you relate to a person that matters. But the initial connection does take place—the initial connection does start off because you are also Indian, or somebody else is also Indian.

As we talked further, the IMG went on to say that it can be easier to relate to people from the United States than some people from India:

> We have a lot of western culture in us because we're very different from—That's why I said that it's not every Indian that I can bond with, because there are some Indians who were brought up in much smaller towns who have a total different, totally different outlook, and I probably would find myself much more in common with an American than with that particular group of Indians. And you have to understand that India is such a large country that it's impossible to be—to find similarities everywhere.

Indications of social separateness for IMGs can entail some contradictions; i.e., being together and apart, included and excluded. Another IMG of Asian Indian origin explained, "Socially, Indians have created their own groups. If they are there, they don't feel segregated. So I think it's really, they are happy with their business, their practices. And social interaction doesn't matter to them because there are so many Indians everywhere. So you don't feel isolated anymore."

Thus, some IMGs might be becoming a part of the local landscape by becoming a part of a separate community that is rooted there. There are also obvious advantages to meeting people who come from the same country originally, according to some participants. For example, an IMG explained:

> You can relate to like things that are happening in Pakistan nowadays, you've got a lot of Indian physicians down here who can relate to that situation. And we talk about it. And you probably socialize, because they understand your culture more than maybe Americans, or your other American peers. Certain things you do different from Americans, yeah. Religious differences. I don't go to church but I'm Muslim, so I don't socialize on that level with my peers. There are certain things that, yeah, sure, you socialize different.

The impression of separateness can be different in different places within Delano County. For example, in walking the hallways of the hospital, I often passed by physicians, both IMGs and U.S. medical graduates. They were all physicians going about the business of being physicians; in the hospital corridors, I had no reason whatsoever to think that IMGs were somehow socially or professionally separate from other physicians. However, in a home environment, the impression of separateness can be different. Only one of my interviews with an IMG was conducted in an IMG's home. I did not tour the entire home so I cannot speak authoritatively about what was there. Besides the prayer room, there was no reason for me to think that his home should look any different from anyone else's home. Yet I recalled reading a book by Abraham Verghese (1994), an IMG of Asian Indian origin, who wrote that one immigrant's home seemed more like India than would probably have been the case in India. An IMG of Asian Indian origin responded to the Verghese account by telling me:

> That happens to people. A lot of people here, when they come, I guess their image of India kind of gets arrested at the time when they leave the land there. Development might have taken place after that, but it's difficult to relate to the new development. They kind of want it the way they had it in their childhood or younger days. That's one. The other thing is they probably see everything different out there, and they probably at least want to have some part which could be the only place they can control completely and make it India. So the homes are the ones that look like it sometimes.

A U.S. medical graduate also talked about separateness between IMGs and other people in Delano County. As he explained:

> You know, we think a lot about community's prejudice, medical community's prejudice against foreign graduates. In many cases, I think the foreign graduates have as much prejudice as the community does. They come here with a sense of other. They socialize only with people from their country, they go away to participate in religious activities with other people from their country. In our case, most of them wind up going to Filmore because that's kind of a melting pot and there's a little bit of every nationality over there. But they—I know it's hard to come in and make an effort to be a part of things. But it's funny, I can see right here in my own practice, foreign medical graduate notwithstanding, we've got people who are American all the way who come here, who maintain the separateness. We have others who come here and throw themselves into the community fully, and are—I think that the second group winds up being much happier.

An IMG of Asian Indian origin talked about the ambiguity of maintaining separateness while being part of the broader community. Raising the idea of assimilation into life in Delano County, he told me:

It would be good, but I think it is difficult for one to completely assimilate one hundred percent into a foreign culture, howsoever you might try. Because there are certain traits and certain things which you cannot dissolve them in a kind of a, with a one slash of a sword or something. So you have to—It takes times. It I think goes with generations. Like second generation migrant might be different from the first generation. The third generation may be almost indistinguishable from the local crowd. So that's what—It can't be done rapidly.

"Is it a goal?" I asked. "Is assimilation what you would be striving for?"

I guess. Yeah. At the same time there will also be a striving to maintain the best of both, kind of, that's the approach. You will not want—See, we have strong familial ties, we have strong familial values. We like to have a close knit family or a respect for the elders in the family. There should be certain things which, you know, go certain ways, which is dissolving in the current American society to some extent, not entirely. Say if you compare to American society maybe at the beginning of the century, they used to be—You know, where the son lived at their parents' house even twenty years, that was okay. He was probably—Now, I think it's almost like they get nervous that he's not moving out, he's not doing something of his own. Which we have this, like, the son—Sometimes the grandfather, the son and the grandchild live together in a family. That may not necessarily happen, but there are certain things which [are] taken care of. The payoff is that, you know, everyone gets looked after and all. But we do like those values, and I probably would if I can possibly do it. The same time, I wouldn't stop my child from doing what the other kids are doing here, just because he is not one of them. He has to be one of them if he's to survive.

The children of IMGs often excel in school, and it remains to be seen whether IMG families become long, established families over generations in rural, needy areas. It is unclear whether the sons and daughters of IMGs are any more likely than other children to remain in rural, needy areas after graduation from high school or college. Many rural areas, including Delano County, experience a brain drain when some of their brightest students do not return once they have an education.

Another concern is the physician's own sense of commitment to the area. The waiver physician who recently left Delano County immediately after completing his obligation had obviously not established a long-term commitment to the local area. A few participants told me that IMGs who are new to the area need to leave an impression that they want to be in Delano County. For example, a nurse practitioner and I were discussing press releases that are used to introduce new physicians to the community. She told me that she wants more information about new physicians in the press releases:

> And not just that they went to medical school at, you know, so and so. A little bit—You know, they selected [this part of the state] because, you know. . . Because they were—You know, they loved the beauty of the region or something like that. Because, you know—For instance, like the Native American population here, one of the reasons—I think this is the prettiest place on the face of the earth. I mean, it's—And there's nothing prettier than going down [name of river] on a foggy morning like this morning. And so, you know, something that they positively say that helps that connectiveness. How can I help connect to this person? Don't just tell me that they're out there, but give me something that they will reach out for.

Community Involvement

Participants often told me that IMGs should be more involved in the community in order to do well in Delano County. However, I often found such a concern to be confusing because there was also separateness in the general community in several ways, such as by race, social class, and religion. Most people could not be expected to make inroads into every white, black, Native American, and Hispanic population, so it was difficult to see exactly which population should be an IMG's point of entry into the general community.

I met some IMGs who were very popular physicians but who described themselves as having only limited involvement in community activities. For example, an IMG told me:

> Like I said earlier, I have not immersed myself in the culture of this community. Part of that is our upbringing, and part of this is sort of not wanting to reach out and kind of realize that—part of that is not wanting to reach out and realize that there's nobody that wants to reciprocate that—How do you put that? Reciprocate that gesture. You know, part of it is we're introverts anyway. The other thing is not wanting to say, hey, you know, we're here and we're glad to be here, and then have folks kind of say, well, you know, yes you're here but, you know, keep to yourself.

I also met a number of IMGs who described themselves as being very active in the general community. For example, another IMG said:

> Here you know your neighbors like your best friend and it just goes on from there. They'll take you out to church things, like the fish fries and the chicken fries and whatnot, I go there every second or third month. One of my neighbors

or one of my friends will just say hey, there's a chicken fry or fish fry, let's go there, and stuff like that, we'll go out there. Pig pickings, I don't eat pork, but still, I go there.

An IMG of Asian Indian origin told me about her plans to do more to help people in the area:

I want to start a soup kitchen shortly, and that's one of my goals. I have a few goals that are nonmedical here in Hamilton. . . . And it's not necessarily just a—for church members, it's just, I can use the church as a center point. The other goal I was having, the next two years that I hope to break ground on is to start a women's center that'll, you know, teach job skills and interviewing skills, Internet skills and that kind of stuff, nutrition and dietetics and . . . just an all comprehensive women's center, just center for the development of women in general. So that's another big plan I have for Hamilton.

Such outreach has obvious benefits not only for the community but for the physician, too. Altruism might erase the perception of greed, to the extent that such perceptions exist. An actively involved physician gains familiarity with the local contexts of health care, erases some of the social distance between doctor and patient, and gains further insight into how patients think. Furthermore, active involvement in community activities could further the perception that a physician is not simply passing through town but, rather, really wants to be in Delano County.

One of the first IMGs in the area offered some advice about doing well as an IMG in Delano County:

You should be friendly to everybody and I think you ought to accept everybody like friends, not foes. And you shouldn't feel like you're different than other people here. You should feel a part of the community. You don't want to isolate yourself because you're a foreigner. So I think if you are nice to other people, you're open to them and don't kind of isolate yourself from other people, you will be accepted. The key is yourself, initiation comes from you. You don't expect to be accepted by other people. You need to make yourself like, be part of the community. So there is no problem. But if you try to isolate yourself, then the problem acceptance. So I think the problem comes when foreigners or foreign medical graduates try to isolate themselves. They don't go openly in the community and introduce themselves and open themselves to other people.

Complicating matters is the difference by specialty in community outreach. The county has five IMGs who are family practitioners, and thirteen IMG internists; community activity is an integral part of family practice, but not as important in internal medicine.

It occurred to me that being active in the community was simply good advice for any physician, even if it was not always clear which community (e.g., white, black, Native American, Hispanic) should be the focus arena of such activity. Then again, the area is becoming highly networked across communities, so a physician who makes an effort in one community could conceivably leave a positive impression in other communities for making an effort.

A lawyer shared his thoughts on the idea of IMGs' community involvement:

> Well, I certainly think that involvement in civic affairs of the community would go a long way to assisting an international physician in solidifying his position, let's say, in the community, and give him an opportunity to meet patients and give them an opportunity to see him at work in another field where they could begin to make an analysis of whether they would like to have him as their physician. So involvement in community affairs is, I think, important for not just international physicians, but I think really for most people. They should be involved in community affairs, whatever, you know, method that takes.

In another interview, a senior citizen shared similar thoughts, albeit with slightly different nuances about IMG activity in the general community:

> Well, I think the thing you need to do is not just to mingle with people of your culture. Come into the community and be a part of the community. Take part in community activities. Be sincerely interested in what's going on and be a part of what's going on. That would include the recreational facilities. We have lots of things here to do. Little Theatre. All the performances up at Berry. Just mingle with people and be a part of the people. Be a part of our culture.

I began to ask, "Do you think that's something that foreign physicians are doing, or is that something—"

"I think they are. I really do. I really do. But there are getting to be so many of them, they too are beginning to congregate with themselves a little bit. That might not be an honest observation, but that's the feeling I get. And I can understand that. They say birds of a feather flock together. [laughs]"

The above considerations about community activity omit a key issue, which is that children are an important avenue for increased community involvement. For example, an IMG of Asian Indian origin reflected on the idea that his children, when they were still in school, led to his family's involvement in school activities: "When kids grow, we don't have that many contacts with everybody now, the same people. Now we have contact with different people, so things still change. But we were very active in the community things, my wife, myself. She was very active in the school, community, this and that."

In another interview, the wife of an IMG of Asian Indian origin told me that she would be more active in the community if she had children:

> Some things I'm sort of cut off from because the exposure—there is less community expose because we don't have children and we're not involved in PTA or this or that, you know. But our friends who's been in this area and they have children and they've been accepted very nicely, you know. I think acceptance goes both ways. You can't just expect, you know, that you have to be accepted without you doing something to get accepted.

Another key issue is that physicians tend to be busy people who do not necessarily have much time to be active in the community. According to an IMG of Asian Indian origin:

> See, I'm too much focused into doing what I'm doing, so whatever I tell you may not be a generalization. Because, you know, if you ask me about other cultural things and how you get integrated in the system, I'm a person who I have no time for anyone else, so I don't really bother about all these thing. [laughs] I would rather somebody not bother me with any social stuff.

Another IMG of Asian Indian origin said:

> Well, I still think, though, that your work like sort of dictates a large portion of where your world is, especially if you're a physician. So I think it does make for a basic dissatisfaction with the area when you feel like work life is one place and your social life is another, or your religious life is another. And that's what I think a lot of people encounter, and that makes for dissatisfaction both from the person who's from another area who's here, and also with the community, who looks at you and says, well, you just work here, you don't ever socialize here, or we don't ever see you outside of work. So I think that is a large part of the problem.

In another interview, an IMG of Asian Indian origin explained:

> I'd love to be more active in the community. Sometimes it just seems a little overwhelming right now probably because I've just taken over and it's a time when I'm trying to establish my practice and right now the practice has been dominant, you know. My profession has kind of dominated the scene and no, I would say I'm not really contributing—not, apart from what I work in the office, no, I haven't really been doing a whole lot of my own. I'd like to at some point, you know, once I think things settle down just a little bit more.

Changing Role of the Rural Physician

As was already noted in the Quincy chapters, medicine in rural America has undergone substantial changes. It is no longer the norm for physicians to be actively involved in their patients' lives beyond the clinic. For example, when I talked with an IMG of South Asian origin about the importance of community involvement, he explained:

> Well, what you're talking about is health initiatives which are—which are—which literally are not needed in the U.S. anymore. Those health initiatives are needed in the majority of the world, which are community health initiatives to the point, you need them in certain issues, like problems with drugs maybe, and other—Because you don't need community health to that extreme so that you have a physician, every practicing physician to be involved in the community? That doesn't work anymore in the U.S. You have a system or a population here which has evolved over the years, that they have clean running water, at least most of them. You still have problems in some pockets or places. They have good sanitation, they've got running water, they've got immunization to all the babies. These are the—they're breastfeeding their children, they're sending them to school, and stuff like that. Which is needed in third world countries, and I'm speaking about the public health measures, these are public health measures. This is not the domain of physicians anymore. It's the domain of planners and—physician planners and whatnot, which are mostly state run or federally funded or whatnot here in the U.S.

In addition, the physician workforce itself has changed, incorporating more women, blacks, Native Americans, and immigrants. Such changes in the physician workforce may have influenced the role of the rural physician in terms of community involvement; e.g., different groups of people may have different time constraints, obligations, or activity spaces that would impede community involvement. Conversely, changes in the need to be involved in community activities might also have opened up opportunities for a more diverse physician workforce. In other words, differences in the role of the rural physician may lead different people to become rural physicians than in previous years.

A U.S. medical graduate added his thoughts on changes in rural physicians' involvement in community activities. Reflecting on what it was like over thirty years ago to move to Hamilton, he told me:

> I mean, everybody was knocking themselves out to make me feel welcome. And not because I had any connections, I didn't. But in no time I had been visited by everybody in the medical community, my wife had been visited by all the wives, a strong effort was made to include us in everything. It was overwhelming. This doesn't happen anymore. We've brought in lots of physicians in the last year, in

the last five or six years, some foreign graduates, some not foreign graduates. Nobody pays much attention to anybody, and I don't know what that is. And part of that is the Generation X and the different—A lot of them don't want to be included, they want to be involved with their family and maybe one other couple and that's all. They're not interested in becoming—in knowing everybody and interacting with the whole community, that's just not what they're about. And so I don't know. And of course, everybody works all the—Thirty years ago no doctor's wife would work, that would be totally unheard of, and now that's not the case. There are a lot of couples who some of them—We've got a lot of these couples where there are two physicians who are married and they both—they all—People don't have the time that they used to have. But it's—I don't think that they're excluded, it's just that nobody's breaking their neck to include them.

Separateness Revisited

In my research on rural areas, I have often come across people who assume that "rural" is necessarily underserved, poor, and closed to change. However, places and people are continually changing. Life in this one rural area is not self-contained within precise borders but instead is influenced by changes in other parts of the United States and the world. Such changes include a reduced social role for many rural physicians, and increased exposure to people from other countries. The foreign has become less foreign, the different less exotic, and the Other has become distinguishable and indistinguishable at the same time. The lines between virtually everything are both clear and unclear. The issue of the separateness of IMGs in Delano County does not lend itself easily to one right answer. Nothing in this study does.

It might not matter if IMGs are separate or not separate from the rest of people in Delano County. What does matter though is the perception of difference or sameness, which could affect a physician's sense of belonging in the area, and possibly retention. Significantly, the issue of IMG separateness is ambiguous, including —in the words of participants—no "really noticeable drawing of the line," and "a sharply demarcated line." Such apparent contradictions are instructive in considering the heterogeneity of IMGs, and the complexity of individual experience.

PHYSICIANS IN THE GLOBAL MARKETPLACE

The global context for local events has been a key, albeit indirect, consideration throughout this entire work. The borders of the United States may appear as sharply delineated lines on maps, but between the lines, there are deep connections and even blurred distinctions with other countries.

Technological innovations, advances in telecommunications, the growth of transnational corporations, improvements in transportation, the flow of capital, and—for purposes of this work—the flow of people are key resources behind a shrinking world. Such resources are not rooted interminably in one place but, rather, part of a global marketplace. The migration of IMGs leads some countries to lose one of their most precious resources, physicians. Meanwhile, the influx of IMGs can be problematic for people who are concerned about whether the United States could otherwise take care of its own citizens. In the words of a U.S. medical graduate in Berry:

> I think if we were looking after our demand as we should have here, there would be no need for international graduates. I really think that's kind of a slap in the face for us, when we say we need them, and admit that we need them. It means we haven't done our job. And you hear me saying, the way things are going, that need is going to get greater rather than less because we aren't doing our job.

Immigrant doctors have become an integral part of the local health care landscape, reflecting changes in the antennae of Delano County and, more generally, the entire United States. Rural places like Delano County are now linked through immigration patterns with places that used to be imaginary or unknown locally (e.g., places in India, Nigeria, or the Philippines). If such newfound linkages with other parts of the world constitute a slap in the face, then the entire United States—and indeed the entire world—is in for a major bruising. It is difficult, if not impossible, to be self-sufficient in a world which has so many flows of people, commodities, and ideas across national boundaries. To be sure, IMGs are not alone as immigrants who fill an important need in the United States. So too do teachers, computer scientists, architects, engineers, mathematicians, accountants, theologians, and other highly skilled immigrants. The provision of highly skilled labor may make IMGs acceptable to some people, according to a community member:

> If that guy is willing to pull up stakes and leave his country, his heritage, everything he knows, in some cases maybe even down to religion, but definitely leaving the culture and environment that he was raised in, and come to a completely strange area, and he's willing to make that sacrifice to come out there partially to do some good, and partially, I think, also to better himself, we should stand in their way? I mean, they want to come in. We're sitting here doing absolutely nothing about illegal aliens coming in, promoting them up the ying yang, and every way we possibly can, and we're going to turn down a guy that's going to come in here and contribute?

Even if IMGs contribute substantially to reducing medical underservice, the influx of IMGs into rural needy areas contradicts the original intent of residency training for immigrant doctors. Originally, immigrant doctors were allowed to come to the United States for graduate medical education that they could then bring back to help people in their home countries (Stevens et al., 1978). Now the "exchange visitor" visas, such as the J-1, are part of an immigration pathway. Many IMGs strongly prefer to practice medicine in rural, needy areas like Delano County over their home countries where opportunities may be limited. Moreover, some of the medical schools in less developed countries have primarily served as sources of physician export (see Ronaghy et al., 1976). A few IMGs even told me that India had a policy of discouraging outmigration of physicians, and therefore they traveled to Indonesia to take medical exams that would allow them to practice in the United States. Even if a country, such as India, wanted to reduce physician export, individual medical schools still had a local culture in which students looked to the United States and other highly developed countries as a preferred destination.

In one interview, I told an IMG of Filipino origin about a telephone call that I had received from another IMG of Filipino origin who wanted my help in finding work so that he could stay in the United States. Explaining about the telephone conversation, I said, "He was concerned about getting a job for his J-1 waiver so he could stay in the country. He couldn't go back to the Philippines because there wouldn't be jobs there, because they don't have the infrastructure, he thought, to support the physician jobs." We were eating lunch in a Greek restaurant that served Italian food, and I had the microphone set between us on the table. The IMG responded:

> Yes and no. I think, you know, like I said, there's a shortage of physicians in the rural areas. Now, when I went to medical school, my feeling was I wanted to stay in the place where I grew up, which was Manila, which was the capital of the Philippines. Unfortunately in Manila, there are thousands of doctors. There's too many doctors in Manila. If I wanted to really establish my own practice and have enough patients come to see me, I would have had to go to the more rural areas. In the Philippines, there's this big thing about going back to where you grew up. If we had a province that I could call, you know, this is my hometown like a lot of my classmates did, you know, I could have just gone back there and say, okay, I'm going to move in here, move back there, and establish my own practice and have a reasonable expectation of having a successful practice. Now, not having any roots elsewhere, other than Manila, I figured that was going to be very tough. So, it is possible for a person to go back and start a practice. It's going to be a lot more difficult in the urban areas, but it's doable. The other thing is, after coming here and seeing the technology here and infrastructure and all that, all the systems in place for a physician going out of practice and joining a practice—You know, when I got out of residency and came here, I didn't have to have capital, I didn't have to hire people to work for me, I didn't have to rent an office, I just moved in, joined them, started seeing patients the first day. In

> the Philippines it's not like that. It's rarely like that. My impression is you have to build your own clinic, you know, rent your own space, hire your own secretary, hire your own nurse, you know, there's not a lot of collusion, you know, joining group practices. So while it is possible, it is very difficult. Especially after coming here and seeing what there is here, the perception then becomes, you know, it's going to be twice as difficult to go back home and do those things. Again, it is possible, it's just a lot more difficult. It's not that you can't become a doctor in the rural areas, you can, it's—The risks you take are going to be a whole lot more than you would here. You know, I didn't have much risk, I just signed a contract and then moved here and started working. Now in the Philippines, if I wanted to go to a rural area which I was not from, then I have to take the risk of moving over there, setting up my own practice and wait for two or three years before, I said, well, you know, it's really taking off, or it's really not taking off.

Therefore, it might actually be easier for IMGs to set up practices in rural America than in some parts of the Philippines, or perhaps even in other countries. In a physician's office in another clinic, an IMG told me:

> So when I did my residency, at that time I had an option to go ahead and do a fellowship or just complete my subspecialty training and then go back to Pakistan, versus staying here for a while. And the things that make that decision for me, obviously if you look at need, my country is a lot more needy than this country, clearly, in terms of health requirements or, yeah, sure, I should go back there and work. It really depends on what I can do there, unfortunately in third world countries there's just not enough incentive for you to go back because you have to take care of the family and make enough money and whatnot. And there's not enough structure. There are not many jobs available. Because health care unfortunately is dependent on structure. You have to have hospitals, you have to have resources so that you can be employed and work gainfully. And in third world countries, there are not many. As a matter of fact we have—when I would finish medical school and did my first year of training there, I didn't have a job. That's why I came to—[laughs] I could find a job in the U.S., I couldn't find a job in Pakistan, believe it or not. So there are too many doctors there for the facilities. So I had a choice of going back to no job or finding a job here.

A similar viewpoint was expressed by one of the first IMGs in Delano County:

> Well, I wanted to go [to the United States] for post-graduation, which I couldn't do in India. Financially I couldn't afford it and I always wanted to for post-graduation so I came here. Then I wanted a [training in a particular specialty] and then, you know, when you learn so much, those days we couldn't go back and practice because medicine wasn't as advanced as it is now. So if I went that

> time in, for example, '82 or '80, I couldn't practice what I learned here. So then I decided to stay here. And I liked it here. Because, you know, it's difficult once you get used to this system to go on a very primitive level again.

In this global context, it can be both easy and difficult to consider IMGs separately from U.S. medical graduates. On the one hand, there are different life experiences that affect the social and professional decisions of immigrants in particular. For example, limited opportunities in a home country and exposure to medical advances in the United States can have powerful impacts on IMGs' career decisions to move to or stay in Delano County. On the other hand, Delano County attracts physicians from different parts of the United States and different parts of the world. The influx of IMGs reflects the local area's increasingly expansive connections with other parts of the world. Delano County can pull from a global marketplace of physicians, albeit within the laws and constraints of the United States and the state. It is almost as though the national boundaries of the United States can be likened to a hologram. From some perspectives (e.g., legal jurisdictions, formal definitions of IMGs), the boundary lines are clear, but look from a different angle (e.g., attachments to places, perceptions of nationality), and the lines between places can become fuzzy or even disappear altogether.

The best way to sum up so many complicated issues is to refer to the words of a pharmacist interviewed for this study. After he had strayed off topic in our interview, he explained, "Well, life is not, unfortunately, a cut and dried affair that I can lay out and say this is a hundred questions and a hundred answers." He was right. In this study at least, there have been more answers than questions, and the answers have almost never been cut and dried.

Part Four

CONCLUSIONS

Chapter Ten

Conclusions

Several years ago, while I was settling on a research question for this study, a doctoral student in the University of North Carolina's Department of Health Policy and Administration (HPAA) relayed to me a suggestion from one of his professors: The best research questions are ones that have a yes or no answer. Later, I also learned that another professor in HPAA would talk about the "Journal of Irreproducible Results" to illustrate some of the problems with poor statistical research. The student and I laughed and joked that some people actually published studies that could not be repeated exactly. In only a few years, this study changed how I view research. Questions that had once seemed worth asking now seemed overly simplistic. Is the answer yes or no—are international medical graduates (IMGs) accepted in rural America? Where are IMGs more accepted, and where are they less accepted? How does acceptability vary by spatial and demographic characteristics? These were the sorts of questions that concerned me at the beginning of this study, but the findings were so nuanced, and the places so different, that straight comparisons or blanket statements now seem naïve.

In both study areas, I learned more about the openness of places to IMGs, while also learning about the uniqueness of places, and the differences in my community entry. Below, I briefly revisit the major issues that surfaced in the Quincy and Delano County study areas.

QUINCY

I recall meeting with an IMG near the end of my fieldwork in Quincy to discuss some of the major findings from this study. This and other meetings held near the end of fieldwork were meant to help me verify the accuracy of my findings. During our meeting, the IMG asked me to summarize the thoughts of U.S. medical graduates toward IMGs. I responded awkwardly but tried to act self-assured, feeling perplexed by my own inability to provide a thorough and succinct answer. I replied that, "if pushed," I would say that IMGs are well-accepted by U.S. medical graduates in the area. I told him of two extremes—one physician who said that we should be "dern glad" to have IMGs, and another physician who expressed a concern that IMGs are not assimilating well into local culture. Yet I felt uncomfortable with my response because there had only been eight U.S. medical graduates in my sample, each with a different personality, different level of openness to me, and different experiences with IMGs. Even though this was not statistical research, my inclination was still to think in terms of succinct answers about human behavior.

Despite only spending two months in Quincy, I managed to conduct over fifty interviews, and participated in a number of community activities, including health care meetings, informal social gatherings, and attendance at a church and at a puja. Typically, I spent two days at a time in Quincy, sleeping overnight in the Motel 6 and packing my schedule with meetings, when possible. To complete my fieldwork in Quincy in the planned one month or (at most) month and a half, I would gauge my progress by the number of interviews conducted per trip. Three interviews was a success. Anything less was a disappointment. My research in Quincy was full of conflicting approaches—conduct as many interviews as possible per trip, but value depth of insight in each interview; try to integrate into the community, but leave in a month; explore complexity, but search for precise answers to research questions.

Meanwhile, the issue of the role of IMGs in Quincy appeared to be a sensitive topic. Participants often wanted to cast themselves or their town in the best possible light. To people in Quincy, it seemed acceptable to talk publicly about problems for IMGs with communication, but not as acceptable to admit to a preference for American doctors. Time and again, townspeople would tell me that they think that IMGs are fine doctors, but "I have trouble understanding what they say." Most IMGs also told me that communication was a concern, as did some of the strongest advocates for having IMGs. My transcriptionist complained about IMGs' accents, although problems with audio quality also added to her concerns. I was surprised by the extent of the problem of communication since I had very little difficulty understanding IMGs. Late in my fieldwork in Quincy, I came to a startling realization that some of the concerns about communication were overstated. Admitting to problems with communication seemed to be much easier than admitting to bigotry. People could not be expected to admit openly to prejudices against IMGs, particularly on tape to a university researcher.

Nonetheless, the concentration of IMGs in Quincy helped create an interesting dynamic for acceptability. IMGs constituted about half of the local physician workforce, and practiced primarily in subspecialty care. Such subspecialization could be a reflection, in part, on the age of Quincy's IMGs, typically in their forties or fifties. A younger workforce might be less specialized, reflecting more of the changes at the federal, state, and local level in emphasizing primary care. IMGs in Quincy provided care in a broad range of specialties (e.g., oncology, cardiology, gastroenterology) that otherwise might not be available locally. The benefits of having IMGs did not always appear so clear-cut, however. Some participants expressed a concern about the extent of IMG concentration in the area, in part because the proportion of immigrants in the physician workforce was starkly different from the proportion of immigrants in the general community. According to the health services literature, it is often best to recruit rural health providers locally, if possible, or at least from the same region (e.g., the Southeast) or from other rural areas in the United States. Such providers might share similar cultural and social backgrounds with patients, and might have longer retention in needy areas (Xu et al., 1997; Gupta and Konrad, 1992; Crandall et al., 1990; Hafferty and Goldberg, 1986). However, the retention of IMGs in Quincy has been phenomenal, especially among physicians of Asian Indian origin. Since it was rare for any IMGs to leave the area, the assumption in health services research that it is best to recruit locally seems at odds with the long-term staying power of IMGs in Quincy.

As more and more IMGs moved to and remained in Quincy, fewer U.S. medical graduates moved to the area. Perhaps IMGs were more willing to move to Quincy because they were more willing to practice in rural, needy areas. Consequently, the IMGs in Quincy might play an extraordinarily valuable role in addressing medical underservice simply through their locational choices. However, a few critics of IMGs claimed that the size of the IMG community posed a problem for the recruitment of U.S. medical graduates. In several interviews, participants contended that Asian Indians have a tendency to refer to and hire other physicians from India. At the same time, some participants claimed that recruitment efforts actually favored U.S. medical graduates. Several participants in the medical community said that the hospital has made efforts to hire more U.S. medical graduates, but members of the hospital administration told me otherwise.

It seemed as though the town had reached two different, uncertain tipping points in terms of acceptability. The first tipping point, *in favor of acceptability*, came about after the first few IMGs had moved to the area. They earned strong reputations as physicians, and thereby opened possibilities for other IMGs to do well in Quincy, too. More recently, the town might have reached a second tipping point *against acceptability* because of concerns about the size of the IMG community. Hospital politics, such as disputes over hiring decisions or referrals, was one indication that the size of the IMG community had become controversial. Other indications of such controversy included the perceived separateness of IMGs of Asian Indian origin, negative stereotypes about Asian Indians (e.g., hierarchical approaches, attitudes toward women, lack of investment in the local community), and the sensitivity of the issue of "foreign doctors" in some discussions with community members and physicians. However, the two possible "tipping points" presupposed a clearly drawn distinction between IMGs and U.S. medical graduates that often did not exist. For example, people did not always know who was an "American doctor" and who was a "foreign doctor." The social and professional status of physicians further transcended distinctions between Americans and foreigners.

Numerous issues surfaced that made the issue of IMG acceptability seem like a small concern for Quincy. For example, people who expressed a concern that the town had too many IMGs also commented favorably on a hospital survey about their individual IMG physician. Furthermore, concerns about IMGs seemed paltry in comparison with the high degree of trust placed in primary care providers. Since most IMGs in Quincy were subspecialists, the referral of a trusted primary care provider was often enough to make a concerned patient accepting of an IMG.

Put another way, IMG acceptability did not simply exist as an isolated event. Rather, acceptability was influenced by numerous *mechanisms* or causal forces, such as the role of primary care providers who made referrals to IMGs, the role of pioneer IMGs, and the role of each individual physician. Retention, competence, work ethic, familiarity, the role of the hospital, and geographic clustering of IMGs were also among mechanisms influencing acceptability.[1]

Meanwhile, such mechanisms were also interrelated with one another and with numerous abstract contexts, such as communication, discrimination, Americanness, and social separateness. For example, the clustering of IMGs in Quincy has arguably reduced the potential for discrimination because IMGs are a familiar sight there. At the same time, some local residents felt that IMGs do not assimilate well into local culture, and that their influx creates a loss in opportunities for U.S. medical graduates. Thus, the interrelations between contexts, mechanisms, and the event of acceptability are exceedingly complex, and do not lend themselves easily to quick summations. Concerns about the roles of women in different societies, the social construction of race, and differences in religion complicated people's perceptions of IMGs even further. In short, the findings revealed a multidimensionality to the issue of IMG acceptability. Such multidimensionality led to far deeper findings than would have been possible if the aim of the study had been to learn about precise social and spatial variations.

DELANO COUNTY

About five weeks after leaving Quincy, I began fieldwork in Delano County. Issues that had seemed covered many times over in Quincy now seemed new. Participants seemed more open in discussing the role of IMGs, and the interviews were livelier and yielded more depth about contexts (e.g., race, gender roles, globalization), mechanisms (e.g., medical clinics, pioneer IMGs, competition, competence, retention), and events (e.g., acceptability, trust, appreciation). Community entry came much easier. It seemed as though every corner led to another helpful contact who introduced me to other helpful contacts.

Perhaps my greatest asset was time. The interlude between my fieldwork in Quincy and Delano County gave me an opportunity to reflect more on my research. Also, my meetings in Delano County were scheduled at more distant time intervals because of a personal obligation that kept me from staying more than one day at a time in the area. I knew that my work would take at least a few months so I felt less rushed and more patient in scheduling interviews, and had more time to absorb what I was learning. Nonetheless, my schedule was often packed with meetings. In only four months, I interviewed nearly seventy people, attended numerous health care meetings, three church services, Diwali (the Hindu New Year's Festival), and various other events.

In conducting such an in-depth study, I felt the need to "cover my bases" by interviewing people from a broad range of professional and social backgrounds. I followed advice about making sure that my sample was comprehensive and did not omit important people; e.g., make sure that you interview at least one or two people from each major health profession that interacts with IMGs; make sure that your sample includes several wealthy business leaders because they can close a town to outsiders;[2] contact IMGs who have left the area to see how their responses might vary from people who still live there. The sample swelled further in size, and I tried but failed to set up telephone interviews with additional IMGs who had moved away from Delano County. Complicating matters, the area had large percentages of whites, blacks, and Native Americans, and I wanted to be able to defend my work by saying that each group was well-represented in this study. Thus, my work in Delano County reflected an ongoing transition in my thinking about research. On the one hand, I no longer gauged my progress by the number of interviews but, instead, by depth of insight. On the other hand, I conducted some interviews largely to shield myself against criticism from people who look at research primarily in terms of numbers. The result was an expanding study, with almost no time to revisit participants for follow-up interviews.

Further adding to the magnitude of the study, participants frequently confided personal and sensitive information, and interviews tended to be fuller and richer than had been the case in Quincy. Moreover, Delano County may have been more open to me as an outsider than to someone with strong local ties. After all, I was not part of local conflicts between whites, blacks, and Native Americans. Then again, neither were many IMGs, which may have made the area more open to them, too. People seemed to be telling me what they really thought, even if that meant disclosing racial preferences in choosing a doctor, talking about the mistreatment of an IMG, or discussing the early exclusion of IMGs from the medical staff. Meanwhile, participants also talked positively about IMGs. I learned that two of the first IMGs in the area won people's praise through the quality of their work, thereby opening doors for other IMGs to do well in Delano County, too. I also learned about the high level of appreciation and trust placed in individual IMGs, with some of the same names surfacing again and again as exemplary physicians.

My research was now full of different nuances and intricacies about acceptability, including complicated and seemingly contradictory findings about competition, competence, retention, and race, among many other issues. The richness of the Delano County findings seemed to have less to do with IMG acceptability per se, and more to do with life in Delano County. We have all seen or heard interviews on television or radio in which specific guests made for particularly lively conversation. The same can be said about individual participants in both study areas. Yet it was more than just having interesting participants but, rather, coming to extraordinary places to do this research. Some places make for more exciting "guests" than do others. Delano County was certainly an exciting place to do research.

With three or four races (Native Americans, whites, blacks, and Hispanics) in the area, networking across communities, and variability in people's social networks, this would not have been a good place to try to find out "right" answers. Instead, Delano County was a proving ground for conducting a study that emphasized nuances and contextualization. My role as a researcher added to such complexity, since I was *in the place*, seeing the area through my limited perspective as an outsider.

Race was a key issue behind so much of the complexity in Delano County. Race was at once a central issue while also an ill-defined, socially constructed term that had different meanings to different people. It was impossible to know who was white, black, or Native American simply based on physical appearance. However, some participants confused "race" with "nationality," and considered Asian Indians to be of a separate race. Race played itself out in separate social networks that were further divided by perceived class distinctions. The possibility of social separateness for IMGs (e.g., participation in social activities in Filmore) fit in well with the existing separateness of the area; that is, the convergence of different social networks helped give Delano County its identities as a place. Amid internal divisions in Delano County, several participants said that it is to IMGs' advantage to practice in a "tri-racial" area because people are used to difference. Race, gender roles, religion, Americanness, and perceptions of separateness were among many abstract contexts that made this study area much more complicated than originally expected.

However, such findings belie what should have been the case if this had been a statistical study. The findings in Delano County could have been, at best, a control for Quincy. In Quincy, IMGs constituted about half of the physician workforce, and the overwhelming majority of IMGs were subspecialists. By contrast, most of the IMGs in Delano County practiced in primary care; the percentage of IMGs was about average for the country, around 20 percent of the physician workforce. Another important contrast surfaced in the ages of physicians in the two study areas. Most of the IMGs interviewed for this study in Quincy tended to be in their forties and fifties, but most of the IMGs interviewed in Delano County were in their thirties.

Some of the same issues that surfaced in Quincy surfaced again in Delano County, albeit with different nuances. For example, problems with communication were major concerns in both areas. Whereas the line between problems with communication and problems with discrimination was blurred in Quincy, I did not have any such indication in Delano County. Trust in primary care providers was another major issue in both areas. However, in Delano County, referrals to IMG subspecialists were not as frequent an issue; not only did IMGs constitute a lower percentage of the physician workforce in the area, but most of the IMGs practiced in primary care. Trust also surfaced in other ways in Delano County. For example, organizational trust was important in increasing the acceptability of the few IMGs who had joined established medical practices alongside U.S. medical graduates. By contrast, in Quincy, physicians were more likely to be in solo practice.

Further contrasts surfaced between study areas in terms of retention. IMGs rarely left Quincy, but Delano County participants had many different perspectives on the retention of IMGs. For example, one U.S. medical graduate in Hamilton said that he would not hire IMGs because, as a rule, they did not have a strong enough commitment to the local area or the state. Although some participants claimed that IMGs are more likely to be mobile, other participants claimed that IMGs have longer staying power. Still others claimed that IMGs vary by country of origin in terms of retention, or that variation in retention takes place primarily on an individual level. Further complexity was found on every issue studied, more so than had been the case in Quincy.

My longer and greater experience in Delano County contributed further to my sense and knowledge of the area. Delano County and Quincy were so different, and the findings so nuanced, that simple comparisons on acceptability seem to be the equivalent of comparing apples and oranges. Some contrasts and similarities can be noteworthy (e.g., systematic exclusion of the first IMGs in one town but not in another; different perceptions on retention) but subtlety is at the core of this study. To reduce the complexity of the findings to precise answers that can be conveyed neatly in separate categories would contradict such subtlety.

CONCEPT MAP

At the outset of this study, my thinking focused on the differences in IMG acceptability from one jurisdictional category to another, as between Hamilton and Quincy. Specifically, certain findings would apply more frequently to one town than another, and then I would postulate the reasons behind such spatial differences. However, I came to realize that a focus on spatial variation would be stifling because it would impede my ability to explore other geographic concepts more fully. In my view, this study has taken geography in new directions, providing new insights into social theory, concepts such as othering and place, and contributions beyond academia.

As my thinking about theory grew through the course of research, I realized that I needed to incorporate other theoretical ideas; hence, a "concept map" summarizing key geographic concepts and their interrelations with one another (Figure 10.1). The concept map is a logical extension of the framework that helped form the basis for my theory, but also includes some new additions, such as "identities of places" and "boundaries." These concepts were added out of necessity. Place matters. Boundaries blur, and yet people cross uncertain boundaries all of the time. Such issues are far too important to omit, and therefore the framework needed to be extended.

The original framework in this study was influenced by critical realism, building on the ideas of events, mechanisms, and contexts. In the course of this study, my thinking about these three layers evolved in order to fit them even further into a geographic perspective. For example, the left side of the concept map (Figure 10.1) is consistent with the diagram of a realist framework shown earlier in Figure 2.1, and now includes local interpretations of abstract *contexts* such as race and gender; *mechanisms* that are based within a place, such as the role of a hospital or the role of pioneer IMGs; and the event of acceptability or othering, considered as "geographies of exclusion."

Every concept, including ones that I added, could be linked conceptually with every other concept in the diagram. It may appear as though every concept exists as a separate, self-contained entity. In reality, the distinctions between concepts are blurred, hence the clouds surrounding concepts.

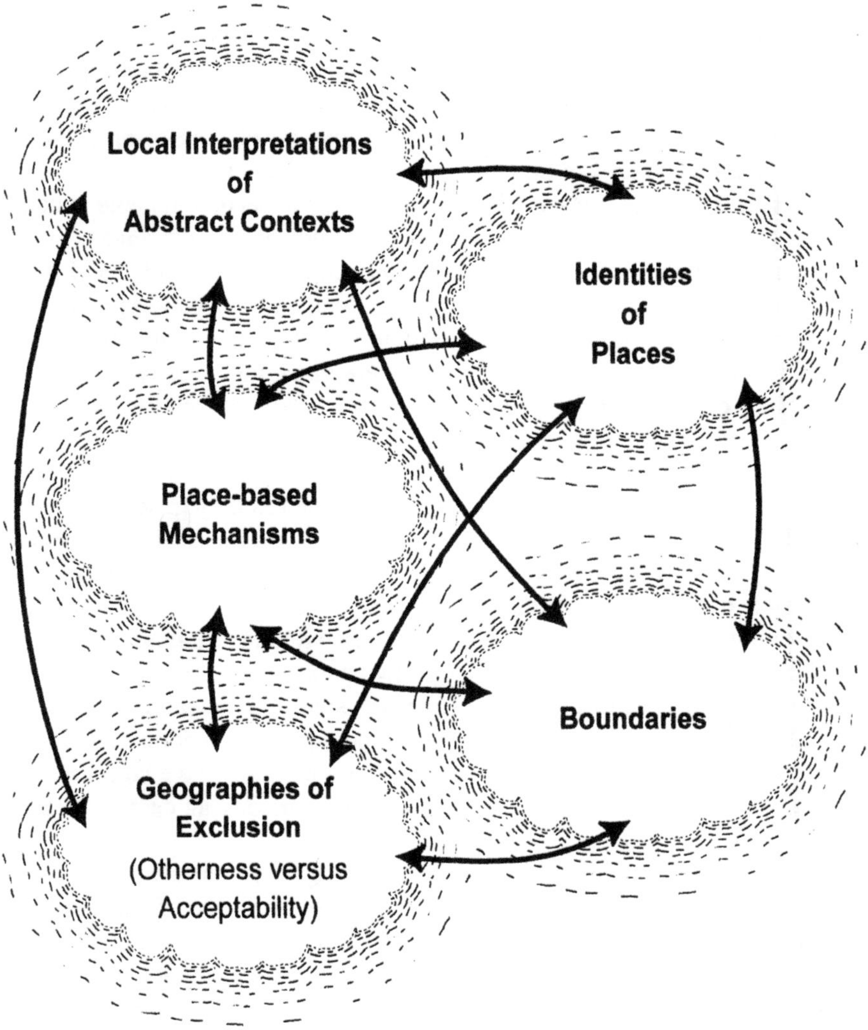

Figure 10.1. Concept Map

Without the use of this concept map, this study could conceivably be reduced to much more concrete dualisms in an equation. For example, acceptability could be the dependent variable, to be measured on a scale or reduced to a simple "yes" or "no" for an equation. Various contexts and mechanisms could be simplified, too. Thus, race, gender, age, physician specialty, or immigrant community size could be among many possible, independent variables. Different data could be input into the equations used in studying acceptability in each town. The results could then lead to straight comparisons between towns, resulting in many concrete lessons about IMG acceptability, such as that IMGs are more (or less) accepted in areas where they practice in specific specialties, or that older IMGs have a stronger (or weaker) sense of belonging in rural towns than do younger IMGs. In other words, the complexity of the study could be erased in favor of precise, dualistic answers.

Nonetheless, some differences between towns have become notable in considering IMG acceptability. For example, in Quincy, the IMGs tended to be about ten years older than their Delano County counterparts. Such age differences could conceivably have a measurable, positive or negative impact on acceptability, and could be the basis for comparisons of the results from the two towns. Similarly, the IMGs in Quincy were much more likely to work in subspecialty care than were their counterparts in Delano County, who were more likely to fill primary care positions. Other potentially measurable differences that could be included in forming a simple equation about IMG acceptability include differences in racial composition (e.g., by general population or by physician workforce), group versus solo practices (including the extent to which IMGs practice alongside U.S. medical graduates), differences in the levels of retention of IMGs, the prevalence of church-related activities in the community, and the towns' locations relative to urban areas. In fact, it would be all too easy to single out one or two particular differences between towns as general rules to take away from this study. At the very least, such straightforward comparisons could serve as the basis to conjecture about the implications of the study for other areas. Why, then, do I have so much reluctance to emphasize such straightforward comparisons as central to this work?

The answer is that such comparisons only scratch the surface of IMG acceptability, and cast an overly simplistic shadow on the issue of causality. In other words, surface-level comparisons only go so far. They can also be wrong. For example, it would be overly simplistic to assume that a handful of measurable variables (e.g., age, specialty) account for all of the different findings in the two study areas. There is no magic bullet and no simple answer that can explain away extraordinary complexities and subtleties. IMG acceptability is not a matter of the impact of "A" on "B," but, instead, of many different, place-specific mechanisms, social and spatial contexts, blurred boundary distinctions, and identities of places. There is a need to look beyond straight spatial comparisons and go to a much deeper, more insightful level of analysis. Here is where the concept map becomes particularly important.

A concept map is often used as a pedagogical tool (Novak, 1998, 1991). The similarities between pedagogy and the major advances of using the concept map also extend to its greatest application, i.e., as a tool for critical thinking. To understand what I mean, consider another model, Perry's schema, which is also a model used in pedagogy (Perry, 1970). Perry's schema indicates the step-by-step transitions of students as they learn about critical thinking. At stage one of the schema, students think of the world through the dualism of "right" and "wrong" answers. Eventually, at the bottom of Perry's schema, students no longer see the world in dualistic terms. Rather than reducing everything to "right" and "wrong" answers, students ideally realize that this is how life will be, and they will have to use their best judgment in an ambiguous world (Perry, 1970). It is my contention that the same basic ideal of transitions from "right" and "wrong" answers to ambiguity applies in research, too.

Like higher levels in Perry's schema, the use of the concept map would be inconsistent with the dualism of definitive right and wrong answers. For example, consideration of the complex linkages between boundaries and mechanisms would be inconsistent with level one of Perry's schema. Observers need to consider the extraordinary ambiguity of the interrelationships between different concepts in order to learn more about IMG acceptability. My role as a researcher—and, by extension, as a teacher—is to help people think more critically about the issue of IMG acceptability.

What are some of the implications of using the concept map? Obviously, some simplistic notions about IMG acceptability can be eliminated rather easily, such as contentions that IMGs can be categorized easily as a "problem" in U.S. health care. For example, Mullan and colleagues (1995) have contended that IMGs take away jobs that otherwise might go to U.S. medical graduates, and that IMGs add to a physician surplus by practicing in places that have too many physicians. However, the distinctions between the abstract contexts of foreignness and Americanness have now become so blurred that it is no longer easy to think of IMGs in dualistic terms. The many local interpretations of race, gender, religion, and language are among many complicated issues that render such dualisms (e.g., foreigner versus American) inconsistent with the more complex realities of life. Furthermore, each place has different causal forces or "mechanisms" upon which acceptability is contingent. Acceptability can be contingent upon the size of immigrant communities, familiarity with immigrants, or the role of individual hospitals. Thus, to cast IMGs en masse as a "problem" makes as much sense as clinging to level one of Perry's schema.

Each part of the concept map can lead to additional complexity. For example, consider the idea of overlapping geographic exclusions. People are not the only ones who can be othered; many rural towns can be othered, too. Rural physicians often have a lower professional status than their peers who practice in urban areas (Crandall et al., 1990). Medical colleges often encourage their students to practice in places considered to be more "prestigious," such as large teaching hospitals in urban areas. Meanwhile, rural physicians face stereotypes that the care that they provide is not as good as the care provided in urban areas. The quality of individual physicians, access to state-of-the-art technology, and peer contact are among many concerns expressed by critics of rural health care (Crandall et al., 1990). Alongside the otherness of rural places, IMGs are othered within rural places, too. The idea of multiple, overlapping layers of geographic exclusions applies everywhere.

The layering of geographic exclusions adds to the difficulty of assimilation for IMGs. Everyone faces otherness in different ways in different places. There is no such thing as a place free of geographic exclusions, or of a person who has a natural or learned predisposition to avoid all possible exclusions. We are all the Other. An immigrant who works hard to be like everybody else, even to the point of participating in specific activities, speaking a certain language in a specific way, practicing a particular religion, or congregating with well-established and respected townspeople, still faces otherness. There are simply too many contexts and mechanisms that influence otherness for geographic exclusions to be erased so simply. There are always local, nuanced meanings to contexts, such as a person's *perceived* race, gender, religion, or language. There are always place-based mechanisms, such as the size of a particular community or the role of a medical clinic, which can trigger geographic inclusions or exclusions. Meanwhile, people cross unseen boundaries and face at least some sort of uncertainty in their own daily lives. Everyone's sense of inclusiveness varies from one place and interaction to another, while also varying over time.

The importance of time to the concept map, and to the place of IMGs, cannot be underscored enough. Every concept in the concept map varies over time. For example, the many local interpretations and social constructions of race undergo frequent changes, rather than remaining constant. The meanings of race in a particular town for one generation cannot be expected to remain identical for another generation. Yet it is unclear how often changes in the meanings of race become significant enough to change the openness of a town to Others from different races. Besides the many other contexts and mechanisms (e.g., foreignness, communication, size of the immigrant community) that can influence otherness, so too does time.

An overnight, dramatic change in the meanings that people attach to race is theoretically possible, but such changes are more likely to take place over an ill-defined but extended period of time. Just as the transition from the simplest level of Perry's schema to higher levels of critical thinking can be difficult and traumatic, so too can the transition from geographic exclusiveness to inclusiveness. Typically, a person or group cannot be expected to lose the status of Other in a place overnight. Instead, people experience difficult transitions in places that are becoming more inclusive. At the risk of oversimplification, a person who loses the status of Other for a particular issue (e.g., having a strong accent), still retains otherness in other ways (e.g., having a particular physical appearance; or even being excluded from a particular conversation). Thus, there are degrees and facets of otherness that cannot be measured, and yet there is no rule that a person can avoid extreme exclusion just by being patient and waiting for months or even years to pass. Too many issues occur simultaneously to allow otherness to be reduced to just one issue. Rather, otherness is a reflection of many contexts and mechanisms and their interactions within and beyond specific places.

The meanings of race and racism are not the same at different times, and always undergo some change and modification through local interpretations and constructions. Meanwhile, each place undergoes changes, influenced not only by internal but also external activities. For example, the civil rights movement had an impact on people's perceptions of race in Quincy and Delano County. One participant in Delano County even said that changes over time in the acceptability of IMGs are a reflection of broader changes in civil rights throughout the United States. Yet the changes in perceptions of race did not take place at the same time everywhere, and the tremors of the civil rights movement are still being felt in different ways in different parts of the United States. The openness of Quincy and Delano County to IMGs is at least a partial reflection of such ongoing tremors, while at the same time influencing perceptions of race in other areas.

Complicating matters even further, place is a *process* rather than a static entity (Massey, 1997). The meanings that people attach to a place, or to its inclusiveness, vary over time. Meanwhile, people's perceptions of their own places change, too. A place that excludes IMGs at one time can be open in another; the subtleties of discrimination change, too. In short, the concept map becomes even more complicated in considering the simple idea that places and people change.

Researchers often overlook changes over time in place identities, as though the exact "boundaries" of each place have actually become more important than the places themselves. However, the world becomes exceedingly complex in light of the idea that people cross unseen boundaries that are virtually everywhere. Geographic boundaries can even be found on the human body, in a public gathering, or in a physician's office. Places do have boundaries, but those boundaries are often ambiguous and changing, and not easily displayed clearly on a map.

Place is deeply interwoven with IMG acceptability. For example, place is behind so many key issues, such as the nuances of contexts, mechanisms, and events in the two study areas; the rationale for not focusing on straight comparisons of acceptability between study areas; and the personalities or identities of Quincy and Delano County.

In many geographic studies, place is not even a consideration. Despite the contributions of researchers like Massey (1996, 1997), Tuan (1974), Kearns (1993), and Gesler (1999), the issue of place is often relegated to an incidental role, a mere backdrop for data analysis. The meaning of places is often overlooked in favor of their spatial boundaries, typically characterized by clearly drawn lines on a map. It is as though human beings exist on a meaningless surface, which is filled with splashed-on colors to show percent white, percent male, percent over age sixty-five, or other sociodemographic or economic characteristics. Thus, the central focus in much of human geography has often been on such characteristics, and not on human behavior *in place*.

Having said that, a focus on "place" (rather than space) can be misconstrued as a focus on uniqueness in all possible circumstances, with no room for generalizations. My preference instead is to find more of a middle ground, to emphasize that generalizations are useful for surface-level comparisons in studying the social world; but to really learn about life, we need to learn about places, in the same sense that we need to learn about individual people to learn about human behavior.

Of course, the question of generalization often does come up in research on human behavior. The concept of generalization has a statistical meaning in which precise, repeatable answers or approaches can apply from a subset to a larger whole. Certainly, I have made some informal generalizations (such as contrasts in the role of communication in the two study areas, age differences among physicians, and my personal sense of the openness of each town to newcomers) but not in a statistical sense. The impossibility of disentangling research findings from the complexity of each place makes statistical generalizations about IMG acceptability difficult. To extend the findings in terms of a concise, repeatable truth about human behavior to other places would not make sense.

THE PLACE OF "FOREIGN DOCTORS" AFTER SEPTEMBER 11, 2001

Earlier, I mentioned that dramatic changes in geographic exclusions typically do not take place overnight. This observation was simply based on my own research findings; that is, geographic exclusions are a process instead of an either/or event. In Quincy and Hamilton, geographic exclusions generally did not suddenly appear or vanish, as though guided by a force of wind. Barring any catastrophic events, a highly regarded IMG did not suddenly become out of place or forced to leave. Even though IMGs in the study area weathered major political and social changes (e.g., civil rights struggles or backlashes, economic recessions, political changes at the local, state, and national levels), none of these changes appeared as make-or-break events for IMG acceptability locally. In other words, the local acceptance of IMGs within Quincy and Hamilton did not automatically rise or sink with the direction of political or social currents in the United States. Yet the events of September 11, 2001, created many new local landscapes for immigrants in the United States.

A question that surfaced in this study, "Can I trust a foreigner?" now entered into the national consciousness in the United States. This question, like so many others, was often unspoken in people's lives, while being asked again and again after the terrorist attacks in Washington, New York, and Pennsylvania. Other important questions also tended to be unstated or discussed cautiously, yet remained inescapably relevant to this study and to the lives of people in America. "Which foreigners can I trust?" "Who is a foreigner?" None of these questions had simple answers, and yet people throughout the United States were now trying to answer them. These were not questions for lengthy academic discussions but instead were encountered and answered in an instant, as though by a natural, psychological reaction. Consider some examples. On the national news, it was reported that there were actually cases of murder and assault as payback for terrorism; for example, an Asian Indian was killed in a case of mistaken national identity. An IMG in Texas was detained by the U.S. government, after his last name matched the last name of one of the September 11 hijackers. What could his adopted hometown have thought of him then? Meanwhile, subtle events took place, too. For example, a woman with black hair walked into a grocery store, and encountered a look of hatred from a stranger. "Is it because this person thinks I'm Arab?" the woman wondered, the same question that many other people throughout the country may have been asking themselves, too. However, these images reflect mainly the fear that surfaced in the aftermath of the attacks. If Eutaw, Alabama presents any indication of the place of IMGs after September 11, 2001, the answer might be that small towns are even more welcoming than before. As Khowla Seljuki, wife of an IMG, explained on Public Broadcasting Network's *Newshour*:

> Right after September 11, initially, I was a little scared to go out because my scarf and my Muslim outlook. But when I went out, people were more friendly to me here in Eutaw. In the grocery stores and everywhere, they were more friendly, and the people whom I barely knew, they were coming to me and they were, like, talking to me and asking me that, "if you need any help, if somebody gives you any trouble, just call and tell us," but nobody gave us any trouble.

Without reopening the study, I can only conjecture about the impact that September 11 had on the IMGs in Hamilton and Quincy, or in other parts of the United States. All of the IMGs that I met, many of whom had worked so hard to gain the trust and respect of others in their adopted hometowns, have a job to do. Everyone else does, too. It is not a new job for anyone. For IMGs, it is the same job that they have been doing all along, taking care of patients. For patients, it is simply that, to be patients of whichever doctor is their doctor, IMG or U.S. medical graduate. Ideally, nothing has changed for IMGs in terms of acceptability. But something has changed nonetheless. The old question that I was asked so many times, "Where are you from?" could now be laced with new, misplaced fears. If the Eutaw example is not repeated elsewhere, towns that had no IMGs could be more reluctant to hire, much less accept, their first doctors from abroad. Doctors who are perceived to be Arab, or perceived to be Muslim, could face more uncertainty from the general public, not to mention from their peers. Whereas IMGs already had to prove themselves, now there could be a new, or at least a renewed, fear of outsiders to overcome, too.

As people go about their daily lives, there is something to be said for the calming influence of time. The differences in the tone of the general public are already noticeable since the early days after the attacks of September 11, 2001. For many people, there had been an anger that seemed boiling to the surface, but feelings often have a way of settling down. Perhaps the terrorist attacks will be a defining event for IMG acceptability in some towns and not in others. Without further distance in time, it is hard to know at this point if the terrorist attacks are a defining moment or not for the acceptability of IMGs. Each place will no doubt change over time, with this global event being rethought locally for the place of IMGs.

Perhaps the most evident changes are already taking place nationally. In the aftermath of the attacks, the U.S. Department of Agriculture (2002) withdrew its participation in the J-1 visa waiver program. The stated reason was concerns about ensuring adequate background checks for national security. However, only a few months later, the U.S. House of Representatives passed legislation for an expansion of the J-1 visa waiver program from twenty to thirty waivers per state (H.R. 4858). In this ongoing policy dynamic, concerns about the influx of new IMGs are not fuelled so much by economic considerations but, instead, national security. It is unknown whether the numbers of new IMGs will increase or decrease in the coming years. It is also unknown how these latest policy decisions will affect the future acceptance of IMGs in rural America. Indeed, the greatest impacts of September 11, 2001, on the place of IMGs may always remain intangible.

POLICY IMPLICATIONS AND RECOMMENDATIONS

Readers expecting grand policy recommendations about the need to increase or decrease the supply of IMGs will be disappointed. A cliché helps explain my reluctance to tell people what to do: The more I learn, the more I realize that I do not have the answers. What I can do though is make several recommendations that could conceivably have a small influence on the acceptability of IMGs in rural America.

First, and perhaps most importantly, policy makers should consider the concept map in thinking about policies. Over and over again, debates in policy circles have focused on simplistic notions about IMGs as a group that "reduces local physician shortages" or "exacerbates national oversupply" (Mick et al., 2000). It is time to move beyond such a simple, dualistic approach to policy and consider instead the multiple layers of complexity surrounding IMGs and their experiences in the United States. As policy makers consider the concept map, the "list" of possible contexts and mechanisms will not be identical from place to place. Indeed, the meanings of "race," "gender," "religion," or other contexts are so different over time and place that it would make little sense to list such contexts in a table. However, simply by considering such complexity, policy makers can build further on critical thinking in making decisions about IMG policies. In short, the best policy makers are those who really *think* in order to make appropriate decisions about health care. This concept map can serve as a valuable tool for the countless policy makers who are thinking far beyond level one of Perry's schema.

A second recommendation, consistent with previous work by Fiscella et al. (1997) and Cole-Kelly (1994), is that IMGs in residency programs can benefit from learning about cross-cultural health care. The specific issues to be considered would obviously vary based on the needs and experiences of IMGs in each residency program. In many cases, preparing for difficulties in communication (e.g., understanding idiomatic expressions, being understood by patients) could help IMGs adjust more quickly than they already do to practice in rural areas. Issues such as gender roles, discrimination, race relations, and traditional beliefs about health care could also be part of IMGs' preparation during graduate medical education. Such education should also take place in small towns for community members and medical staff so that they, too, can recognize and learn further from cultural differences in order to improve the experiences of IMGs. Such educational programs would not necessarily need to be formalized within individual towns but could, instead, be logical extensions of community outreach by churches, schools, and hospitals to the general community.

Third, the J-1 visa waiver should be coordinated across the state and federal waiver-requesting agencies (U.S. General Accounting Office, 1996).

Such coordination could serve to reduce paperwork so that placements can occur more quickly, thereby benefiting both employers and waiver physicians. At the same time, it remains to be seen whether interagency coordination could be useful in improving placement decisions so that IMGs are matched more closely with specific towns. It also remains to be seen how such coordination should be used in ensuring that employers do not take advantage of the vulnerability of waiver or H-1B physicians. Such issues warrant review and consideration.

Fourth, efforts to improve IMG acceptability do not need to be explicitly related to health care. For example, many of the spouses of IMGs are highly educated but have limited employment opportunities in rural areas. Public or private investments in rural America can lead to more employment opportunities, social activities, and greater contact with others who have similar educational backgrounds. As a result, spouses who have previously made "sacrifices" in their careers might have more opportunities in rural America. Educational investments can also further the likelihood that IMGs will feel accepted in rural areas. For example, IMGs of Asian Indian origin often expressed a strong concern for family. Improvements in the quality of schools could influence IMGs' sense of belonging in their adopted towns. Education can also be useful in exposing communities to new ideas, including further openness to different cultures.

Fifth, policy makers and community members can now have a stronger idea of some of the unanswered questions surrounding IMG acceptability. For example, further research can focus on issues such as the role of the happiness of the spouse in the recruitment and retention of physicians from different cultural and geographical backgrounds, the career choices and commitment to rural areas for IMGs' children who choose to become physicians, the experiences of IMGs from particular medical schools or specific countries of origin, and considerations of IMG acceptability in other countries. By focusing on these and other issues in future studies, policy makers and community members can have an even stronger understanding of the experiences and contributions of IMGs.

Finally, this book can be particularly useful in adding a human face to complex policy considerations. I feel that there is often a disconnect between policy makers and people in rural areas. It is my sense that a similar disconnect exists between policy researchers and rural America. Most health services research has a "top-down" approach to policy, in which the researcher or funding agency decides in advance which data sets will be explored, and the potential "answers" for the study. Researchers then make claims about human behavior, without even leaving their offices. By contrast, the methods used in this study were designed to emphasize rural Americans' perceptions and experiences. Such methods included interviews with a broad range of community members and health providers, firsthand accounts, participation in local activities, and suggestions by contacts about the direction of the study. As a result, in-depth considerations of doctor-patient and doctor-community interactions can hopefully flow upward from rural America to policy makers.

The policies that are most directly related to the issue of IMG acceptability include: the J-1 visa to allow IMGs to pursue residency training; the J-1 visa waiver to stay in the country in exchange for practice in an underserved area; the H-1B visa that enables application for permanent residence; legal requirements for permanent residence and citizenship; and a broad range of health workforce policies at the local, state, and national level that influence the distribution of providers into needy areas (e.g., underservice designations, community health center regulations, rural residency rotations).

Behind the many policies lie human experiences with those policies. Statistical studies or maps of geographic distributions conceal the fact that a waiver physician in Delano County worked long hours in a rural clinic, taking care of the poor and the elderly. The hard work of people in a Quincy clinic that is staffed almost entirely by IMGs also does not show up in a statistic or a map. Against this backdrop of real life, policy makers and other observers often dismiss IMGs as "the problem," based primarily on concerns that IMGs exacerbate national physician oversupply. However, once a human face is presented, it becomes extraordinarily difficult to brand an entire, diverse group of people as "the problem."

Certainly, others may arrive at additional insights and policy implications about IMG acceptability that may not have occurred to me. In other words, this is not a closed book but an open one, to be read and referenced in decision making. IMGs can be better prepared for life in rural areas; community members can ideally reach out more easily to individual IMGs after seeing some of the issues that might be faced in their lives; and recruiters can know more about the cultures and experiences of people living in their communities. As a result of all of these issues, people can be in a much stronger situation to design their own strategies for increasing the acceptance of IMGs.

NOTES

1. These examples of mechanisms and contexts are simply meant to remind the reader of what was discussed, rather than to serve as a comprehensive or formal list. As explained earlier, there is a gray area between mechanisms and contexts, and not everything fits neatly in one category or another.

2. I saw no indication that wealthy business leaders played a special role in Delano County's attitudes toward IMGs.

Appendix: Interview Guide

Note: I have tried to reconstruct the final interview guide from shorthand into questions written-out for discussion with participants from diverse backgrounds. I did not standardize questions but instead followed the flow of conversation. The exact phrasing, placement, or inclusion of a question varied from interview to interview. If a respondent answered a question that I was going to ask, I did not ask it.

1. Could you please tell me a little about what you do?
2. Where are you from? What is your hometown? Do you think that the answer to this question matters to people in the area? Explain.
3. How long have you lived in this area?
4. Question for physicians: Did you have any initial expectations or concerns about [town name]—things you or your family thought you might or might not like? [Probe for how well expectations were met.]
5. Question for physicians: What led you to move to [town name]?
6. Where do people need to be from in order for most people to think of them as belonging to this area? How open do you think this area is to people who come from outside of the area that you described?
7. Do you have any thoughts on the role of church in making newcomers feel more a part of the community? The role of schools? [Elaborate.]
8. Question for physicians: Could you reflect on the happiness of the spouse as an issue of importance for physicians, particularly international medical graduates?
9. Suppose that I am an international medical graduate[1] coming to [town name] to practice, and I asked you about mistakes that other international medical graduates make when they move to the area. Are there common mistakes that people make? What advice would you give me? What could

I do to make myself fit in this town as: (a) a community member, and (b) a physician?

10. I just used the term "international medical graduate." [2] To see if we are thinking about the same issues, could you define the term, "international medical graduate?"
11. Have you ever been the patient of a physician from another country? If so, could you comment on the experience? Did you have any initial expectations or concerns about the physician—things you or your family thought you might or might not like? [Probe for how well expectations were met.] If not, suppose that your doctor referred you to an international medical graduate. What questions would you ask?
12. Why do you think physicians from other countries decide to practice in this town?
13. Trust is an issue that surfaces in thinking about doctor-patient interactions. If you were to go to an international medical graduate, or if you were to go to a U.S. medical graduate, would there be any difference in the level of trust that you would have in what the doctor tells you?
14. Question for physicians: In your view, are there any groups of people in this area who have more difficulty or ease than others in their acceptance of international medical graduates? [Probe for differences by education, income, race, age, rurality.]
15. Another issue that surfaces in talking about physicians is communication, in two directions. One, the patient understanding the physician, and two, the physician understanding local dialects and sayings and regional expressions. Are there regional expressions or sayings that someone from outside the area might have difficulty understanding? [Probe for impact on communication with international medical graduates.]
16. In your view, do concerns about communication affect compliance? In other words, if you have problems communicating with your physician, would you be more or less likely to take prescriptions, follow advice, and return for follow-up visits?
17. In the book *My Own Country*, Abraham Verghese writes about his surprise in learning that a pharmacist thinks less of him for being a physician from another country. Have you had experiences in [town name] that reflect such problems with pharmacists, nurses, doctors, or other health care professionals?
18. Do you think that physicians from other countries are as competent as physicians from the United States? As qualified? [Relate to their personal experience.]
19. In your view, do people in [town name] express a concern about seeing a doctor of a different race? Of a different ethnic or cultural background?

[Probe to see if this is a frequent or uncommon concern.] If yes, what is your view of their concern?

20. Are there areas where the community can improve in terms of its treatment of international medical graduates? Likewise, are there areas where international medical graduates need to improve so that they can be more accepted?
21. A lot of policy makers say that the country has too many doctors, as a whole, and also local areas that need more doctors. They say let's cut back on the number of new international medical graduates coming into the country. In your view, would a cutback in the number of international medical graduates affect health care in [town name]? [Probe for reaction.]
22. Question for physicians: Do you feel on-stage when you go to the grocery store or do other routine activities in public (play with the kids, drive in traffic)?
23. Question for physicians: Do patients contact you a lot after hours, calling you up, for example?
24. Question for physicians: If I were to come back here in ten or fifteen years, would you still be here?
25. I'm asking every participant about age, marital status, educational background, and children. [Go over one at a time, as needed.]
26. In thinking about this interview, is there anything that I missed in trying to learn about people's perceptions of physicians from other countries and in trying to learn about the openness of the area? Are there questions that I should have asked or things you'd like to elaborate more on?
27. Do you have any questions of me or about this study?

NOTES

1. Depending on the participant and the flow of the interview, I would substitute "waiver physician," "physician" or another category for "international medical graduate."

2. At this point, the term "international medical graduate" would have already surfaced in the interview. I used the term "foreign doctor" in talking with people in the general community, and further adjusted terminology according to the wishes and interests of the participant.

Bibliography

Admire, J.B. 1993. Caring for those different than me: Another look at cross-cultural health care. *Rural Clinician Quarterly* (Fall) 3. Reprinted in *A shared vision: Building bridges for rural health care access. Conference proceedings*. National Rural Health Association: Kansas City, 1994, 169–171.

Alderman, D.H. 1997. Integrating space into a reactive theory of the asylum: Evidence from post-Civil War Georgia. *Health and Place* 3: 111–122.

American Association of Colleges of Osteopathic Medicine, American Medical Association, American Osteopathic Association, Association of Academic Health Centers, Association of American Medical Colleges, and National Medical Association 1997. *Consensus statement on the physician workforce*.

American Medical Association (AMA). 1996. AMA Physician Masterfile.

American Medical Association International Medical Graduates Section. 2000. Demographics of IMGs. Retrieved from Internet, http://www.ama-assn.org/ama/pub/category/1550.html, accessed August 18.

Anderson, K.J. 1987. The idea of Chinatown: The power of place and institutional practice in the making of a racial category. *Annals of the Association of American Geographers* 77(4): 580–598.

Arcury, T.A and S.A. Quandt. 1999, Participant recruitment for qualitative research: A site-based approach to community research in complex societies. *Human Organization* 58(2): 128–133.

Area Resource File (ARF). 1998. Office of Research and Planning. Rockville, MD: Bureau of Health Professions, US Department of Health and Human Services.

Atkinson, P. 1995. *Medical talk and medical work*. Thousand Oaks, California: Sage.

Baer, L.D., T.C. Ricketts, T.R. Konrad, and S.S. Mick. 1998. Do international medical graduates reduce rural physician shortages? *Medical Care* 36(11): 1534–1544.

Baer, L.D., T.R. Konrad, and J.S. Miller. 1999a. The need of community health centers for international medical graduates. *American Journal of Public Health* 89(10): 1570–1574.

Baer, L.C, K.A. Baldwin, R.J. Sisk, P.P. Watts, M.S. Grinslade, B. Brockschmidt, M.K. Dinger, L.N. Marion, and J. McCubbin. 1999b. Development of an instrument to measure community acceptance of nurse practitioners and physician assistants. *Journal of Nursing Measurement* 7(1): 63–77.

Barnett, J.R. 1991a. Where have all the doctors gone? Changes in the geographic distribution of general practitioners in New Zealand since 1975. vol. 1: Regional and urban-rural differences. *New Zealand Medical Journal* 104: 314–315.

Barnett, J.R. 1991b. Where have all the doctors gone? vol. 2: Intraurban trends: Changes in the geographic distribution of general practitioners in Auckland, 1980-87. *New Zealand Medical Journal* 104: 337–339.

Barnett, J.R. 1991c. Where have all the doctors gone? Changes in the geographic distribution of general practitioners in New Zealand since 1975 vol. 3: New Zealand and foreign medical graduates compared. *New Zealand Medical Journal* 104: 358–360.

Barnett, J.R. 1991d. Geographical implications of restricting foreign medical immigration: A New Zealand case study, 1976-87. *Social Science and Medicine* 33(4): 459–470.

Bastien, J.W. 1985. Qollahuaya-Andean body concepts: A topographical hydraulic model of physiology. *American Anthropology* 87: 595-611.

Blalock, H.M., ed. 1971. Causal models in the social sciences. Chicago: Aldine Atherton,

CBS News. 1999. A doctor in the house? *60 Minutes*. R. Hartman, producer. Aired November 7.

Cawley, J.F. 1996. The evolution of new health professions: A history of physician assistants. In *The US health workforce: Power, politics, and policy*, ed. M. Osterweis, C.J. McLaughlin, H.R. Manasse Jr., and C.L Hopper, Washington, DC: Association of Academic Health Centers, 189–207.

Chehrazi, A., M. Maggio, R. Aronson, and R. Deasy. 1999. J-1 waivers for physicians—the current state of the art. In *1999–00 Immigration & Nationality Law Handbook: Volume II: Advanced Topics,* ed. R.P. Murphy American Immigration Lawyers Association, 283–311.

Cloke, P., C. Philo, and D. Sadler. 1991. *Approaching human geography: An introduction to contemporary theoretical debates*. New York: Guilford Press.

Cole-Kelly, K. 1994. Cultures engaging cultures: International medical graduates training in the United States. *Family Medicine* 26 (10): 618–624.

Conte, S.J., A.W. Imershein, and M.K. Magill. 1992. Rural community and physician perspectives on resource factors affecting physician retention. *Journal of Rural Health* 8: 185–196.

Council on Graduate Medical Education. 1998. *Eleventh report: international medical graduates, the physician workforce, and GME payment reform*. Washington, D.C.: US Department of Health and Human Services, Public Health Services, Health Resources and Services Administration; March.

Council on Graduate Medical Education. 1999. *Fourteenth report: COGME physician workforce policies: Recent developments and remaining challenges in meeting national goals*. Washington, D.C.: U.S. Department of Health and Human Services, Public Health Services, Health Resources and Services Administration; March.

Council on Graduate Medical Education. 2000. *What is it? What has it done? Where is it going?* Rockville, MD: US Department of Health and Human Services, Public Health Services, Health Resources and Services Administration; March.

Crandall, L., J. Dwyer, and R. Duncan. 1990. Recruitment and retention of rural physicians: Issues for the 1990s. *Journal of Rural Health* 6: 19–38.

Cravey, A.J. 1998. *Women and work in Mexico's maquiladoras*. Lanham, MD: Rowman & Littlefield.

Cutchin, M.P. 1997. Physician retention in rural communities: The perspective of experiential place integration. *Health and Place* 3: 25–41.

Cutchin, M.P. 1999. Qualitative explorations in health geography: Using pragmatism and related concepts as guides. *The Professional Geographer* 51(2): 265–274.

Dear, M. and J.R. Wolch. 1987. *Landscapes of despair*. Princeton, NJ: Princeton University Press.

de Blij, H.J, and P.O. Muller. 2000. *Geography: Realms, regions, and concepts 2000*. New York: John Wiley and Sons.

Devers, K.J. 1999. How will we know "good" qualitative research when we see it? Beginning the dialogue in health services research. *Health Services Research* 34 (5) (Part II): 1153–1188.

deVise, P. 1973. Misused and misplaced hospitals and doctors: A locational analysis of the urban health care crisis. Commission on College Geography Resource Paper No. 22. Washington, DC: American Association of Geographers.

Dorn, M., and G. Laws.1994. Social theory, medical geography and body politics: Extending Kearns' invitation. *Professional Geographer* 46: 106–110.

Eisenberg, D.M., R.C. Kessler, C. Foster, F.E. Norlock, D.R. Calkins, and T.L. Delbanco. 1993. Unconventional medicine in the United States: Prevalence, costs, and patterns of use. *New England Journal of Medicine* 328: 246–252.

Entrikin, J.N. 1991. *The betweenness of place: Towards a geography of modernity*. Baltimore, MD: Johns Hopkins University Press.

Ernst, R.L., and D.E. Yett.1985. *Physician location and specialty choice*. Ann Arbor, MI: Health Administered Press.

Fiscella, K., M. Roman-Diaz, B-H. Lue, R. Botelho, and R. Frankel. 1997. 'Being a foreigner, I may be punished if I make a small mistake': Assessing transcultural experiences in caring for patients. *Family Practice* 14(2):112–116.

Fowkes, V. 1993. Meeting the needs of the underserved: The roles of physician assistants and nurse practitioners. In *The roles of physician assistants and nurse practitioners in primary care,* ed. D.K. Clawson, and M. Osterweis. Washington, D.C.: Association of Academic Health Centers, 69–83.

Gesler, W.M. 1992. Therapeutic landscapes: Medical issues in light of the new cultural geography. *Social Science and Medicine* 34: 735-746.

Gesler, W.M., S.T. Bird, and S.A.Oljeski. 1997. Disease ecology and a reformist alternative: The case of infant mortality. *Social Science and Medicine* 44: 657–671.

Gesler, W.M. 1999. Words in wards: Language, health and place. *Health and Place* 5: 13–25.

Gesler, W.M. 2000. Hans Castorp's journey-to-knowledge of disease and health in Thomas Mann's *The Magic Mountain. Health and Place* 6: 125–134.

Giddens, A. 1984. *The Constitution of Society*. Berkeley, CA: University of California Press.

Gilbert, M.R. 1998. "Race," space, and power: The survival strategies of working poor women. *Annals of the Association of American Geographers* 88(4): 595-621.

Good, C.M. 1987. *Ethnomedical systems in Africa*. New York: Guilford Press.

Gould, P. 1993. *The slow plague: A geography of the AIDS pandemic*. Cambridge, MA: Blackwell.

Gupta, G.C., and T.R Konrad. Allied health education in rural health professional shortage areas of the United States. *JAMA* 268: 1127–1130.

Hafferty, F.W. and H.I. Goldberg. 1986. Educational strategies for targeted retention of nonphysician health providers. *Health Services Research* 21:1; 107–125.

Hall, E.T. 1969. *The hidden dimension*. Garden City, NJ: Doubleday.

Harvey, D. 1990. *The condition of postmodernity: An enquiry into the origins of cultural change*. NY: Blackwell.

Helman, C. 1984. *Culture, health and illness: An introduction for health professionals*. Bristol, England: John Wright and Sons.

Holloway, S.R. 1998. Exploring the neighborhood contingency of race discrimination in mortgage lending in Columbus, Ohio. *Annals of the Association of American Geographers* 88 (2): 252–276.

Hunter, K.M. 1991. *Doctors' stories: The narrative structure of medical knowledge*. Princeton, NJ: Princeton University Press.

Jackson, P. 1989. *Maps of meaning: An introduction to cultural geography*. Boston: Unwin Hyman.

Jansen, B. (Associated Press). 2000. Tech visa quota bill stirs up senators. *The Herald Sun*, September 16, 1a.

Jones, K., and G. Moon. 1987. *Health, disease and society: An introduction to medical geography*. New York: Routledge and Kegan Paul.

Joseph, A., and D. Phillips. 1984. *Accessibility and utilization: Geographical perspectives on health care delivery*. New York: Harper & Row.

Kearns, R.A. 1993. Place and health: Towards a reformed medical geography. *Professional Geographer* 45: 139–147.

Kearns, R.A., and W.M. Gesler, eds. 1998. *Putting health into place: Landscape, identity, and well-being*. Syracuse, NY: Syracuse University Press.

Kearns, R.A., and A.E. Joseph.1993. Space in its place: Developing the link in medical geography. *Social Science and Medicine* 37: 711–717.

Kleinman, A. 1978. Concepts and a model for the comparison of medical systems as cultural systems. *Social Science and Medicine* 12B: 85–93.

Kleinman, A. 1980. *Patients and healers in the context of culture: An exploration of the borderland between anthropology, medicine and psychiatry*. Berkeley: University of California Press.

Kleinman, A.1988. *The illness narratives: Suffering, healing and the human condition*. New York: Basic Books.

Kobayashi, A., and L. Peake. 1994. Unnatural discourses: 'Race' and gender in geography. *Gender, Place, and Culture* 1(2): 225–243.

Konrad, T.R., E.S. Williams, M. Linzer, et al. 1999. Measuring physician job satisfaction in a changing workplace and a challenging environment. *Medical Care* 37(11):1174–1182.

Laws, G., J. Radford. 1998. Place, identity, and disability: Narratives of intellectually disabled people in Toronto. In *Putting health into place: Landscape, identity, and well-being*, ed. R.A. Kearns, and W.M. Gesler, Syracuse, New York: Syracuse University Press, 77–101.

Litva, A., J. Eyles. 1995. Coming out: Exposing social theory in medical geography. *Health and Place*1(1): 5–14.

Maggio, M. 1998. Understanding H-1B specialty worker visas. *Legal Report*, Summer.

Marston, S.A. 2000. The social construction of scale. *Progress in Human Geography* 24 (2): 219–242.

Massey, D. 1984. Spatial divisions of labour : Social structures and the geography of production. London: Macmillan.

Massey, D., and P. Jess. 1995. The conceptualization of place. In *A place in the world*. New York: Oxford University Press, 45–85.

Massey D. 1996. Politicising space and place. *Scottish Geographical Magazine* 112: 117–123.

Massey, D. 1997. A global sense of place. In *Reading human geography*, ed. D. Massey, T. Barnes, and D. Gregory. New York: Arnold, 315–323. Reprinted from *Marxism Today*, 1991.

Mayer, J.D., and M.S. Meade. 1994. A reformed medical geography reconsidered. *Professional Geographer* 46 (1): 103–106.

McPheron-Alex, T. 1993. Cultural diversity in rural health. *Rural Clinician Quarterly* Fall 3. Reprinted in *A shared vision: Building bridges for rural health care access. Conference proceedings*. Kansas City: National Rural Health Association; 1994: 171–172.

Mick, S.S., and S.D. Lee. 1997a. The safety net role of international medical graduates. *Health Affairs* 16: 141–150.

Mick, S.S., and S.D. Lee. 1997b. Addendum 2 to final report: Nonmetropolitan and metropolitan location of IMGs and USMGs in US states' counties characterized by measures of potential need or under service. A report to the Council on Graduate Medical Education and the Bureau of Health Professions, Health Resources and Services Administration, DHHS. Ann Arbor, MI: Department of Health Services Management and Policy, School of Public Health, University of Michigan,

Mick, S.S., S.D. Lee. 1999a. Are there need-based geographical differences between international medical graduates and US medical graduates in rural US counties? *Journal of Rural Health* 15 (1): 26–43.

Mick, S.S., and S.D. Lee. 1999b. International and US medical graduates in US cities. *Journal of Urban Health* 76 (4): 481–496.

Mick, S.S., S.D. Lee, and W.P. Wodchis. 2000. Variations in geographical distribution of foreign and domestically trained physicians in the United States: 'safety nets' or 'surplus exacerbation'? *Social Science and Medicine* 50:2, 185–202.

Mick, S.S., and M.N. Pfahler. 1995. Review and synthesis of the literature on foreign medical graduates / international medical graduates, 1980-1994. Washington, DC: US Department of Health and Human Services.

Miller, R.S., M.R. Dunn, and T. Richter. 1999. Graduate medical education: A closer look. *JAMA* 282 (9): 855–860.

Mohammad, R. 1999. Marginalisation, Islamism and the production of the 'other's' other. *Gender, Place and Culture* 6:3, 221–240.

Moos, A.I., and M.J. Dear. 1986. Structuration theory in urban analysis: 1. Theoretical exegesis. *Environment and Planning A* 18: 231–252.

Mullan, F. 1997. National Health Service Corps and inner-city hospitals. *New England Journal of Medicine* 336:1601–1604.

Mullan, F., R.M. Politzer, and C.H. Davis. 1995. Medical migration and the physician workforce. *JAMA* 273;1521–1527.

Nast, H.J., and S. Pile. 1998. *Places through the body*. New York: Routledge.

Novak, J.D. 1991. Clarify with concept maps: A tool for students and teachers alike. *The Science Teacher* 58: 45–49.

Novak, J.D. 1998. *Learning, creating, and using knowledge: Concept maps as facilitative tools in schools and corporations*. Mahweh, NJ: Lawrence Erlbaum Associates.

Parker, R., and T. Tuxill. 1967. The attitudes of physicians toward small-community practice. *Journal of Medical Education* 42: 327–344.

Patton, M.Q. 1990. *Qualitative evaluation and research methods*. Newbury Park, CA: Sage Publications.

Perry, W. 1970. *Forms of intellectual and ethical development in the college years*. New York: Holt, Rinehart, and Winston.

Politzer, R.M., J.M. Cultice, and A.J. Meltzer. 1998. The geographic distribution of physicians in the United States and the contribution of international medical graduates. *Medical Care Research and Review* 55: 116–130.

Pulido, L. 2000. Rethinking environmental racism: White privilege and urban development in southern California. *Annals of the Association of American Geographers* 90(1):12–40.

Pulsipher, LM. 2000. *World Regional Geography*. New York: W.H. Freeman and Company.

Radley, A. 1994. *Making sense of illness: The social psychology of health and disease*. London: Sage.

Random House Unabridged Dictionary. 1993. Second edition. New York: Random House.

Ricketts, T.C., L.A. Savitz, W.M. Gesler, D.N. Osborn eds. 1994. *Geographic methods for health services research: A focus on the rural-urban continuum*. Lanham, MD: University Press of America.

Robinson, J.C. 1999. *The corporate practice of medicine: Competition and innovation in health care*. Berkeley, California: University of California Press.

Rohrer, J.E. 2000. Rigor at the expense of relevance equals rigidity: Where to next in the study of medical care utilization? *Health Services Research* 34 (6): 1307–1310.

Ronaghy, H.A., K. Zeighami, and B. Zeigham. 1976. Physician migration to the US—Foreign aid for US manpower. *Medical Care* 14(6): 502–511.

Rose, G. 1993. *Feminism and geography: The limits of geographical knowledge*. Minneapolis: University of Minnesota Press.

Said, E.W. 1978. *Orientalism*. New York: Random House.

Sayer, A. 1985. Realism and geography. In Johnston RJ (ed.), *The future of geography*. Methuen: London, 159–173.

Sayer, A. 1992. *Method in social science: A realist approach. 2nd edition*. New York: Routledge.

Sayer, A. 2000. *Realism and social science*. Thousand Oaks, CA: Sage.

Sibley, D. 1992. Outsiders in society. In Anderson K, Gale F (eds.), *Inventing places: Studies in cultural geography*. Melbourne: Longman Cheshire/Wiley Halsted Press, 107–122.

Sibley, D. 1995. *Geographies of exclusion: Society and difference in the West*. New York: Routledge.

Skultans, V. ed. 2000. Special issue: Narrative illness and the body. *Anthropology and Medicine* 7 (1).

Smith, S.J. 1993. Residential segregation and the politics of racialization. *Racism, the city and the state*. In *Racism, the city and the State,* ed. M. Cross, and M. Keith, New York: Routledge, 128–143.

Spitzer, W.O., D.L. Sackett, J.C. Sibley, R.S. Roberts, M. Gent, D.J. Kergin, B.C. Hackett, and A. Olynich. 1974. The Burlington randomized trial of nurse practitioners. *New England Journal of Medicine* 290: 251–256.

Stevens, R., L.W. Goodman, and S.S. Mick. 1978. *The alien doctors: Foreign medical graduates in American hospitals*. New York: John Wiley and Sons.

Takahashi, L.M. 1998. Concepts of difference in community health. In *Putting health into place: Landscape, identity, and well-being*, ed. R.A. Kearns and W.M. Gesler. Syracuse, NY: Syracuse University Press, 143–167.

Taylor, D.H., and A. Esmail. 1999. Retrospective analysis of census data on general practitioners who qualified in South Asia: Who will replace them as they retire? *BMJ* 318: 3306–3310.

Tuan, Y.F. 1974. Space and place: Humanistic perspective. In *Progress in geography: International reviews of current research,* Vol. 6, ed. C. Board, P. Haggett, and D.R. Stoddart Vol. 6. London: Edward Arnold.

Tudor Hart, J. .2000. Three decades of the inverse care law. *British Medical Journal* 320 (7226): 18–19.

Tudor, Hart, J. 1971. The inverse care law. *Lancet* 1 (7696): 405–12.

U.S. Census Bureau. Census 2000. Profile of General Demographic Characteristics: 2000. Retrieved from Internet, http://www.census.gov, September 3, 2002.

U.S. Department of Agriculture. 2002 USDA Participation in J-1 Visa Waiver Program. Retrieved from Internet, http://www.usda.gov/news/releases/2002/03/fsj1visa.htm. Statement updated March 22, 2002. Accessed March 28, 2002.

U.S. General Accounting Office. 1996. Foreign physicians: Exchange visitor program becoming major route to practicing in US underserved areas. GAO/HEHS-97–26. Washington, DC: US General Accounting Office.

Valentine, G. 1999. Imagined geographies: Geographical knowledges of self and other in everyday life. In *Human Geography Today*, ed. D. Massey, J. Allen, P. Sarre, 47–61.

Verghese, A. 1994. *My own country: A doctor's story*. New York: Vintage Books.

Williams, G. 1984. The genesis of chronic illness: Narrative re-construction. *Sociology of Health and Illness* 6: 174–200.

Wilton, R.D. 1996. Diminished worlds? The geography of everyday life with HIV/AIDS. *Health and Place* 2: 69–83.

Xu, G., J. Veloski, M. Hojat, R.M. Politzer, H.K. Rabinowitz, and S.L. Rattner. 1997. Factors influencing primary care physicians' choice to practice in Medically Underserved Areas. *Academic Medicine* 72 (October Supplement 1): S109–S111.

Index

acceptability: definition of, 1, 4–5, 166–167
adherence, 76–78, 100, 241–242, 251
American Medical Association, 7, 12
Appalachian Regional Commission, 10
appreciation, 166–169, 253, 275, 276
Argentina, 46, 51, 119, 190
assimilation, 62, 94–95, 101, 252, 256–257, 272, 274, 282

Berry, 115, 117, 119, 120–124, 126, 167, 169–170, 173, 187–188, 195, 198, 200, 205–206, 220, 223, 227–228, 244–245, 260, 264. *See also* Delano County
Bhaskar, Roy, 17
Bolivia, 234
Bombay, 129–130, 141, 150
Buddhism, 219
Bulgaria, 119, 131–132, 253

Canada, 3, 46, 49, 88, 119, 158, 178, 186, 187, 247
Caribbean, 51, 119
causality, 18–19, 280
China, 25, 188, 244–245
Christianity, 36–37, 95–100, 101, 102, 103, 104, 116, 122, 123, 142, 170, 176, 190, 199, 201, 203, 218, 219–228, 255, 258, 272, 275, 280, 287
community health center, 6, 53, 118, 149, 170, 250, 289
competence, 59–63, 64, 140, 146, 172, 177–181, 253, 274, 275, 276
communication: doctor-patient, 22, 45–46, 54, 56, 60, 62, 64, 67–79, 83, 84, 86, 99, 100, 168, 170–171, 177, 179, 181, 182, 185, 186, 190, 199, 201, 202, 229–243, 251, 253, 272, 274, 277, 282, 284, 287
competition, 100, 105, 134, 145, 149, 162–166, 275, 276
concept map, 278–284, 287
context, 6–13, 15, 19–23, 24, 25–26, 27–28, 29, 31, 64, 67–109, 185–267, 274, 275, 277, 278, 279, 280, 282, 283, 287
Council on Graduate Medical Education, 6, 10, 11–12
critical realism, 13, 15, 17, 18–23, 24, 25, 31, 278
Cuba, 44, 190

Delano County, 113–267, 271, 275–278
Dominican Republic, 179, 190

Educational Commission for Foreign Medical Graduates, 9
emergency room, 56, 93, 118, 202, 231, 241

family practice, 50, 63, 64, 103–104, 119, 147, 148, 173, 259
Filmore, 114, 124, 127–128, 133, 140, 144, 218, 223, 253, 256, 276
foreign medical graduate (FMG). *See* international medical graduate
formality, 80–81, 100, 133, 150, 246, 247–248
France, 119, 197
Free Clinic, 75, 82

gender, 4, 6, 15, 21–22, 29, 30, 67, 81, 89–95, 100, 120, 199, 207–218, 241, 243–244, 252, 275, 277, 278, 279, 281, 282, 287
geographies of exclusion: overview of, 27–29
Germany, 44, 192
Guam, 191
Guatemala, 119, 166, 190

Haiti, 119
Hamilton, 5–6, 113–267, 275–278, 284, 285, 286; south Hamilton, 115, 116, 119, 120, 126, 173, 175, 186, 200, 226, 245, 246, 250. *See also* Delano County
hierarchy: social, 80–82, 95, 209, 246, 248–249
Hinduism, 51, 92–93, 95, 97–99, 127, 205–206, 211, 212–213, 218, 219, 221–222, 223, 225, 227–228, 275
Hispanic, 39, 75–76, 101, 115, 176–177, 189–190, 218, 227, 250, 253, 258, 260, 276
Honduras, 44, 51, 53

IMG. *See* international medical graduate
India, 7–9, 35, 38–39, 46, 50–53, 55–56, 58–59, 68–70, 73, 80, 81–82, 83, 84, 92–102, 106–107, 119, 127, 128–131, 133, 135, 136–13, 139, 141, 146–147, 158–159, 165, 166, 178, 179, 181, 186, 192, 193–194, 196, 204, 205, 210–218, 222–223, 226, 230, 237–238, 247, 248, 249–252, 254–256, 264, 265, 266–267, 273–274
Indonesia, 265
international medical graduate: defined, 3; pioneer, 53–58, 133–145, 146, 167, 170, 173, 174, 189, 203, 230, 251, 274, 275, 278. *See also* individual country names
Internet, 39, 219, 259
inverse care law, 12
Ireland, 129
Islam, 95, 97, 99, 255, 285–286
Italy, 44, 45, 51, 53

J-1 visa waiver, 10–12, 28, 50, 147–153, 156–158, 160, 161, 166, 167–168, 249, 257, 265, 286, 287–288, 289
Jamaica, 51
Japan, 25, 51, 55, 70
Judaism, 136, 221

Knox County, 35–109
Korea, 9, 55, 233

Lebanon, 119, 137

malpractice, 60–61
Massey, Doreen, 15, 24, 25, 27, 284
mechanism, 17, 19–22, 23, 24, 26, 27–28, 29, 49–65, 108, 133–184, 274, 275, 278, 279, 280, 281, 282, 287
Medicare, 10, 11, 12
Mexico, 9, 162, 176, 190

national security 7, 11, 12, 284–286
Native American, 115, 116–117, 119–124, 126, 132, 169–170, 179, 184, 187–189, 193–203, 204–206,

218, 227, 237, 238, 250, 253, 258, 260, 262, 275, 276
Nigeria, 97, 119, 127–128, 130, 191, 192, 264
nurse practitioners, 23, 61, 73, 81–82, 131, 132, 151–153, 156, 168, 170, 181–184, 194–195, 201, 202, 206–207, 210, 221, 230, 232–233, 248, 257–258
nurses, 22, 41, 45, 46, 52, 53, 61, 62, 63, 68–69, 76, 77, 78, 81, 83, 87, 90, 94–95, 103, 106, 138, 144, 186, 192, 207, 208, 209, 211, 214, 217, 224, 230, 231–234, 236, 266. *See also* nurse practitioners

obstetrics and gynecology, 50, 85, 88–89, 119, 147, 199, 203, 207–208, 210
otherness. *See* geographies of exclusion

Pakistan, 9, 46, 51, 53, 58, 106, 119, 168, 171–172, 180, 198, 213, 255, 266
pediatrics, 50, 119, 147, 168, 180–181, 208–209
Philippines, 9, 51, 53, 54, 55–57, 58, 97, 119, 144, 159, 168, 244–245, 264, 265–266
physician assistants, 23, 73, 81–82, 132, 147, 164–165, 181, 184, 205
physician oversupply, 3, 7, 10, 11, 13, 281, 289
physician shortage, 4, 6, 25, 49, 56, 163, 265, 287
Pierce, 124, 132, 143, 176. *See also* Delano County
Poland, 119
positivism, 17–18, 19, 23, 24, 29–32, 44, 284
pronunciation, 46, 68, 70, 83, 230, 235, 238, 239
Puerto Rico, 46, 190–191

Quincy, 5–6, 35–109, 271–274, comparisons with Delano County, 113–114, 117, 119, 129, 144, 147, 148, 160, 172–173, 174, 177, 185, 190, 191, 192–193, 201, 203, 207, 212–213, 214, 218, 219, 223, 224, 226, 229, 231, 234, 235, 238, 246, 247, 248, 249, 251, 252, 262, 275–278. *See also* Knox County

race: social construction of, 84–89, 193–207, 274, 276–277
recruitment, 3, 45, 49–53, 54, 88, 91–92, 136–137, 145, 146–150, 155–156, 163, 168, 178, 190–191, 192, 193–194, 217–218, 250, 273, 288
referral, 11, 35, 56, 59, 63–65, 81, 84, 105–106, 137, 164, 172–175, 176, 180, 245, 273–274, 277
religion, 6, 21, 22, 26, 28, 36, 51, 54, 57, 67, 92–93, 95–100, 101, 127, 199, 211, 212, 218–228, 241, 243, 252, 256, 258–259, 262, 264, 274, 277, 281, 282, 287. *See also* Buddhism, Christianity; Hinduism; Islam; Judaism
retention, 14–15, 22, 39, 49–53, 54, 90, 91, 155–162, 166, 217–218, 263, 273, 275, 276, 277–278, 280, 288
Russia, 44, 159

Sayer, Andrew, 17, 19, 20, 21
senior citizens, 44, 56, 62, 74, 78–79, 95–96, 168, 171, 172, 174, 181, 187, 189, 191–192, 201–202, 213, 219, 226, 231, 233, 234, 235–236, 237, 245, 246–247, 250, 260, 289
September 11 2001, 7, 11, 12, 284–286
social theory, 13–16, 17–32, 278
South Africa, 166
Spain, 44
Spanish, 9, 39, 75–76, 176–177, 190, 227
spouse: of physician, 89–95, 97, 128, 129–130, 131, 144, 145, 149, 154–156, 159, 162, 164, 165, 192,

207, 212–218, 233, 234, 251, 261, 262–263, 285, 288. *See also* gender
stereotype, 65, 79–84, 144, 217, 243–252, 274, 282
structuration theory, 21
Switzerland, 136

Taiwan, 119, 143, 233
traditional medicine, 72, 99–100, 176
trust, 22, 59–65, 67, 76, 85, 91, 95, 122, 145, 169–184, 190, 202, 209, 220, 253, 274, 275, 276, 277, 285–286
Tuan: Yi Fu, 15, 24–25, 26, 284

United Kingdom, 13, 25, 44, 51, 81, 88, 89, 106–107, 181, 186, 187, 188
U.S. Department of Agriculture, 12, 286

Vietnam, 55

Wilson, 123, 126, 132
Wizard of Oz, 14

Yankee, 46, 124, 191

About the Author

Leonard D. Baer is a lecturer in the Department of Geography at Lancaster University in England. He received his Ph.D. from the University of North Carolina at Chapel Hill, and his master's degree from Virginia Tech. His work has previously appeared in *Social Science and Medicine*, *The American Journal of Public Health*, and other journals. This is his first book.

www.ingramcontent.com/pod-product-compliance
Ingram Content Group UK Ltd.
Pitfield, Milton Keynes, MK11 3LW, UK
UKHW040154091026
15587UKWH00018B/266

9 780739 104934